D1326479

GLOW

Your Complete Four-Week Guide to Healthy, Radiant Skin

KATE O'BRIEN

GILL BOOKS

Gill Books
Hume Avenue
Park West
Dublin 12
www.gillbooks.ie

Gill Books is an imprint of M.H. Gill & Co.

978 07171 7938 1

Designed by www.grahamthew.com
Photography by Rob Kerkvliet of A Fox in the Kitchen
Photos on pp. 52, 103 and 256 by Jaclyn Visbeen
Photo on page 86 courtesy of VOYA, www.voya.ie
Skin illustration on p.8 © Science Stuff / Alamy
Styled by Orla Neligan of Cornershop Productions (www.cornershopproductions.com), assisted by Clare Wilkinson
Copy-edited by Emma Dunne
Proofread by Jane Rogers
Printed by Liberdúplex, Spain

PROPS
Avoca: www.avoca.ie
Meadows & Byrne: www.meadowsandbyrne.com
Marks & Spencer: www.marksandspencer.ie
Article Dublin: www.articledublin.com
Dunnes Stores: www.dunnesstores.com
TK Maxx: www.tkmaxx.ie
Kathryn Davey Fabrics: kathryndavey.com

This book is typeset in 12 on 15pt Mr Eaves Sans.

The paper used in this book comes from the wood pulp of managed forests. For every tree felled, at least one tree is planted, thereby renewing natural resources.

A CIP catalogue record for this book is available from the British Library.

5 4 3 2 1

'NATURE GIVES YOU THE FACE
YOU HAVE AT TWENTY; IT IS UP
TO YOU TO MERIT THE FACE
YOU HAVE AT FIFTY.'

– COCO CHANEL

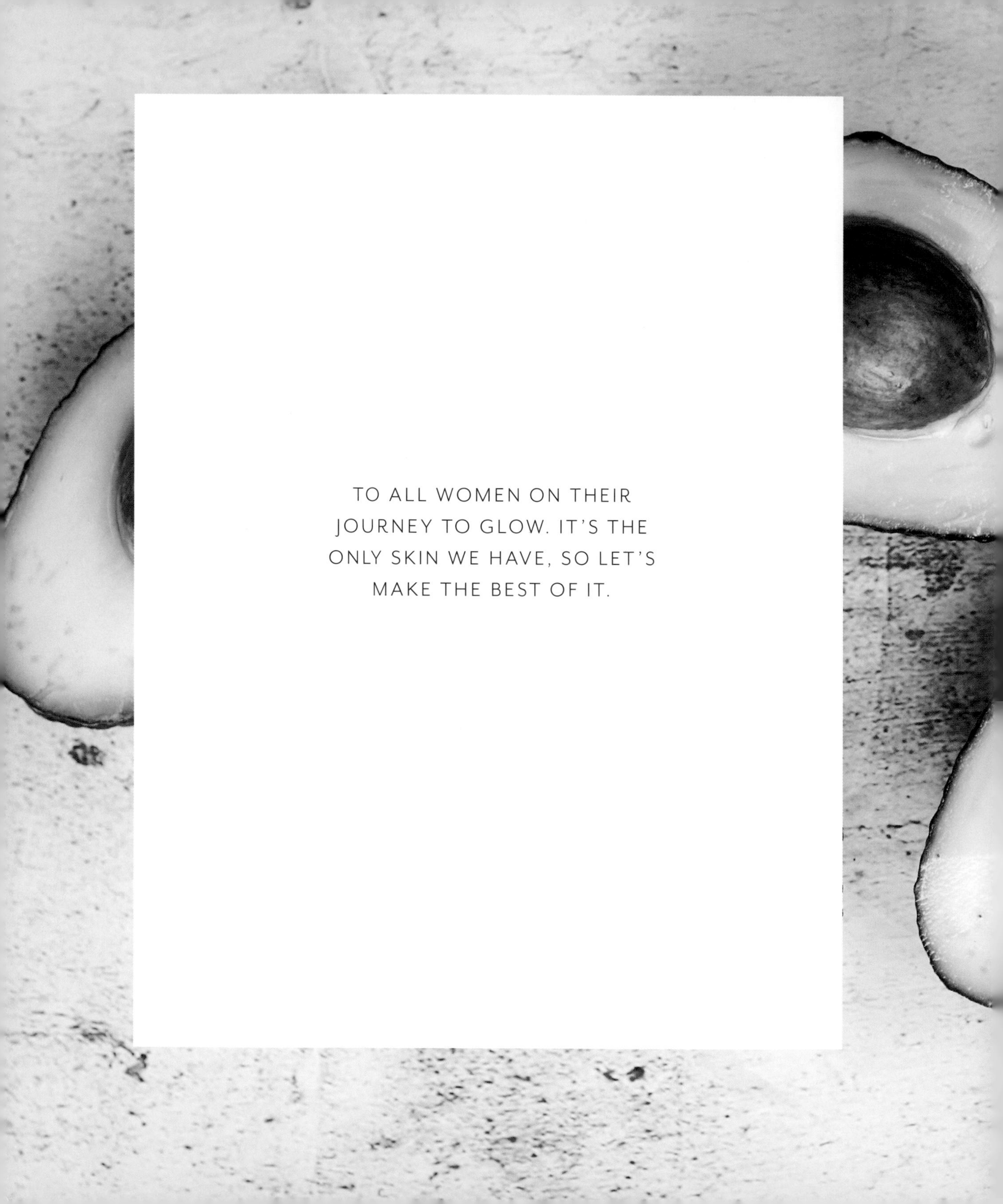

TO ALL WOMEN ON THEIR
JOURNEY TO GLOW. IT'S THE
ONLY SKIN WE HAVE, SO LET'S
MAKE THE BEST OF IT.

This book would not have happened without the patience of my supportive family, Mike, Liam, Raif and my immensely talented foodie daughter Maya Duncan (15), who brought many of these recipes to life and who, in all honesty, sweated the hard stuff in the kitchen ensuring the recipes look and taste as delicious and healthy as they sound.

To Alexandra Soveral and her delightful team at Alexandra Soveral London for their contribution and ongoing support. Thanks to Melissa Sansone and Dr Gross Skincare who helped my skin GLOW during my own four weeks to radiant skin. Also to the kombucha queen Dearbhla Reynolds and seaweed expert Prannie Rhatigan for your expert contributions to GLOW.

Thanks to Orla Neligan, Clare Wilkinson and photographer Rob Kerkvliet, who shared their creative expertise and helped keep me sane through the days of shooting (Clare, your blackberry rose kombucha is fab!). Jaclyn Visbeen, you are amongst the very few who bring out the best of me on camera!

Finally, thanks to the hugely supportive team at Gill Books, especially Sarah Liddy, Catherine Gough, Teresa Daly and Ellen Monnelly, who were ever-present and helpful along the way.

CONTENTS

INTRODUCTION 1

PART 1: THE SCIENCE 5

The Skin We're In 7
What Skin Needs 19
Skin Stressors 39
Gut and Skin 53
Sleep and Skin 59

PART 2: FOUR WEEKS TO GLOW 69

GLOW Foods 71
Kitchen Essentials 95
Better Skin Tips 99
The Plan 105
Week One: Cleanse 107
Week Two: Heal 119
Week Three: Nourish 127
Week Four: GLOW 135

PART 3: THE RECIPES 141

Breakfasts & Brunches 142
Herby Edamame Omelette 143
Five Ways with Oats 145
– Maya's Granola 145
– Overnight Oats with Seasonal Berries 146
– Oaty Breakfast Bars 149
– Oaty Banana Smoothie 150
– GLOW Banana Bread 152
Salted Caramel Smoothie Bowl 155
Summer Surprise Smoothie 156
Avocado on Toast – Three Ways 158
Buckwheat Pancakes with Caramelised Banana Bites 160
Shakshuka 163

Dressings, Dips & Spreads 164
Mustard Dressing 165
Zesty Apple Cider Vinaigrette 165
Tahini Dressing 166
Guacamole 167
Walnut Basil Pesto 168
Cashew Cream 168
Pea and Edamame Houmous 170
Mango, Pomegranate and Cucumber Salsa 171
Tzatziki 171

Soups 172
Quick Homemade Vegetable Stock 173
Creamy Squash and Red Pepper Soup 174
Courgette and Almond Soup 177
Quick Miso Broth with Edamame 178
Spinach and Broccoli Soup with Flaked Almonds 181

Salads & Sides 182
Spring Medley 183
Quinoa, Pomegranate and Feta Salad 184
Orange, Walnut and Quinoa Salad 186
Beetroot, Edamame and Orange Salad 188
Sautéed Spinach with Edamame 189
Minted Farro and Three Bean Salad with Goat's Cheese 191
Cannellini Bean Salad with Marinated Alaria 192

Mains 194
GLOW Frittata **195**
Sweet Potato, Pea and Courgette Cakes **197**
Broccolini Risotto **198**
Nachos with a Twist **200**
Shepherdless Pie **202**
Salmon – Three Ways
– Citrus Turmeric Salmon **205**
– Flax and Sesame Crusted Salmon with Spinach and Tahini **206**
– Moroccan-Style Salmon **208**

Seasonal Bowls 210
Spring: Asian-Style Salmon Bowl **211**
Summer: Cauliflower and Baby Spinach Bowl **214**
Autumn: Root Veggie Bowl **217**
Winter: Warming Squash, Red Pepper and Chickpea Curry Bowl **218**

Snacks & Sweet Things 222
Apple, Pear and Blackberry Crumble **223**
ChocNOlate Chip Cookies **226**
Citrus Delight Cake **228**
Orange and Almond Muffins **229**
Chocolate Orange Energy Balls **231**
GLOW Trail Mix **232**
Walnut Brownies **234**
Berry Sorbet **236**
Mint Choc-Chip 'Ice Cream' **236**

Juices 238
Earthy Goodness **242**
Zesty Cleanser **242**
Skin Soother **243**
Intense C **243**
Pineapple Punch **244**
Double Green **244**
Sunshine Skin **245**
Vital Skin **245**

GLOW Teas 246
Lemongrass, Ginger and Mint **247**
Nettle and Ginger **248**
Lavender and Rosemary **248**
Fennel and Mint **248**
Ginger and Turmeric **252**
Matcha Mint Latte **252**
Green Tea with Mint **254**
Orange and Mint Iced Green Tea **254**
Rosebud Brew **255**
Kombucha **257**
– Pineapple Crush **260**
– Booch Mojito **260**
– Blackberry Rose **262**

KATE'S TRUSTED BRANDS **265**

SELECT BIBLIOGRAPHY **268**

INDEX **270**

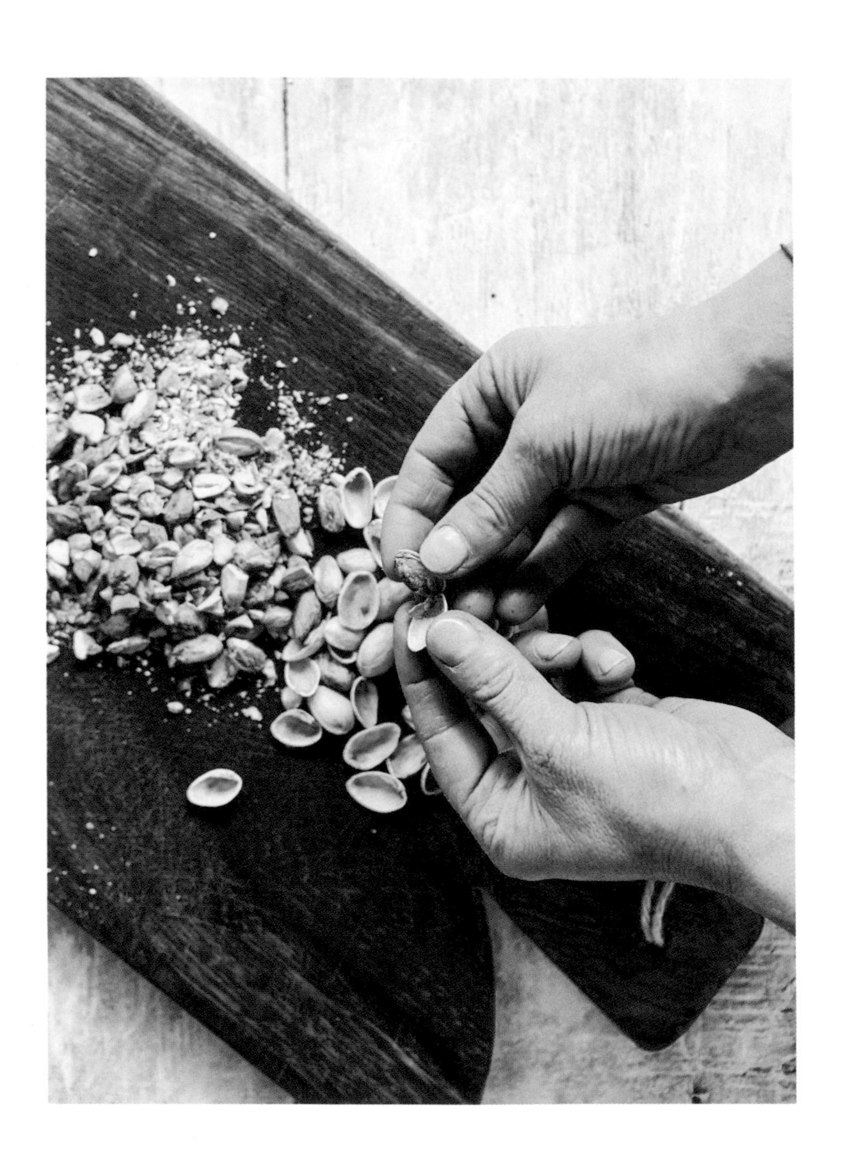

INTRODUCTION

◊

Skin is a powerful outward expression of what is happening inside, with that elusive healthy glow being utterly dependent on internal balance in the body. This equilibrium can be assured with *GLOW: Your Complete Four-Week Guide to Healthy, Radiant Skin*. This comprehensive guide cuts through the misinformation, offering scientifically grounded facts about how skin really works at a cellular level to help you create strong new foundations for better skin – for life.

This step-by-step guide is designed to be followed for four weeks for optimum results, with simple meal planners, easy-to-follow shopping lists and more than sixty fresh, tasty and seasonal recipes that don't require a science degree or chef's hat to prepare. Most important, the meals taste delicious – from Salted Caramel Smoothie Bowl and Citrus Turmeric Salmon to vibrant Nachos with a Twist and an autumnal Root Veggie Bowl, and lots more in between.

Each week focuses on a different aspect of skincare, from cleansing and exfoliating to healing, nourishing/balancing and ultimately the GLOW, with simple tried-and-tested recipes and corresponding skin masks and scrubs. This said, there is no pressure to prepare these, as plenty of great skincare products are available on the market. However, if you really want to make a difference to the health of your skin, you need to ensure that the products you use are packed with active skin goodness, and *GLOW* outlines exactly what you need at various stages of your life and why you need them too.

With the latest statistics from the Global Wellness Institute (2017) showing that beauty is the goliath of the global wellness industry, accounting for US$1 trillion of its US$3.7 trillion, this book could not be more timely. The trend for juices, beauty drinks and supplements is at an all-time high, fuelled by the concept of beauty from within. Almost every kitchen has a stylish blender and almost every woman is worried about how she looks and how the passing years and toxic load of daily life are impacting her skin. She wants her best skin and she wants it *now*. She wants to use more natural and organically produced products but doesn't know which to choose – and if truth were told, she's not really sure what she needs in the first place. She researches as best she can but panics when shopping for skincare, as it all becomes so confusing!

Having dedicated many years to seeking the soundest skincare advice and writing about it in various publications worldwide, I have been fortunate to interview some of the world's leading cosmetic scientists and dermatologists, as well as prominent skincare manufacturers and celebrities. And the prized nuggets of information gleaned from them, in conjunction with my professional qualifications in both nutrition and cosmetic science, have resulted in this revitalising skin-centric GLOW plan. I am immensely passionate about natural products, especially oils, and am fortunate to have sampled the best – and the very mediocre rest. I know what works for skin of every age and stage in life, and I am very proud that, finally, I can share the knowledge I have accrued over the past fifteen years here in these pages. This said, what I am not, and could never claim to be, is an expert cook. All of the recipes in the plan, without exception, are easy to cook and most are relatively quick to prepare too, which is essential given the chaotic pace of life today.

GLOW is not about deprivation, nor is it a diet book. In fact, the word 'diet' doesn't even deserve a mention. As you will see, there are no calorie counts in the recipes. All of this is deliberate, as I firmly believe that the current focus on dieting is leaving many well-intentioned people fixated on counting calories and not enjoying the food they are eating. The recommended foods and recipes in this plan are designed to give your skin the fuel it needs to repair, nourish and truly glow and to give your body the energy and nutrition it needs to thrive.

However, in sticking with the plan you might find that your clothes get a little looser along the way. While this is not the focus, it does follow naturally, as all of the recipes are super nutritious and packed with only good ingredients. All that is missing is the empty energy, stress and exhaustion that comes with processed foods – these same foods that science is now proving bring us down mentally and physically, adding years to our faces and bodies.

Many books promise results in seven to ten days, some even less. If weight loss is the aim, some difference should be noticed after one week when sticking with the plan, but to affect skin at the cellular level takes more than a few days of facemasks and dedicated skin smoothies. A minimum of four weeks is required for real change at a deeper level. This equates with lasting change and better skin and, as the meals and techniques outlined are designed to fit into busy lives, better skin can continue to be yours.

As you browse the recipes, you will see the plan is meat free. It is also low in dairy products and many of the recipes are gluten free. Not that red meat, chicken and milk-based foods don't have a role in health – they undoubtedly do; but for these four weeks, the emphasis is firmly on the numerous benefits of oily fish, eggs and the range of primarily plant-based GLOW foods that are overflowing with essential skin-loving goodness and destined to make your skin thrive.

Most important, the recipes should be enjoyed, just as vibrant skin should be cherished. And this vibrant skin also reflects a positive mindset because the mind exerts a huge influence on how we look (as the skin and the nervous system are very closely intertwined). So while you work through the four weeks, use this time to slow your pace of life a little, to listen to and nurture your body.

GLOW doesn't promise perfect skin – no book, or product for that matter, can – but what it does commit to is helping you make the best of what you have, whatever your age. Ultimately it's the difference between a good complexion and an amazingly fresh and radiant one. By combining nature's most active skin-nourishing foods with a targeted step-by-step skin routine, peppered with deeply nourishing scrubs and masks, this can be yours in just four weeks. As beauty guru Sali Hughes says in her book *Pretty Honest*: 'The only thing worse than feeling like crap is looking like crap too' – so join the revolution.

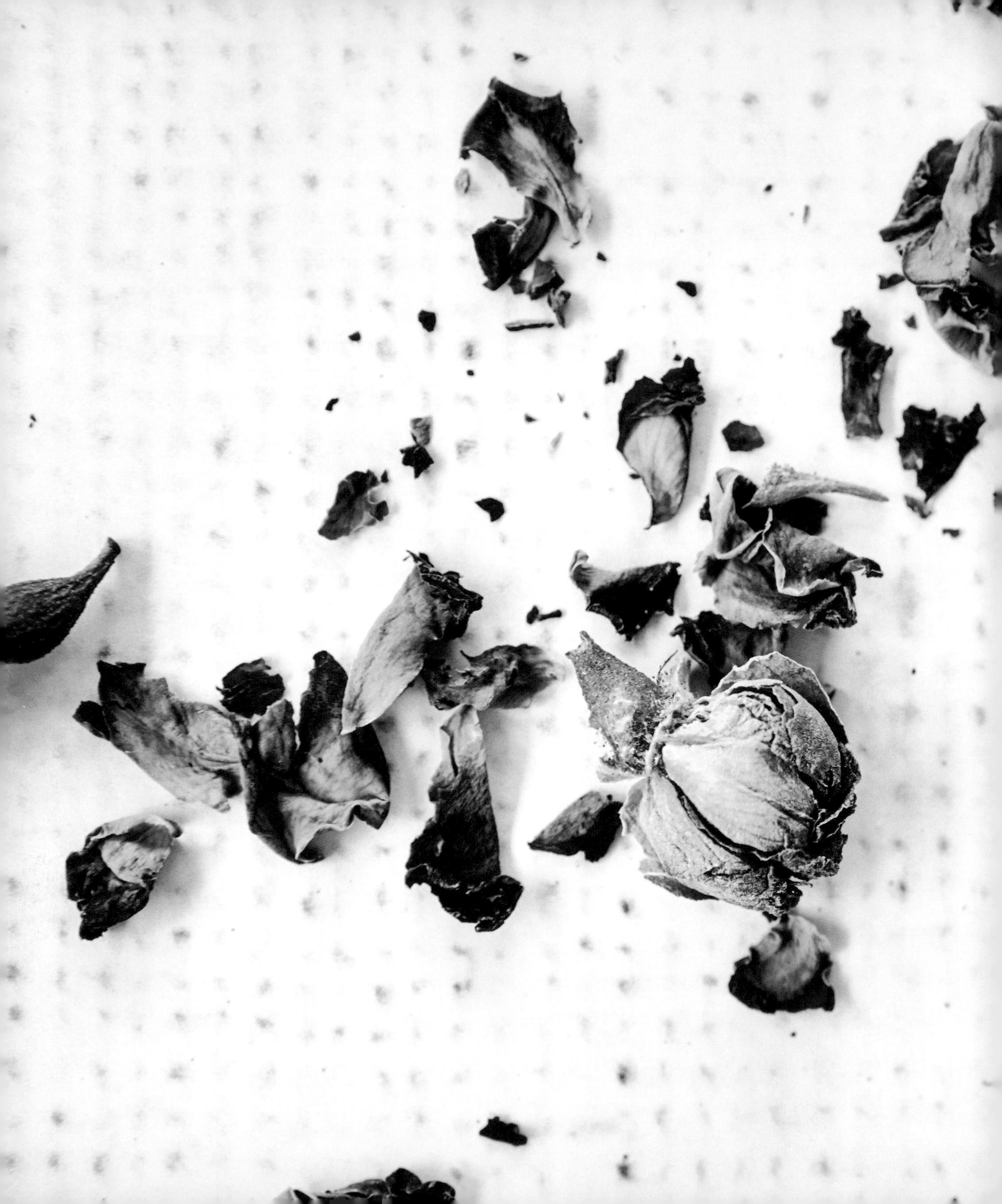

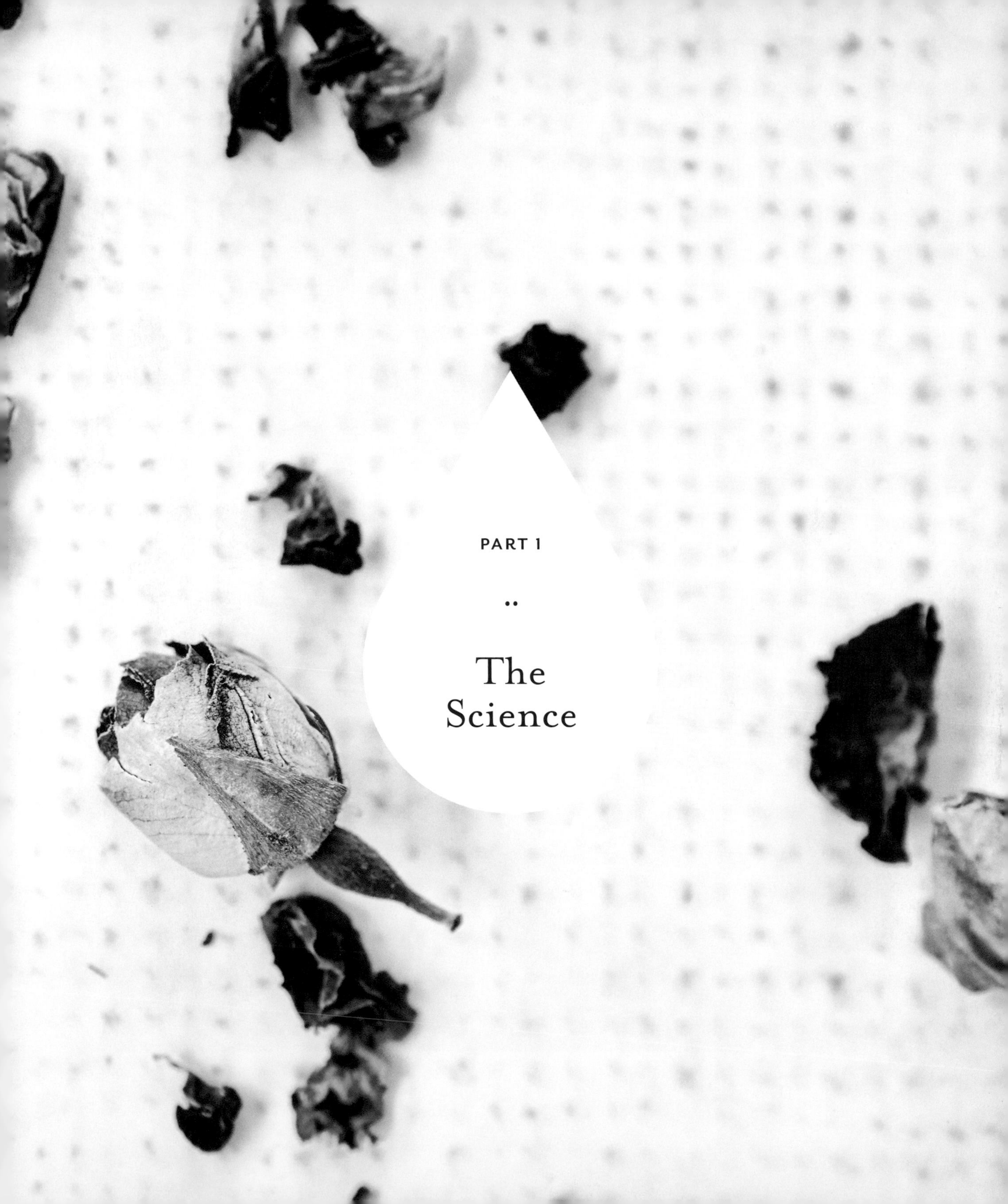

PART 1

The Science

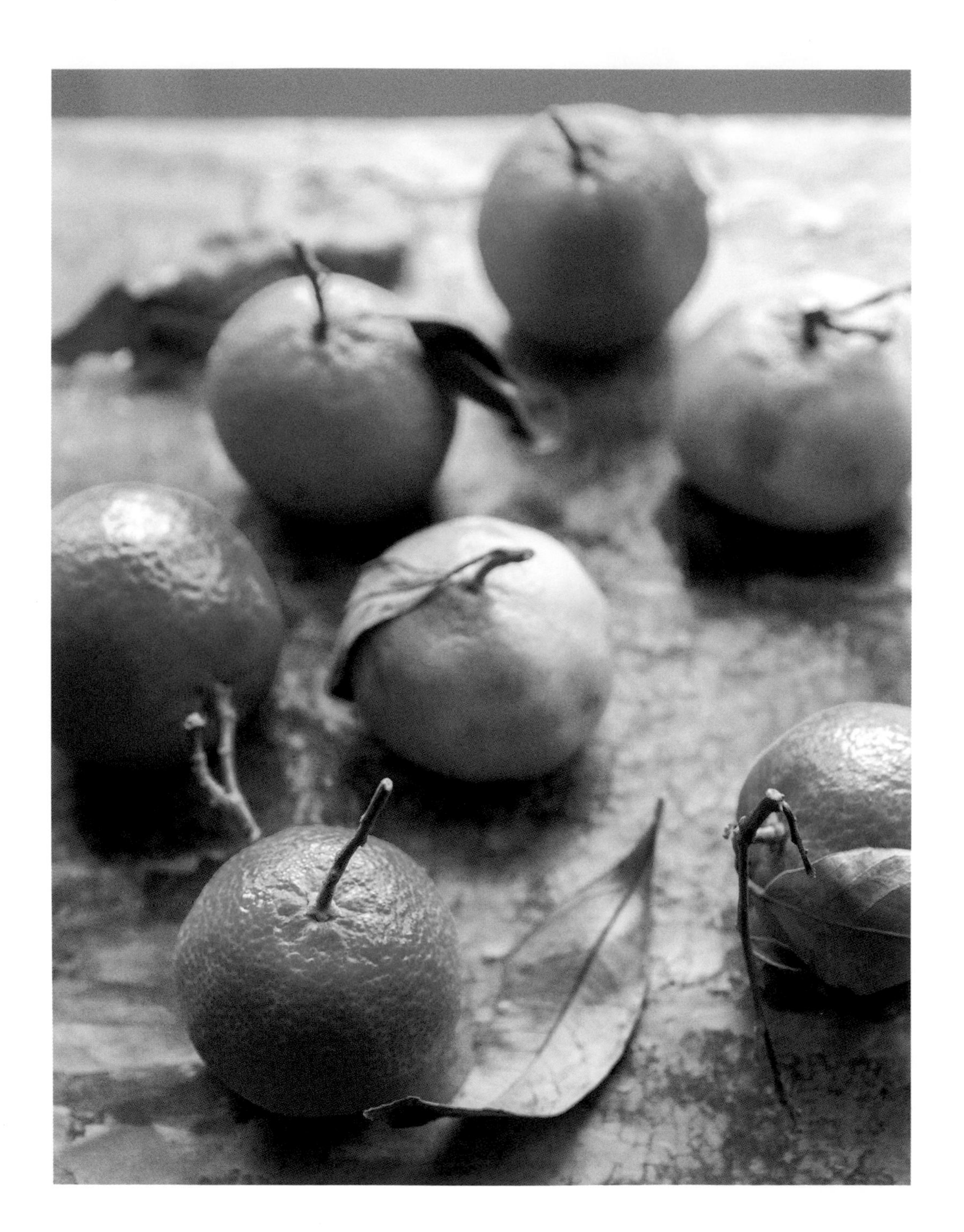

THE SKIN WE'RE IN

◊

The skin is the body's largest organ, with numerous functions far deeper than simply being our outside selves. Through its network of sensory nerves, the skin communicates pressure, pain, temperature, odour and sexual stimuli to the brain, which responds via the blood system to maintain relatively constant body temperature and water content.

Most of us know that fresh, bright and healthy skin can shift that 'just OK' feeling up a gear to one of real self-assurance and confidence. However, for many that 'just OK' all too easily becomes our every day. But we can change this: all it takes is a little effort and a combination of skin-nurturing foods, the best skincare advice and regular treatments to rejuvenate dull, lacklustre skin, leaving it deeply nourished and glowing.

THE BIOLOGY

Like a freshly ironed sheet covering a newly sprung mattress, the skin of a newborn is soft, smooth and entirely blemish free. As the mattress ages, the sheet starts to sag. This sheet is the skin's epidermis. Just 0.02 mm thick on the face, it comprises cells called keratinocytes glued together by an extracellular matrix. The epidermis is continually regenerated by stem cells at its base that spawn new keratinocytes, which migrate through the epidermis before sloughing off to reveal even fresher cells underneath.

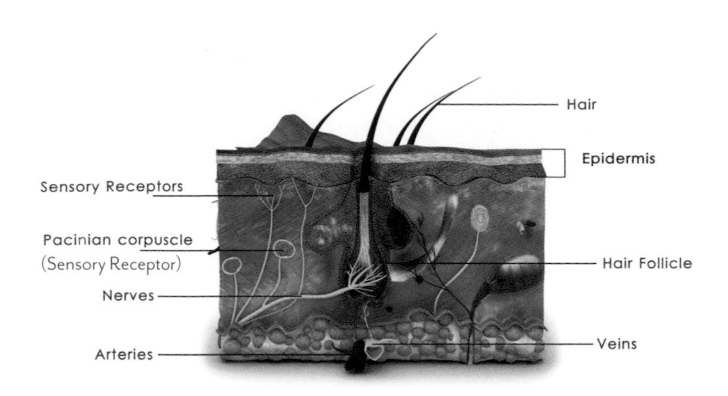

The thick mattress beneath the epidermis is the dermis, a chunky, gelatinous sea of matrix and cells. Woven though this mesh are rope-like protein fibres of collagen (giving skin its firm, tensile strength) and feathery coils of elastin (to maintain resilience). While this network of collagen and elastin provides strength and elasticity, the stuffing is made of large molecules of glycosaminoglycans (GAGs), the most common of which is hyaluronic acid. These absorb water to give the dermis of young skin its jelly-like consistency and smooth, plump feel.

MAKING YOUR SKIN WORK FOR YOU

Daily care for the skin is everything and if you are not prepared to spend the few minutes it takes to effectively cleanse, tone and nourish your skin every morning and night, then read no further. Experts recommend starting age maintenance in the late twenties/early thirties (see Skin through the Decades on page 14) rather than age restoration ten years later.

All skin is different so finding a product that works is entirely personal and can entail much trial and error. Bear in mind too that our skin's needs vary with hormonal fluctuations and the seasons, with richer and more nourishing creams and oils needed during colder, drier periods. So while sticking to some form of routine is wise, it's also good to switch up your regime from time to time. Our skin changes with age too, so what works now might not be as beneficial in the future.

All of this said, the following guidelines are based on three simple steps: **cleanse**, **tone**, **nourish**. When performed twice daily, without fail, this will help us all, regardless of our age and skin type, to look and feel radiantly fresh and bright. It goes without saying that daily sun protection is the final piece of skin armoury (see page 43).

CLEANSE

Cleansing the face every morning and night is an absolute must for healthy skin. For most experts, a thorough cleanse – rather than a quick wipe – is regarded as the most important step in an effective routine. Wipes generally just move the dirt and grime from one part of the face to another, so applying expensive serums and creams over that is just a waste of time and money. Even when time is precious, this step is non-negotiable. Use a cleanser suited to your skin type and how your skin is feeling. If, for instance, your skin feels dry and parched, an oil-based cleanser will give the best cleanse while also locking in moisture.

A few tips to get you started on your journey to better skin:

- **MORNING CLEANSE:** A quick clean using a small amount of cleanser (oil- or water-based) will suffice as there should be no make-up, sunscreen or grime to remove.
- **EVENING CLEANSE:** This is most important to remove make-up, dirt and sunscreen remnants from the day. Oil-based cleansers are generally better at removing oily make-up and sunscreen, as the oil in the cleanser attracts the oil or excess sebum on the skin. Avoid mineral oil, which is a by-product of petroleum distillation (often called paraffin oil or liquid petroleum) – it is of absolutely no benefit and can clog pores. (See Skin Oils, page 27.) Use a clean cloth that has been held under warm water to wipe away cleanser. Rinse and repeat until all traces of make-up and grime are removed.
- **DOUBLE CLEANSING:** This generally works on a two-product system – first, a thick balm is applied to the face to remove make-up and stubborn grime. After washing off, a lightweight gel cleanser is applied, ideally with a cloth, to complete the thorough cleanse. This is especially beneficial for those who wear heavy make-up during the day or live in highly polluted cities, as although specialised make-up removers will take make-up off, they generally don't cleanse the pores quite as well.

EXFOLIATION AND PEELS

A deep, yet gentle, exfoliation once or twice each week helps slough stubborn dead skin cells, encouraging fresh cell renewal, while also allowing the skin to breathe and function more effectively. Choose an exfoliator that works for you, is not too aggressive and has no harsh ingredients. For example, if your skin is hormonally aggravated, choose a creamy or oily product that is gentler on the skin. For sensitive and very dry skin, a gentle exfoliation once a week will generally suffice, while oily and combination skin types should exfoliate two to three times a week using a gentle enzyme- or granular-based product.

Our current obsession with skin peels in their many guises (think peel pads, peel enriched toners, alpha hydroxy acids [AHAs] and so on) can leave skin thin and fragile. Yes, peels have a place, but they are not for everyday use and not for every skin type. So ease off on the scrubbing – be gentle. For specific advice ask your dermatologist.

TONE

A spray of mist or toner on thoroughly cleansed skin gives a dose of moisture to support the skin's protective barrier. Always choose alcohol-free toners (alcohol dries the skin). Those containing natural disinfectants like witch hazel can help remove residual bacteria and are especially useful for oilier and acne-prone skin. Keep a toning mist handy to spritz the skin during the day – while at work, after exercise or when travelling. Let the toner sit on the skin. Don't wipe it off.

Exfoliating toners are a relatively new category of toner, applied in the same way as more traditional types. Often called acid toners, they use acids like glycolic and salicylic to delve more deeply into the skin to slough away grime. These should not, however, replace traditional toners, but can be used, as needed, for a more intensive tone. As with exfoliators, above, they can strip the skin, leaving it very fragile, so be gentle.

NOURISH

Traditional skin creams (as our mothers' generation called them) worked in a superficial way, as the cream simply sat on the surface of the skin creating a barrier that retained moisture. The advent of cosmeceuticals in the 1980s brought cosmetics into the medical science arena, with ingredients scientifically formulated to delve deeper into the skin to nourish and tackle wrinkles, spider veins, pigmentation and many other issues. (See What Skin Needs, page 19.)

SERUMS

Serums are generally more active than moisturisers and are specifically designed to treat and repair the skin. An effective serum will contain the highest level of active ingredients possible, clearly matched to the problem they are trying to address (for example, peptides, hyaluronic acid and vitamin A derivatives in serums designed for ageing skin – see What Skin Needs, page 19). Think of it as a concentrated supplement boost for the skin. They should not be overloaded with additional ingredients (like sunscreens, for instance) as these can weaken the activity of the key ingredients and thus compromise overall performance.

From a practical perspective, one of the benefits of serums is that they are light in texture and absorb almost instantaneously into the skin, making them especially popular in hotter climates. While heavy creams can leave the skin feeling oily and weighty, serums feel luxuriously soft and smooth.

Serums generally fall into two categories: those packed with antioxidants to protect the skin during the day and those designed to repair the skin overnight. While it is worth investing in both, it is equally important to think about what your skin really needs, as this alters with the seasons and life changes. For example, for a boost of hydration, try a hyaluronic-acid-based serum, and for acne reduction and prevention use retinol and vitamin C. Always check the labels, as many poorer quality serums contain large amounts of silicone, a relatively cheap ingredient that lends a silky texture but no added skin benefits. If what you are being sold sounds too good to be true – then it probably is! Read product labels and buy from a trusted manufacturer.

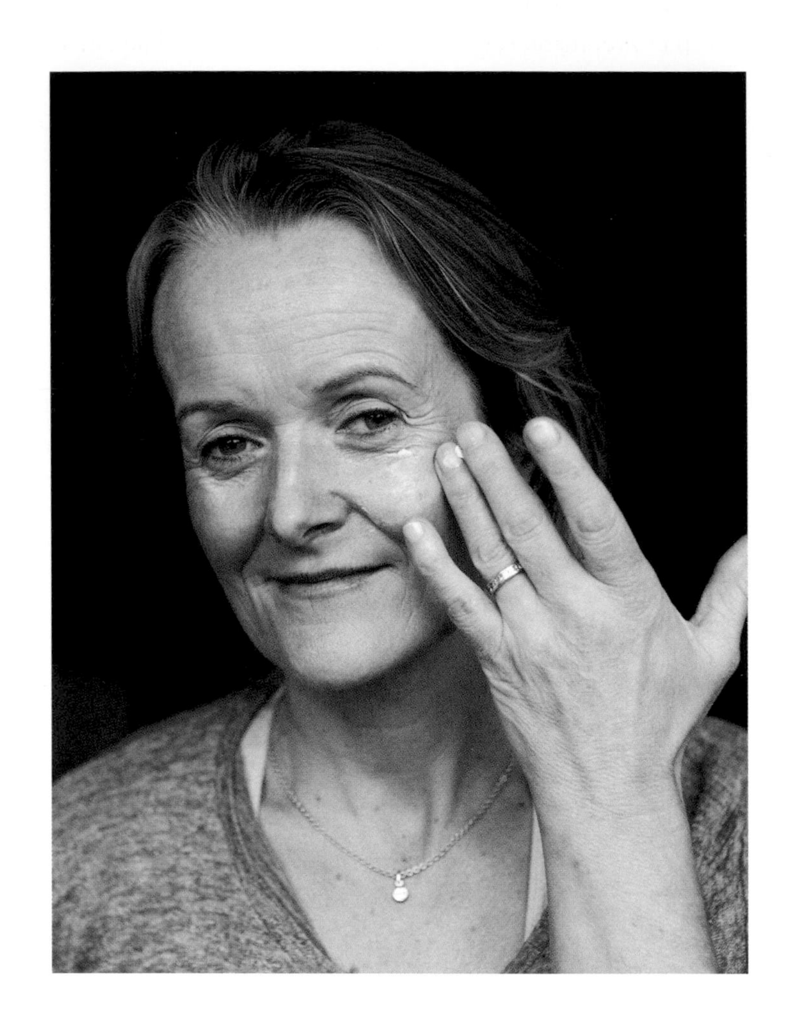

EMOLLIENTS AND HUMECTANTS

Emollients are lubricating agents that help keep skin hydrated by creating a barrier to lock moisture in and keep environmental aggressors out. Mineral oils and squalene are emollients, while more natural emollients include butters (cocoa and shea) and lanolin, which are the recommended options. Emollients are especially beneficial for those with dry complexions, as they keep the skin soft and supple. However, those with oily, congested skin may find this barrier function exacerbates congestion and blocks pores, especially if the product is rich.

A humectant is a substance that bonds with water molecules to increase the water content in the skin itself. Examples include glycerin and hyaluronic acid (see What Skin Needs, page 19). Humectants typically draw water into the skin from the environment, while also enhancing water absorption from the outer layers of the skin. Many humectants can also have emollient properties (hyaluronic acid, for instance) but not all emollients are humectants. The best skin moisturisers will include a combination of both on their ingredients list.

MASKS

Facemasks are ideally used once or twice a week, after a thorough cleanse, when enjoying a bath or long, hot shower, as the steam generated enhances the absorption of the essential ingredients. Quality masks combine repairing and nourishing actives (think vitamin C, hyaluronic acid, nicotanamide and so on – see What Skin Needs, page 19) with deeply nourishing plant oils. Many of today's masks can be kept on the skin overnight (in place of a night cream) to sink deep into the skin. Choose a brand you trust and use as directed on the product. When applying a mask, always include the décolletage, as it is especially sensitive and if not cared for will quickly show the signs of age. (See facemask recipes in Part 2.)

SKIN THROUGH THE DECADES

From the moment we are born we begin to age, but it's only in our twenties that the effects start to become visible in the skin. Skin typically works on a twenty-one-day cycle that begins to slow as we grow older.

- **INTRINSIC AGEING** is the natural skin-ageing process where collagen production slows, skin loses firmness, dead skin cells take longer to shed and skin cell turnover is diminished.
- **EXTRINSIC AGEING** is caused by external factors like sun and lifestyle stressors that exacerbate premature ageing.

While a comprehensive anti-ageing skincare routine is not necessarily needed until the late twenties/early thirties, it is *never* too early for preventive measures like sun protection, meals overflowing with skin-nourishing ingredients (as in the recipes in this plan) and regular exercise.

While every skin is different, the following is a general overview of some of the typical changes our skin undergoes as we move through the decades. None of this is predestined, but, without a doubt, the more we protect and nourish our skin during the earlier years, the better our skin will look and feel as we grow older.

20s

Regardless of skin type, once we reach adulthood, skin becomes a little drier every day. For people with naturally dry skin, some dullness, rough texture, flaking and skin tightness may be evident even at this young age. During the latter part of the twenties, natural biological ageing slowly sets in with biochemical changes in the skin's collagen and elastin fibres and the once neat architecture slowly starts to degrade. Excessive sun exposure during these earlier years will exacerbate skin ageing and can leave young skin looking and feeling at least a decade older.

WHAT YOU CAN DO

Thorough cleansing and adequate sun protection are non-negotiable. Choose light, natural products that are gentle on the skin. Invest in a gentle, light and pure face oil and apply it over cleansed and toned skin and around the eyes at night (See Skin Oils, page 27).Eat enough healthy fats and essential fatty acids (see The Plan, page 105). Drink plenty of water and, if you really want to care for your skin, limit alcohol intake and get adequate sleep and rest.

30s

Subtle changes occur throughout the thirties, which can become more pronounced with stress, late nights, alcohol, lack of exercise and so on. The skin under the eyes slowly starts to thin, leaving fine lines and puffy dark circles.

WHAT YOU CAN DO

The natural rate of skin exfoliation starts to slow, with a reduction in collagen and elastin fibres. Skin starts to lose water and its natural protective barrier weakens. Sun-induced damage can become more apparent, with an increase in dark sunspots and damaged pores.

Keep skin well hydrated with nurturing foods, water and appropriate skincare – think natural healing skin oils and targeted serums (for example, hyaluronic acid or niacinamide – see pages 20 and 27), especially at night, to repair and nourish while you sleep. Vitamin C-enriched products can protect skin from daily environmental aggressors and used in masks it can help bring back the glow. This is a good time to consult a trusted cosmetic dermatologist rather than relying on the sales representative at the local beauty counter. Get it right now – reap the rewards later.

40s AND 50s

For many women approaching their perimenopausal years, the hormone-induced changes to the skin can be quite disturbing, with loss of collagen, slackness, dryness, increased sensitivity and overall skin thinning. The skin's protective barrier grows weaker, leaving skin drier still and more vulnerable to environmental aggressors.

From the age of forty or thereabouts, it's estimated that the skin thins by 1 per cent per year, with a projected 2 per cent reduction noticed in collagen and elastin, while further damage is incurred by skin cells simply drifting into 'senescence' – in other words, just shutting down.

This is also the decade in which existing fine lines begin to morph into deeper wrinkles and the density of the skin decreases, resulting in a loss of overall facial volume and a drawn look. By the fifth decade, this process becomes even more exaggerated.

WHAT YOU CAN DO

Sun avoidance is essential, as is daily use of moisturisers and products enriched with antioxidants, active retinoids, collagen-stimulating peptides and AHAs (if used) to adequately repair, nourish and protect the face and neck from the ravages of hormone loss. More than ever before, essential fatty acids come into their own to deeply nourish even the driest of skin. Think natural, nourishing oils overflowing in essential fatty acids – eat them, drink them and apply them! Use targeted serums and masks, especially at night, to aid repair and deeply nourish.

NOTE: During these years, the increased energy demands of intense exercise can give rise to a skeletal, bony face, or 'runner's face' as it is often called. This is the result of a marked loss of fatty tissue beneath the layers of skin, leading to the deepening of wrinkles, loss of elasticity and the pronounced appearance of facial bones. To make matters worse, hours spent training outdoors exposed to harmful UV radiation incurs further damage on already compromised skin. To help prevent this bony look, ensure your overall energy intake is enough to meet the demands of your exercise routine, follow the daily skincare recommendations outlined here and always protect your skin with broad-spectrum SPF30+ sunscreen, regardless of the weather.

60s +

Through the sixties and beyond, skin succumbs further to age and gravity. It is estimated that a woman will lose up to 30 per cent of facial collagen during the five years after menopause, while hormone-induced facial bone loss can be up to 20 per cent, lending a very dull and shrunken look. The skin's natural protective barrier deteriorates even further, leaving skin drier, more sensitive and susceptible to bruising. While wrinkles and fine lines generally start to settle, gravity takes its toll and skin tone can become increasingly lax with the appearance of jowls and excess folds.

WHAT YOU CAN DO

Ageing skin needs a daily supply of essential fats and naturally nourishing oils, so continue to eat them and apply them liberally. Exfoliate regularly to brighten the skin and to allow better absorption of essential oils and other active ingredients. This is also the time to layer targeted serums rich in antioxidants, peptides, hyaluronic acid and so on, with oils and rich creams, one over the other, especially at night, to aid repair and deeply nourish. Lastly, maintain regular exercise – brisk walking, yoga or whatever you enjoy – which will increase blood flow to the skin and throughout the body.

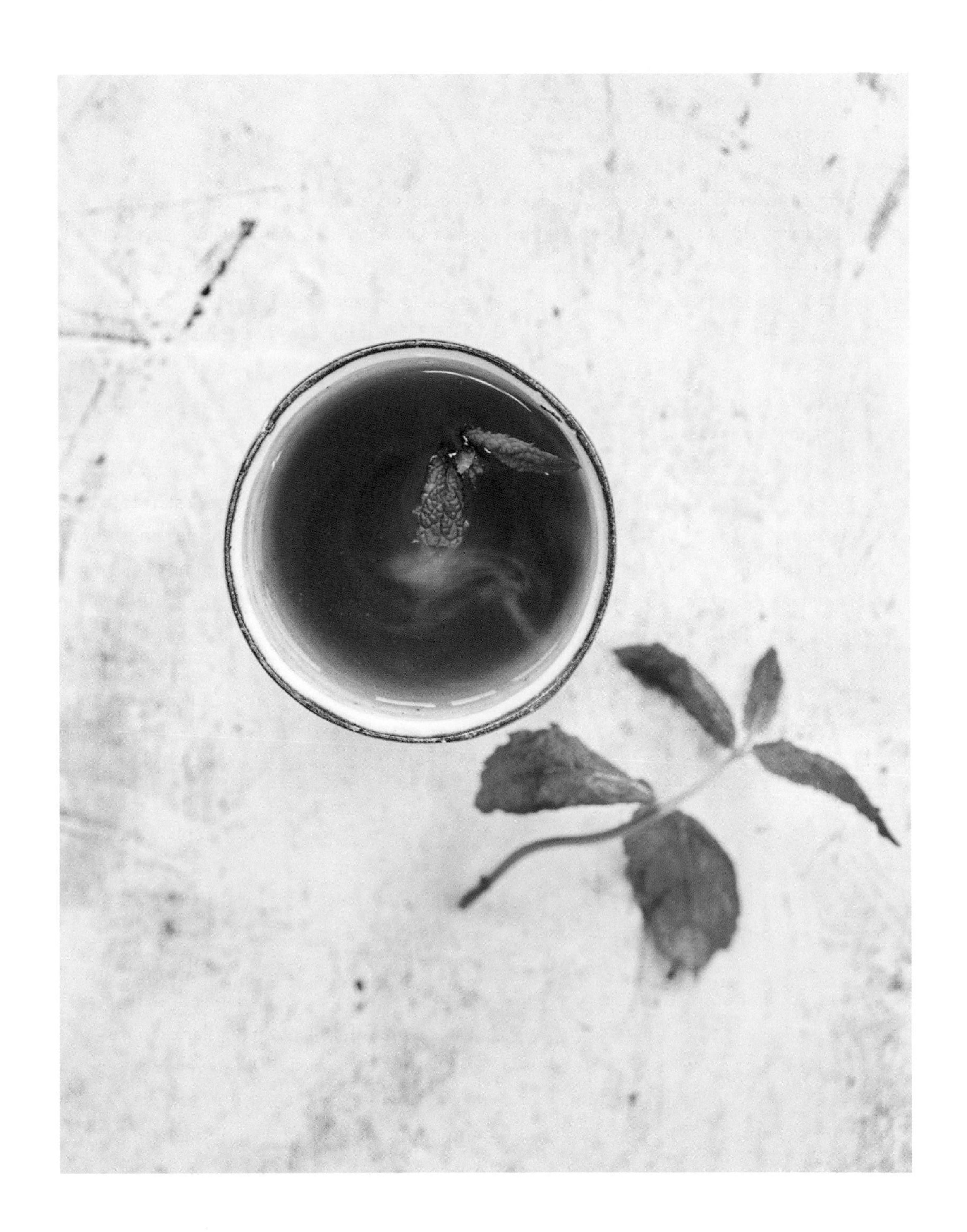

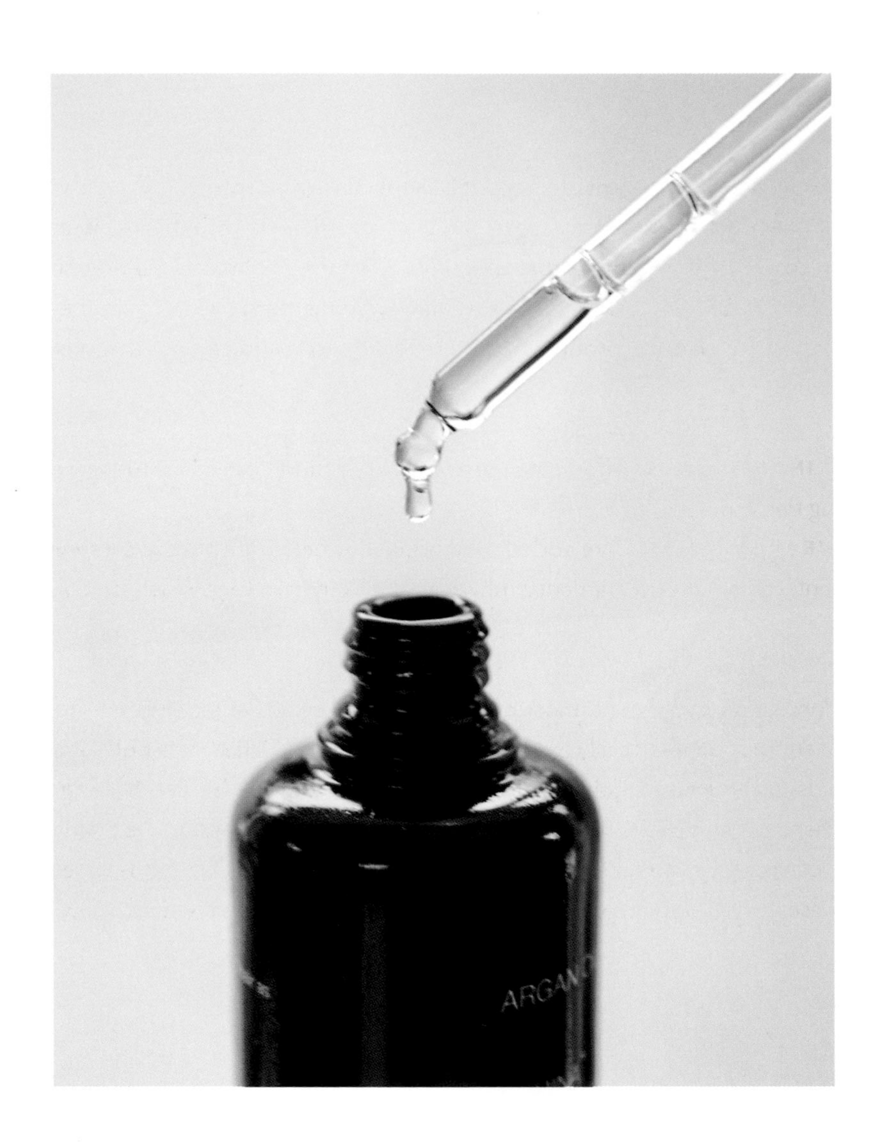

WHAT SKIN NEEDS

◊

Skin needs a network of nutrients to keep it healthy, balanced, protected and working at its best. The GLOW foods outlined on pages 71–92 are overflowing with the nutrients needed to maintain radiant skin from within. What we put on our face also makes a difference, and with advances in skin science, more complex-sounding ingredients are coming to the fore. All of the ingredients in our skincare products are there for a reason and can be categorised as either active or inactive.

- **ACTIVE INGREDIENTS** offer some therapeutic action, be it nurturing, repairing or protecting the skin.
- **INACTIVE INGREDIENTS** are added to a formula to help transport or preserve the active constituents or to alter a particular physical characteristic (e.g. smell or colour) of the product.

While everyone's skin is different, most of the following key active ingredients should be part of your skincare routine, especially from your thirties onwards. This list is not complete, but it reflects what is currently used in the most effective skincare ranges. With each new generation of actives, the benefits multiply, as does the ease of penetration into the skin. The building blocks of most of these ingredients come directly from food, so the more GLOW foods we eat, the more efficiently these actives work to protect and nourish our skin through the day and overnight.

COLLAGEN

Collagen is the fibrous protein-based connective tissue that holds our body together and makes up about one-third of the body's total protein content. It is found in tendons, ligaments, bone, muscle, cartilage and skin, where, with elastin, it forms a mesh that gives the skin structure, strength and elasticity.

Over 70 per cent of our skin is collagen, with the amount peaking in early adulthood and declining thereafter. Factors including sun and other environmental toxins, poor nutrition, smoking, insufficient sleep and stress exacerbate a decline in collagen, leaving the skin weaker, thin and prone to sagging. As collagen is a protein it is broken down by the digestive system into its constituent amino acids that are then distributed where needed through the body.

The key to maintaining healthy collagen levels in the skin is to first minimise the main threats from environmental aggressors, stress, poor diet and insufficient sleep. In addition, eating sufficient protein, unprocessed grains and healthy fats (most especially omega-3-rich fish oils) has been shown to improve collagen metabolism and overall skin health.

COLLAGEN DRINKS AND CREAMS

Collagen-enriched creams and drinks do not immediately translate into higher collagen levels in the skin. Sufficient protein intake is essential for providing the body with the building blocks it requires to replenish skin's collagen in the first place. There is no guarantee that drinking collagen drinks or lathering the face in collagen-enriched creams is any more effective than sufficient dietary protein taken through meat, fish, eggs, cheese, nuts, pulses and grains.

HYALURONIC ACID

Hyaluronic acid (also known as HA, hyaluron or hyaluronate) is a clear, sticky substance that occurs naturally in the body, where its main function is hydration. Scientifically, it is a glycosaminoglycan (or GAG) that helps the body build stronger, more flexible joints. It works as a shock absorber, lubricating the fluid in joint tissues through the body, while at the same time protecting joints from free radical destruction. HA shows similar benefits on the skin, where it works like a massive sponge, pulling moisture from the air into the skin and holding up to a thousand times its weight in water to soften and plump the skin. This basically means that it retains moisturising ingredients in the skin and prevents moisture loss from the skin. Young skin is smooth, elastic and rich in HA, but as our skin ages the natural production of hyaluronic acid slows.

Until relatively recently, synthetic HA molecules were too large to properly penetrate the skin's surface (unless used in injectable HA fillers) so the benefits were very limited. But with the advent of lower molecular weights (think nanoparticles) and cocktails of HA molecules of varying weights, they can now penetrate the deeper layers of the skin to repair and nourish, while also plumping the outer layers and protecting the fragile skin barrier for longer-lasting benefits. Due to its compatibility with the human body, HA is widely used by dermatologists as injectable dermal fillers. Its lightweight, gel-like texture makes it suitable for use in serums, moisturisers and masks for all skin types.

PEPTIDES

Peptides are short chains of amino acids (that make protein) and the fundamental building blocks of collagen, elastin and keratin, all jointly responsible for skin texture, elasticity and tone. Peptides keep skin intact and firm with the ability to bounce back as needed.

Just as there are many peptides, all of which are made from different combinations of amino acids, there are many peptide-based formulae, each with different therapeutic benefits – from smoothing fine lines and hydrating to increasing firmness and preserving the skin's barrier function. Peptides are present in therapeutic levels in quality anti-ageing serums and moisturisers, with many of the newer products combining a number of different peptides and targeting a range of concerns at once. As with other active ingredients, peptides are vulnerable to degradation from light and air so ensure you are buying a trusted brand.

RETINOL

Retinol describes the vitamin A molecule that when broken down creates more potent retinoid particles. Retinol works by stimulating collagen production, increasing cell turnover and exfoliating the top dead layers of the skin to reveal fresh new cells underneath. The latest generation of retinols deliver a range of revitalising effects from treating acne (without drying the skin), refining pores and diminishing dark spots, to smoothing the skin, reducing lines and improving overall texture and tone.

The potency of retinol-based products varies depending on whether prescribed (the prescription-only Retinoic Acid or Retin-A used to treat severe acne, for instance) or purchased over the counter. Retinol also occurs in skincare as retinyl palmitate, retinaldehyde, retinyl retinoate and retinyl propionate, although pure retinol is thought to be far more effective than retinol derivatives.

Although retinol is found in formulae designed for day use, it is best used as part of a night routine, starting slowly with a weaker strength every other night, before building up to a stronger formulation if tolerated. A note of caution, however, as although retinol-based products can help revitalise the skin, they can also dehydrate and so should only be used as recommended by a trusted dermatologist or skin expert. Particularly at a higher strength, retinol is very potent and can strip the skin. If redness or peeling occurs, use should be discontinued. Product stability is a concern and packaging needs to ensure minimal exposure to light and air (clear bottles must be avoided).

ACIDS: AHAs & BHAs

Acids help slough away dead skin cells, lending more radiance to the face. They are found in many skincare products, from face washes and toners to serums, masks and peels. AHAs and BHAs are the most commonly used skin acids.

AHAs (alpha hydroxy acids) are either naturally occurring or synthetic chemical compounds. Many are derived from organic sugars, such as glycolic acid (from sugar cane) and lactic acid (from milk). They work on the skin's surface to enhance natural moisturising properties within the skin. They have also been shown to help reduce the visible signs of sun damage.

BHAs (beta hydroxy or salicyclic acid) work both on the skin's surface and inside the pores to exfoliate and soothe congested and acne-prone skin. BHAs' anti-inflammatory, anti-microbial and natural skin-calming properties help calm skin redness and irritation.

As a general rule:

- **LACTIC ACID:** best for dry or sensitive skin
- **GLYCOLIC ACID:** best for ageing skincare
- **SALICYLIC ACID:** best for congested and acne-prone skin

AHAs act as chemical exfoliators that work primarily by dissolving the bonds between skin cells to facilitate the removal of dead cells, leaving a smoother skin surface. Glycolic acid is the most commonly used AHA. Due to its smaller molecule size and ease of penetration, it helps reduce fine lines, dark spots and acne scars. AHAs can increase photosensitivity, so always wear sunscreen – although you should already be doing so! AHAs come in varying strengths: lower strength for home use (2 per cent max) and varying higher strength formulae applied under expert supervision.

BHAs are oil soluble so they can penetrate to the roots of the pores, instead of operating at the surface level, making them ideal for treating oily and acne-prone skin in particular. As well as treating existing blemishes, BHAs also help neutralise bacteria within the pores, thereby deterring further breakouts. However, as they are heavy duty they can be drying on the skin and irritation may occur, especially in sensitive skin types, so start at a low concentration and gradually build up.

PHAs (polyhydroxy acids) are increasingly appearing in the latest generation of peels. They include ingredients like gluconolactone and lactobionic acid that are believed to be as effective as AHAs but more gentle, helping to slough away dead cells and hydrate the skin without irritation and stinging.

NOTE: AHAs are extremely potent, as they strip skin. If you are using them start very slowly at a low dose, 1–2 times per week, and see how your skin reacts. Do not use daily unless recommended by an expert, as for those with thinner or sensitive skin AHAs can do more harm than good, making the skin thinner and even more sensitive.

VITAMIN C

Vitamin C, or L-ascorbic acid in its purest form, is a powerful antioxidant and skin brightener. Other forms of vitamin C listed on skincare labels include ascorbyl palmitate (which is lipid soluble), magnesium ascorbyl phosphate (MAP), tetrahexyldecyl ascorbate (THDA) and sodium ascorbate.

Vitamin C is water soluble and protects skin from environmental aggressors and free radical damage. It acts by penetrating deep into the skin to stimulate fresh collagen production, while also helping to smooth, brighten and revitalise the complexion – hence the use of these key words in vitamin C-enriched products! Used daily at an appropriate concentration, it can help clear pores and reduce pigmentation.

Vitamin C is available in various concentrations, from less than 1 per cent in moisturisers and serums (although serums can support higher levels) to over 20 per cent in professional treatments. While it is best used as part of a morning routine in toners, serums and moisturisers designed to protect skin against UV and environmental aggressors through the day, it can be safely used as an adjunct to a night routine to boost collagen production through the night.

However, like all antioxidants, it is vulnerable to damage, so choose light, water-based formulations that penetrate fast, packaged in opaque, airtight containers. Alternatively, vitamin-C powders tend to be more stable and can be used straight on the skin or mixed into other products. If the colour of the formula darkens or the smell changes, it has probably oxidised and should be binned.

VITAMIN D

Vitamin D is not technically a vitamin (as vitamins are not produced by the body) so, as it is produced in the skin on exposure to sunlight, it is more accurately described as a hormone. It is estimated that after just twenty to thirty minutes of sun exposure, the skin will produce up to 10,000IU vitamin D, which more than covers our daily needs at all times of the year.

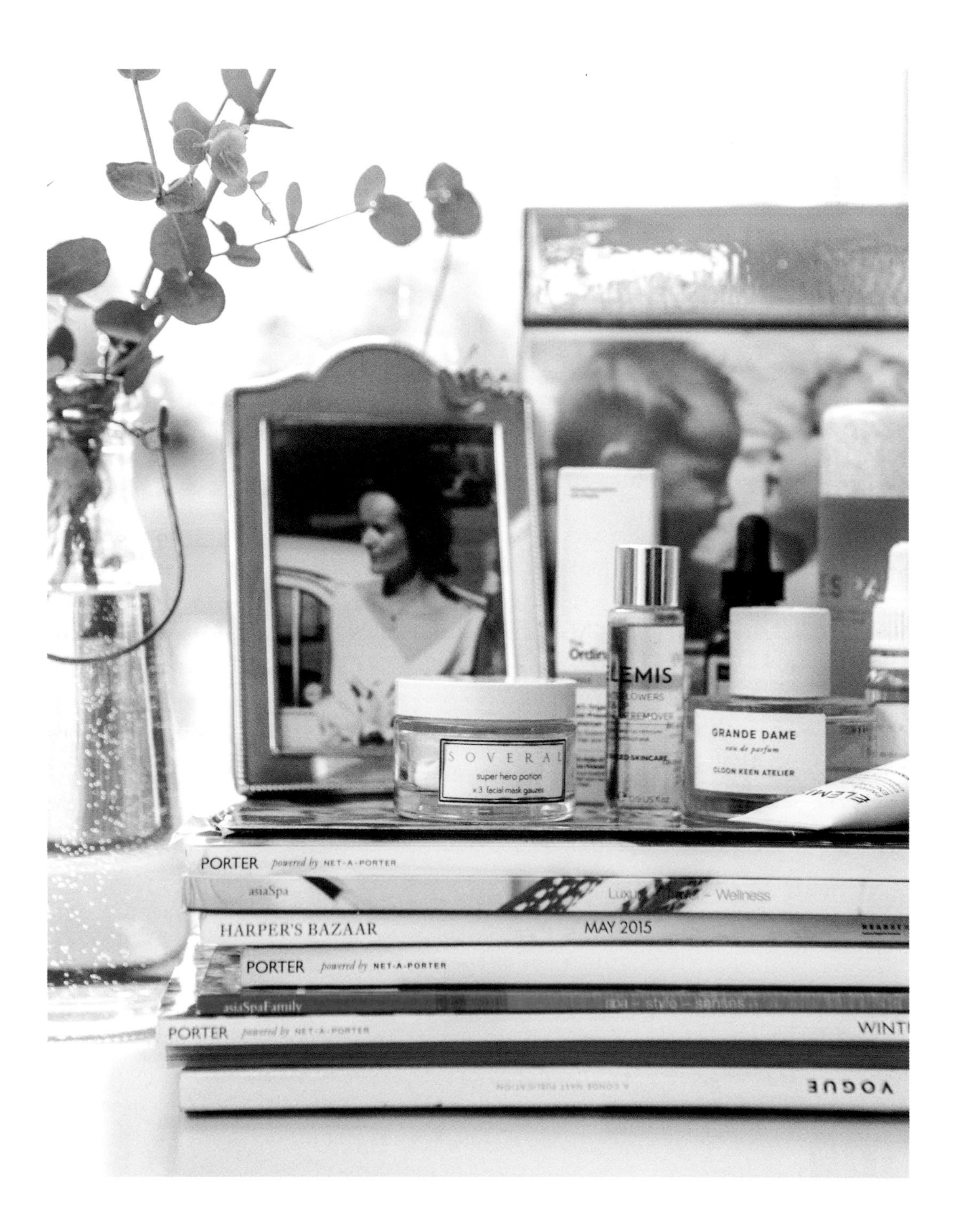
SOVERAL
super hero potion
x 3 facial mask gauzes
GRANDE DAME
eau de parfum
CLOON KEEN ATELIER
PORTER powered by NET-A-PORTER
asiaSpa
HARPER'S BAZAAR
MAY 2015
PORTER powered by NET-A-PORTER
asiaSpaFamily
PORTER powered by NET-A-PORTER

Epidemiological studies have highlighted an association between low vitamin D intake and a number of diseases, including cardiovascular disease, diabetes, certain cancers, cognitive decline and depression. Vitamin D3, the active form of vitamin D, is believed to be involved with over two thousand interactions in the body, including enhancing a healthy immune system, strengthening bones and teeth, enhancing digestion, absorption and essential skin repair and protection. Evidence suggests it also has a role in tackling acne and psoriasis.

We can avail of the benefits of vitamin D through sunlight and food (oily fish, egg yolks, fortified milks and cereals). However, as numerous studies have highlighted the prevalence of vitamin D deficiency, especially in northern Europe, evidence supports the use of vitamin D3 supplements, most especially during the winter months when sunshine is limited.

VITAMIN E

Vitamin E or d-alpha-tocopherol is a fat-soluble vitamin that functions as a powerful antioxidant and skin healer. It has long been used to repair lesions, scars, burns and abrasions. It occurs naturally in human skin but is easily depleted with environmental exposure in the absence of sun protection.

Vitamin E helps protect the integrity of cell membranes and restore moisture in dry and damaged skin. It is a heavy emollient so is suitable as a cleanser, removing dirt, grime and other impurities, while simultaneously working to maintain skin's oil balance (a feat that many other cleanser-type ingredients fail to achieve). It is believed to be more effective in its natural alcohol form (alpha-tocopherol) than the acetate form (alpha-tocopherol acetate), so always read the label and choose the purest product available.

NIACINAMIDE

Also known as vitamin B3 and nicotinic acid, niacinamide is one of the water-soluble B group of vitamins. In addition to its numerous functions throughout the body, studies have shown that niacinamide is an effective skin-restoring ingredient that protects and strengthens the skin barrier, reducing water loss and visibly improving the appearance of enlarged pores, fine lines and uneven skin tone.

NIACINAMIDE AND VITAMIN C

While there has been debate over the simultaneous use of niacinamide and vitamin C, either in the same product or layered separately one after the other, research has shown that the combination of the two can offer enhanced results and a smoother, brighter, more radiant complexion.

SKIN OILS

Oils from plants, nuts and seeds are a concentrated source of minerals, vitamins and essential fatty acids (EFAs) that have long been used as natural healers. From gently cleansing the skin of impurities to keeping it smooth and supple, these botanical oils are the ultimate multitaskers and it seems our ancestors already knew what scientists have subsequently been able to prove: that when applied directly to the skin pure plant oils can dramatically improve the condition of the skin, strengthen nails and give hair a healthy, glossy sheen. They are perfect for super-dry environments too (such as when flying) and the real beauty is that they can be adapted to match our body's changing needs – be they hormonal, seasonal or stress-induced.

While those with oilier complexions have traditionally avoided oil-based products (in the mistaken belief that they make the skin even oilier), it is now accepted that, when used appropriately, oils are the gentlest and most effective cleansers and regulators of oily skin. The skin absorbs oil-soluble substances more easily than it does water-soluble, so when essential oils are diluted with a plant or vegetable carrier oil they can deliver results deep within the skin. Take rose and chamomile, for example – when used over or blended with moisturiser they create a barrier that prevents moisture loss, while also protecting dry skin from external aggressors. Experienced make-up artists apply oils like rose on the face and neck before applying make-up, knowing that, in addition to nourishing the skin, the oil helps prep the skin, ensuring that make-up lasts longer. Natural oils are equally beneficial when used on the hair, keeping it clean and shiny – as Indian women have known for centuries.

NOTE: Rose, used on its own or combined with frankincense and geranium, for instance, works as an intensive skin therapy when applied under regular night cream or a facemask and left overnight to boost collagen and restore firmness – all while we sleep.

For optimum results, the oils must be high quality, as bland mineral oils just sit on the surface of the skin, clogging pores. While it can prove difficult for consumers to check the purity of oils, by buying from a trusted skincare company, you can be more confident about the quality of the ingredients. Finer-grade natural oils tend to be lighter in colour too, but shop around for the best quality.

Many of today's niche brands use oils cultivated by skilled artisans from remote, rural communities in the Himalayas, the Amazon rainforest or the markets of Morocco, where organic is the standard process of agriculture and the seeds and nuts are hand gathered from native trees, immune to the effects of harsh and suspect chemicals. Quality oils can be expensive to produce – like pure rose, for instance, where the flowers are hand gathered at dawn before the volatile oil starts to evaporate – but a little goes a long way and your skin will thank you.

Some top-quality products are certified organic; others may not be, but they can also contain the very best of ethical, natural ingredients, so shop wisely.

Oils are simple to use. They are absorbed better when applied to damp skin, so apply a few drops (a little more if skin feels very dry) on cleansed and toned skin, massaging upwards from the neck and with circular movements over the face to stimulate blood flow (see GLOW Face Blend, page 135). Alternatively, a few drops of oil can be added to moisturiser or a mask before applying to the face.

NOTE: To cleanse with oil, smother the oil over dry skin to remove make-up. Add a splash of warm water to emulsify, forming a milky fluid that removes all traces of dirt without stripping the skin. Rinse with warm water.

TOP PICKS

Argan Oil (*Argania Spinosa*)

The Berber women of Morocco have used the pressed juice of the argan kernel for centuries to combat the dry desert air and reduce the signs of ageing. The oil is sourced from argan trees that grow exclusively in the Souss valley of southwestern Morocco, now a UNESCO biosphere reserve, where locally they are known as the 'Tree of Life'.

Top-quality argan oil is overflowing with vitamin E, essential fatty acids and antioxidants, which together help soften, repair and rejuvenate every skin type. The oil is a wonderfully soothing anti-inflammatory too, thanks to its rare plant sterols. It is light and non-greasy on the skin and is absorbed easily to give a radiant glow while also being great for hair. It has a warm nutty taste and can be drizzled over pasta and salads. Heating destroys its nutrient benefits so use it cold.

You can also use argan oil to make amlou – the heavenly blend of argan, honey and almonds that the Moroccans use in place of jam for breakfast or as a dip for bread. Simply grind 300g roasted almonds, then blend in 250ml argan oil and 125ml runny honey. Experiment with the ratios to find your perfect mix.

Camellia Oil (*Camellia Oleifera*)

Generations of wisdom surround the delicate camellia flower and its deeply nourishing oil, which is believed to have been discovered thousands of years ago by Japan's Oshima Island Girls (or Anko) who harvested the winter bloom for its precious oil. Rich in vitamins, oleic acid and essential fatty acids, camellia (or tsubaki) oil is one of the most treasured secrets of the geisha, who used it to remove their iconic stage make-up and nourish their skin and hair. This legacy has passed through generations to modern-day geisha, who continue to reap the benefits of its skin-enhancing properties.

Marula Oil (*Sclerocarya Birrea*)

Marula is rich in antioxidants and essential fatty acids and a great multitasker for the skin. Native to the miombo woodlands of Southern Africa, the Sudano-Sahelian range of West Africa and Madagascar, it helps lock moisture into the skin, making it especially beneficial as part of a nightly skin regime to keep skin hydrated and maintain moisture in the protective skin barrier. A few drops rubbed through the hair guarantees instant texture and deep nourishment.

Coconut and Monoi Oils

Coconut oil is a non-volatile plant oil full of vitamin E, ferulic acid and other antioxidants to soothe and nourish both the skin and hair. Slathered over the body post-showering, it locks moisture into the skin, while a few drops added to a warm bath make for a soothing night-time ritual.

Monoi oil is a lighter, more fragrant variant of coconut oil traditionally used by ancient Polynesians in worship ceremonies to anoint newborns and purify objects. It is cultivated by steeping Tiare Tahiti (an exotic gardenia) blossoms in pure coconut oil to make a fragrant oil that is liberally applied over the body and hair to nourish, repair and protect.

Prickly Pear Seed Oil (*Opuntia Ficus Indica)*

A member of the cactus family, prickly pear is native to Mexico and now widely grown in semi-arid areas like Morocco. It is known as a miracle plant for its ability to survive droughts and still produce healthy fruits packed with small black seeds from which the antioxidant-rich oil is extracted.

Rich in vitamin E and essential fatty acids, prickly pear oil helps stimulate cell renewal and restore skin's elasticity, keeping it moist and soft. It is suitable for all skin types, even the most sensitive, reducing redness and instantly soothing.

Rose (*Rosa Centifolia* and *Rosa Damascena*)

The ancient Egyptians were the first to harness the benefits of rose for medicinal purposes, but it was the Arabic perfumers who are believed to have perfected the commercial distillation of rose water around the seventh or eighth century, with large areas of Iran, Iraq and Syria now dedicated to its cultivation.

There are two main families of rose: *Rosa centifolia*, also known as Rose de Mai, grown mainly in Grasse, in France, and flowering during the month of May (hence the name), and *Rosa Damascena*, or Damask rose, grown in Bulgaria, primarily for the perfume industry. With both varieties, the flowers are collected at dawn, before being exposed to the sun, to harness optimum vitality. They are then distilled into a deep, pure rose oil or otto that boosts blood circulation and deeply regenerates skin cells.

NOTE: According to perfume expert Roja Dove, it takes approximately 307,000 roses to produce 1kg of oil – to put that into context, it would take one of the best pickers a total of 24 hours to pick enough roses to produce 30ml of essential oil. That is precious.

Rosehip (*Rosa Rubiginosa*)
Vibrant orangey-red rosehips have long been used by the ancient Egyptians, Mayans and Native Americans and are now common-place along European hedgerows during the autumn months.

Their cold-pressed oil is packed with antioxidant vitamins A and E and essential fatty acids and is regarded by many experts as one of the most effective plant oils for repairing and regenerating skin cells. From scar tissue to stretch marks, sun damage, psoriasis, fine wrinkles and irregular pigmentation, it acts directly on affected cell membranes to repair and revitalise.

Sweet Almond Oil (*Prunus Amygdalus Dulcis*)
Sweet almond oil comes from the deciduous almond tree native to an area stretching from Pakistan to Syria, Israel and Turkey. Rich in essential fatty acids and vitamin E, it is one of the most versatile skin oils available and is routinely used on its own or as a base oil to soften and nourish the skin. It is lightweight and non-irritating, making it especially suitable for sensitive skin types. Applied in tiny amounts to the hair, it instantly adds lustre and gloss.

Apricot oil (*Prunus Armeniaca*)
Active ingredients: Vitamins A and E, gamma linolenic acid (GLA) and other essential fatty acids.
Benefits: The light oil from the kernels is absorbed quickly to nourish and soothe the skin and maintain moisture balance.

Avocado oil (*Persea Gratissima*)
Active ingredients: Vitamins A (beta-carotene), D and E and essential fatty acids.
Benefits: Regenerates skin cells and strengthens membranes. Soothes and heals sun damage, scars and dry skin.

Borage seed oil (*Borago Officinalis*)
Active ingredients: Concentrated source of essential fatty acid (GLA).
Benefits: Moisturising plant oil that nourishes and locks in moisture. (Also listed as *Borago officinalis* extract or oil.)

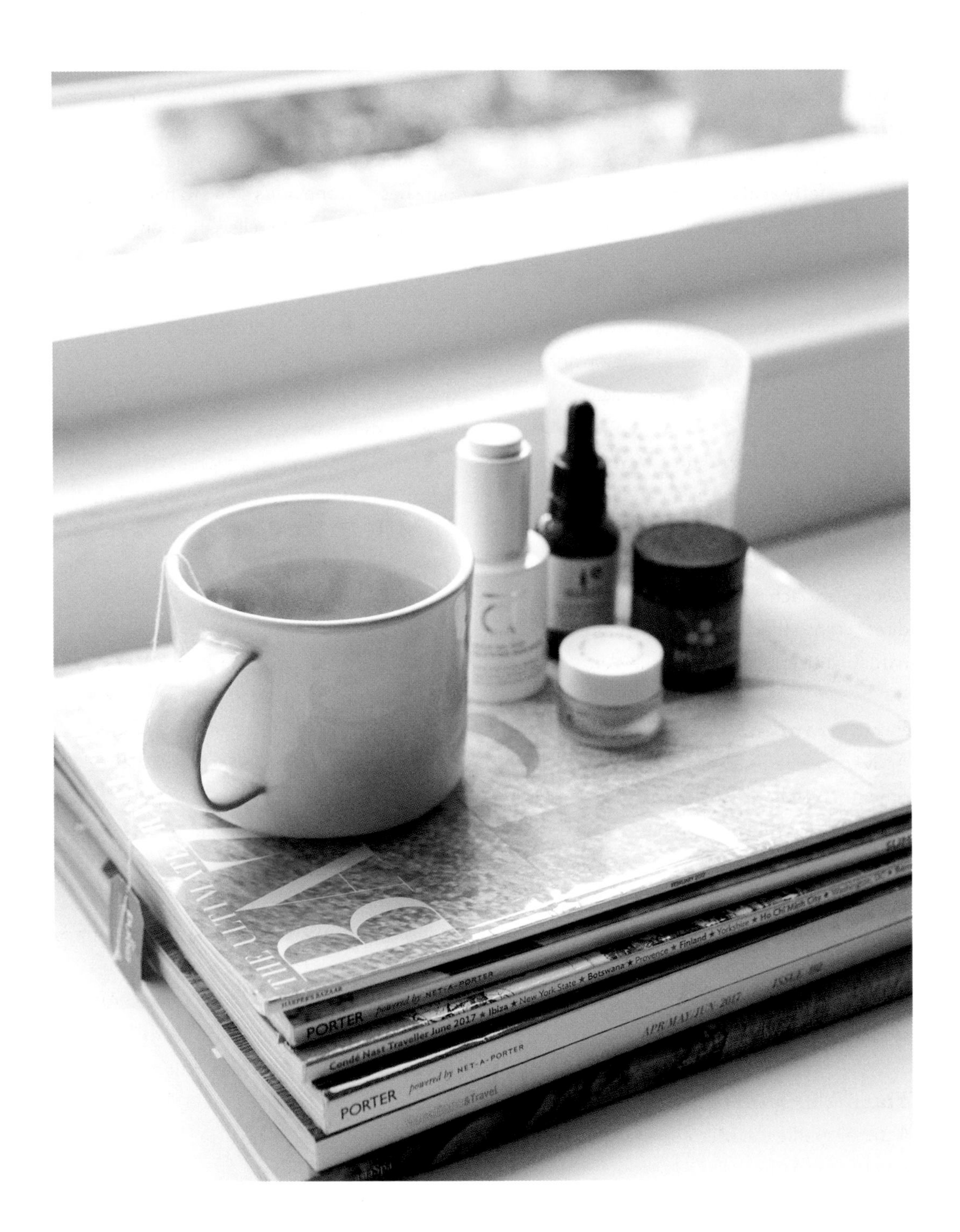
PORTER powered by NET-A-PORTER
Condé Nast Traveller June 2017 ★ Ibiza ★ New York State ★ Botswana ★ Provence ★ Finland ★ Yorkshire ★ Ho Chi Minh City
PORTER powered by NET-A-PORTER

Evening primrose oil (*Oenothera Biennis*)
Active ingredients: Concentrated source of essential fatty acids, especially GLA.
Benefits: Boosts circulation and nourishes skin and scalp. Soothes irritation and helps relieve eczema, psoriasis and dry skin conditions. Powerful hormone regulator and used to help relieve premenstrual tension and other hormone-related imbalances.

Lavender (*Lavandula Officinalis*)
Active ingredients: Linalool and linalyl acetate.
Benefits: Multipurpose healer that can relieve headaches and tension (when rubbed directly onto the temples) and acts as a natural antiseptic healer on the skin.

Peppermint (*Mentha Piperita*)
Active ingredients: Menthol, menthone and other menthol-type compounds that create a cooling effect through the body.
Benefits: Commonly used in toners and products designed to cool and stimulate the skin. Can help relieve scaly skin and dermatitis on the skin and scalp, while also easing hot flushes, sweating, headaches and mild stomach upsets.

Ylang-Ylang (*Cananga Odorata*)
Active ingredients: Methyl benzoate, 4-menthyanizole, benzylbenzoate and other compounds.
Benefits: Stimulates circulation, repairs and nourishes skin and adds shine to hair. A mood balancer that can help relieve tension and anxiety.

USING ESSENTIAL OILS ON THE BODY

In the Bath
Add 6–8 drops of your chosen oil or blend to bathwater. A couple of drops each of clary sage, geranium and cypress oil can help rebalance hormonal aggravations, while a soothing blend of rose and chamomile calms the body and aids restful sleep.

As a Body Oil
Dilute 4–5 drops of chosen essential oils in 10ml of carrier oil (e.g. jojoba or sweet almond oil) or add a few drops of chosen essential oils to your favourite body oil and massage into damp skin after a bath or shower.

As an Inhaler
Essential oils can also be inhaled directly from a tissue or added to a diffuser or vaporiser following manufacturers' instructions. Alternatively, carry a small spray bottle of mist – try peppermint or lavender (see recipe page 120) – in your handbag and spritz the face, head and neck as required.

SKIN SUPPLEMENTS

Our skin needs a wide range of nutrients to nurture, replenish and repair it, and supplements, regardless of format, are not the answer. Feeding the skin from within really is the game changer and this four-week plan is heavy on deliciously nourishing foods and light on non-essential extras. In truth, added supplements should not be needed. This said, if you struggle to get your fill of essential fats or are living through a stressful period in your life and feel your overall health is suffering, some of the following might help add some vitality and balance to dull, lacklustre skin. Be very careful not to overdo it, however, as taken in levels beyond the recommended, certain nutrients can be detrimental and, in many cases, a complete waste of money.

THE INFORMATION provided here is not intended to replace conventional medical treatment. These recommendations are not intended to treat, cure or prevent any disease or symptom. Personalised dosage and usage instructions should be provided by a qualified healthcare practitioner.

ESSENTIAL FATTY ACIDS

Cold-water oily fish – notably salmon, trout and tuna – are packed with omega-3 fatty acids that help strengthen blood cells and plump the skin, boosting the production of essential collagen and elastin. They are also essential components of cell membranes throughout the body. Other sources of EFAs include flax seeds, walnuts, hemp, almonds, eggs and dark green leafy vegetables. Even if you are eating a healthy mix of these foods, if your skin is looking and feeling dull and lifeless then a supplement could help bring back the glow.

KRILL OIL

Krill oil extract is prepared from a species of Antarctic krill (*Euphausia superba*) that shares a similar fatty acid profile to fish, with an efficient delivery mechanism in the body. Krill oil also contains astaxanthin, a powerful antioxidant that helps to protect against free radical damage.

VITAMIN E

This fat-soluble vitamin is a prerequisite for healthy, glowing skin (see page 26). If you are worried that your skin is ageing faster than it should, then it is worth considering a vitamin E boost in natural supplement form, starting with 200IU for at least a month, increasing if needed and recommended by a qualified healthcare practitioner. Simply pierce the capsule and either blend the rich oil with your serum or moisturiser or lather directly over your face as part of your evening skin routine.

TIP: Vitamin E rich oils can be a game changer for healing skin damage and scar tissue. Look for products containing the natural rather than the synthetic form of vitamin E.

LECITHIN

Essential for healthy cell membranes throughout the body, sufficient lecithin can make the difference between soft, plump skin and skin that is dull and lifeless. Sunflower lecithin is rich in choline and other essential fatty acids, and because it's extracted without the need for potentially damaging chemical solvents, it is the most natural option. With no harsh aftertaste, it can be added to juices and smoothies without affecting the flavour.

VITAMIN D

Experts recommend a Vitamin D supplement in the range of 1000IU from spring to autumn and 3000IU from autumn to spring to ensure daily needs are met through the winter months. As vitamin D is oil soluble it can be difficult to absorb in the body so can be sprayed under the tongue, thereby avoiding the gastric route. Consult your healthcare practitioner for further information.

PROBIOTICS

The live probiotic bacteria in our intestines are essential to health. Probiotics are active live microorganisms naturally present in foods and also widely available as over-the-counter supplements. With our stressful lifestyles and dependence on processed foods, our need for these probiotic bacteria is greater than ever. When selecting a probiotic, choose acid-resistant strains, such as lactobacillus species, with a minimum of 4 to 5 billion organisms per capsule. Choose a probiotic with multiple strains of bacteria, coated enterically to protect them from the acid stomach environment and ensure they colonise the gut effectively. (See Gut and Skin page 53.)

BEAUTY POWDERS

Inner beauty drinks and powders are big business now, with no sign of waning. While some contain medicinal-grade extracts accompanied by a wealth of scientific support, the jury is out as to the benefits of many others. Their taste alone can be far from beautiful, with a lot of disguising required to make them palatable!

Many of these inner beauty powders list hydrolysed collagen or marine proteins as their hero ingredient. Science has shown the importance of collagen for keeping skin elastic and supple, but what actually happens when we ingest collagen, regardless of the source, is that as soon as it reaches the stomach it will be used the same way as any other food protein (such as eggs, meat or fish): the stomach will release enzymes to break this protein into its constituent amino acid building blocks that will then be either used by the body or excreted (if not needed).

In essence, we don't actually need to put collagen into our body: we help our body make its own by feeding it the necessary building blocks through the foods we eat every day.

If you're buying a beauty powder then choose a pure natural extract (not naturally derived) with a maximum of six ingredients. Also check for Eur Ph (European Pharmacopoeia) next to an ingredient, as this indicates that the extract is medicinal-grade pharmacopoeia that can safely make clinical or medicinal claims.

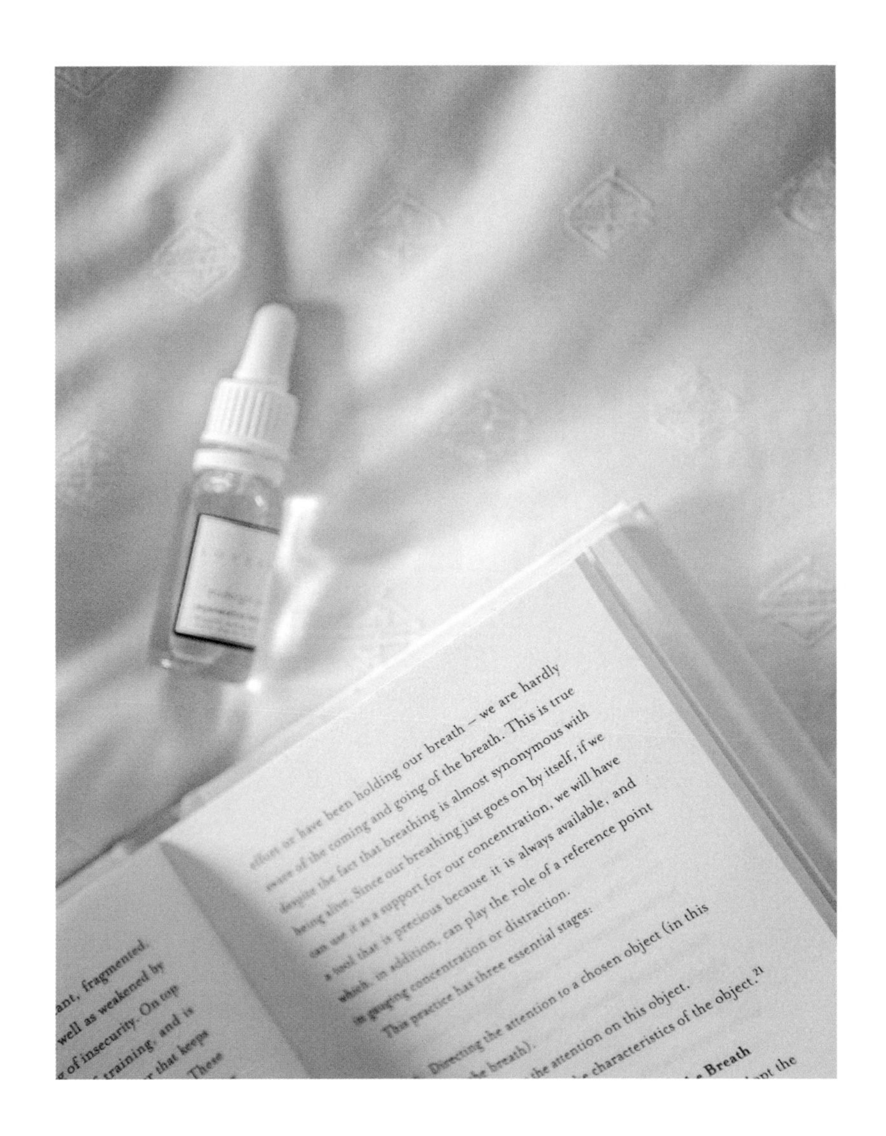
have been holding our breath – we are hardly
of the coming and going of the breath. This is true
the fact that breathing is almost synonymous with
Since our breathing just goes on by itself, if we
it as a support for our concentration, we will have
that is precious because it is always available, and
in addition, can play the role of a reference point
concentration or distraction.
This practice has three essential stages:
Directing the attention to a chosen object (in this
the breath).
the attention on this object.
characteristics of the object.[21]

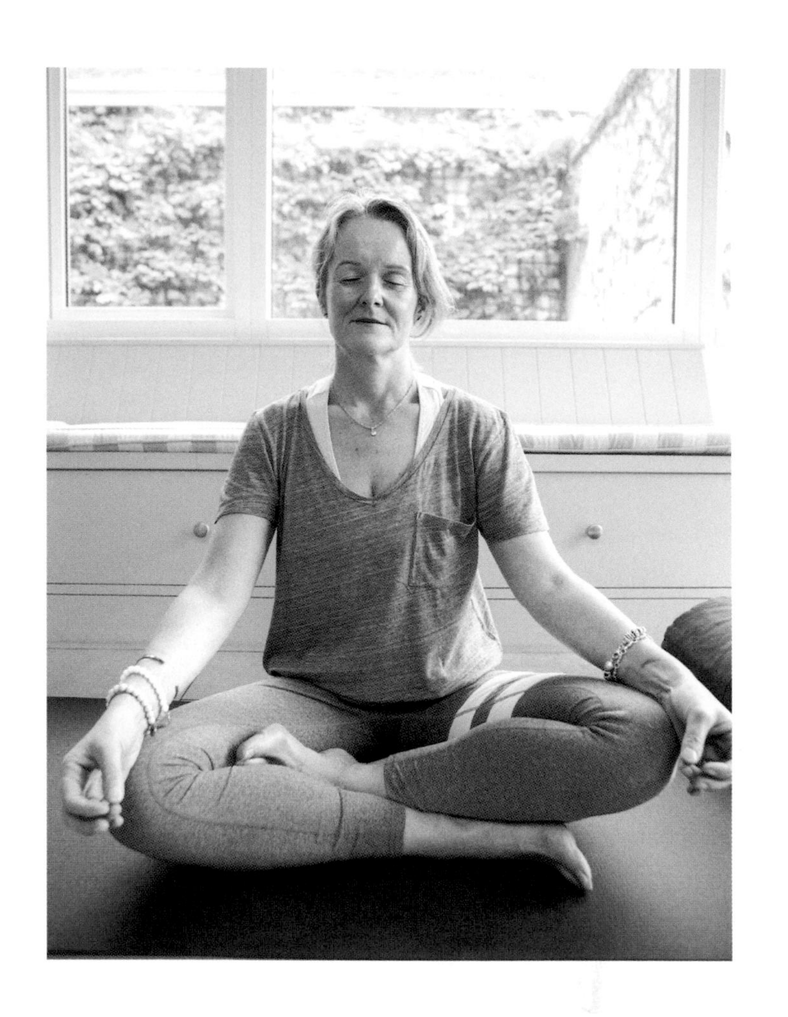

SKIN STRESSORS

◊

The last twenty years have seen profound shifts in our understanding of the impact of our environment and chaotic lifestyles on our skin. A combination of stress, UV damage, pollution, cigarettes, alcohol, late nights, poor diet and lack of exercise take their toll and, given that the skin is our largest organ, it's highly susceptible to these aggressors. This said, our skin also responds very quickly to lifestyle changes, so once you make the decision to give up smoking or sugar, for example, your skin will start to breathe and cleanse relatively quickly and benefits will soon become apparent.

STRESS

The field of psychodermatology explores the intrinsic interaction between the mind and the skin. It has established an indisputable link between stress levels and our skin, and once we appreciate that our skin and nervous systems developed from the same part of the embryo during our development, we can understand why this is so. So whether we are embarrassed, shocked or stressed, our skin, being the most noticeable part of our body to be impacted by psychological factors, responds accordingly by either blushing, flaring up or breaking out.

Science has shown that stress impacts the skin via a cascade of reactions from the brain that promote the release of hormones including cortisol, oestrogen and testosterone (among others), causing blood vessels to dilate, instigating sweating and flushing, and often increasing oil production in the hair follicle – the perfect recipe for acne.

Stress can also trigger neuropeptides (chemicals unleashed from nerve endings in the skin) that can leave skin red and itchy and encourage T cells (the skin's infection fighters) to overreact, making the skin turn over too quickly, resulting in flaking and scaling (think psoriasis and eczema). Elevated stress levels also give rise to glycation that ultimately destroys the smooth, springy bundles of collagen, leading to tissue inflammation and damage (see page 49).

Added to the mix is a more localised stress-induced system, one in which the permeability of the skin's protective barrier becomes more vulnerable, allowing water to escape and bacteria and allergens to penetrate, leaving the skin dry, irritated and problematic.

The collateral damage of this chronic stress cascade is an overload in free radical formation that damages the cells' DNA by shortening telomeres (the buffers at the ends of chromosomes that protect every cell's DNA integrity). Skin cells are thought to be particularly susceptible to this shortening because of their high proliferation rate and exposure to UV and other environmental stresses.

Even our stomach is closely linked with both our brain and skin through a highway of hormones, chemicals and neurons, and studies have shown that people with gut disorders such as irritable bowel syndrome and ulcerative colitis (both conditions exacerbated by stress) have been shown to experience higher levels of skin complaints (see Gut and Skin, page 53).

As the consequences of chronic stress on the skin are now recognised as a medical issue, dermatologists are combining traditional skin treatments with psychotherapy, hypnosis and meditation to soothe the skin by reducing the stress response. So much so that the American Association of Dermatology stated: 'traditional dermatologic therapies should be used in conjunction with stress management therapies to treat stress-related skin conditions'. And as the mind–skin connection gains further credence, beauty companies have seized the opportunity to launch serums and balms formulated to tackle the consequences of stress overload on the skin.

STRESS AND HAIR

Increased exposure to air pollution and other environmental toxins is now believed to contribute to common hair concerns including dry, itchy scalp and dull, lifeless hair. Stress is known to be a key cause of scalp flaking, itching and increased hair fall. With these aggressors at an all-time high, our hair needs every protection possible:

- Minimise air pollution exposure where possible by avoiding busy main roads.
- When in polluted environments keep your hair covered or tie it back.
- Wash hair regularly. Many common pollutants sit on the outside of the hair cuticle and are easily washed off with regular shampooing.
- Use more natural-based products, free from unnecessary chemicals.

BREAKING THE STRESS–SKIN CYCLE

The following are simple techniques that have been proven to help manage our stress levels, even during challenging times.

- **LOOK FOR THE WARNING SIGNS:** Keep a diary to help you look out for signs of stress in your life – irritability, poor concentration, insomnia, mood swings and so on – as acting on these from the outset can prevent stress levels from getting dangerously high.
- **NOURISH YOUR BODY:** It is now widely accepted that alcohol and stimulants such as sugar and caffeine can heighten anxiety levels in the body. All of the GLOW foods outlined in this book – without exception – are designed to keep skin nourished, while also helping to reduce the impact of stress on skin and throughout the body.
- **SKIN TREATMENTS:** Topical products can help relieve outward signs of stress on the skin (eczema, acne, dry skin and so on) when used in conjunction with relaxation techniques and targeted skin treatments delivered by a trusted expert.
- **MAKE TIME TO PRACTISE MEDITATION/MINDFULNESS:** Science has shown that the more we practise mindfulness and meditation techniques, the more in tune we become with our bodies and our lives. And as our brain adapts, so too does our ability to remain relatively calm in difficult situations. A UK study of people with psoriasis found that eight weeks of mindfulness-based cognitive therapy resulted in patients reporting reduced flare-ups and improved quality of life.
- **SELF-CARE:** Neuroscience is showing that by simply making the choice to be kind to ourselves we can alter our brain and body chemistry, with huge implications for our mental and physical well-being.
- **EXERCISE:** Regular moderate exercise floods the body with endorphins that help keep us healthier, stronger and more in control of our lives. This said, studies have shown that

prolonged endurance sports can exacerbate stress, so work with your body and know your limits. If you're new to exercise, invest in sessions with a trusted personal trainer.

- **YOGA:** There's something hugely powerful and grounding about a steady yoga practice that is not evident in many other forms of exercise. Find a qualified and experienced teacher and the benefits will be endless.
- **SLEEP:** Sleeping soundly can add years to your life – and your face (see page 59).
- **SMILE AND DO MORE OF WHAT YOU ENJOY:** Sounds obvious, but it's surprising how rarely we take the time to really enjoy our lives and smile – both of which release endorphins and make us feel (and look) brighter and better.

BREATHE EASY

An ancient teaching dictates that we enter this world on an inhalation and leave on an exhalation, and that in between we have a finite number of breaths. So in our chaotic world, it makes sense to breathe slowly, deeply and calmly. Even if you are not inclined to meditate or practise mindfulness, simply pausing and breathing slowly and deeply for a few minutes every day calms the mind and reduces anxiety.

We are hardwired to breathe fast and high into the chest, so the diaphragm remains tight and the breath doesn't penetrate the body. This cycle then stimulates the sympathetic nervous system, triggering the stress response. Slow controlled deep breathing, on the other hand, stimulates the parasympathetic nervous system (think calm and relax) with instant benefits. This seemingly simple subconscious action of breathing floods the body with oxygen, prompting a cascade of favourable actions through the body. (See breathing exercise on page 67.)

ENVIRONMENTAL STRESS

It is now proven that a combination of UV radiation from the sun, smoking and the plume of chemicals we face every time we are outdoors, especially in cities, takes its toll on our skin. The main consequence of this at the molecular level is oxidative stress and the generation of free radicals in the skin. These free radicals damage healthy cells, compromising their DNA and destroying the delicate lipid structure of the cell membrane. The mitochondria (the power house of every cell) are especially susceptible to free radical damage, with a loss of energy inside the cell and ultimately the progression of skin ageing.

SUN

Both the US Department of Health and Human Services (DHHS) and the World Health Organisation (WHO) have identified UV as a proven human carcinogen. A tan results from injury to the skin's DNA. The skin darkens in an imperfect attempt to prevent further DNA damage and these imperfections, or mutations, can lead to skin cancer. UVA is the dominant tanning ray that causes cumulative skin damage over time. These skin-ageing rays, although less intense than UVB, are thirty to fifty times more prevalent and are present with relatively equal intensity during daylight hours throughout the year. UVB, on the other hand, is the chief cause of skin reddening and sunburn and plays a key role in the development of skin cancer. UVB can burn and damage skin year-round, especially at high altitudes and on reflective surfaces like snow or ice, which bounce back up to 80 per cent of the rays, so they hit the skin twice.

Here are some of the terms commonly used when discussing sun protection:

- **SPF (SUN PROTECTION FACTOR):** The theoretical amount of time one can stay in the sun without getting sunburned (linked to UVB)
- **UVA (AGEING):** Rays penetrate the skin more deeply, causing cell damage and premature ageing
- **UVB (BURN):** Rays that hit the top layer of the skin and are responsible for sunburn and skin damage
- **BROAD SPECTRUM:** Sunscreen that protects the skin against UVA and UVB.

This sector of the beauty industry is prone to much misunderstanding, as the legislation of SPF products is so varied. Amid all the confusion, however, one fact remains clear: we can protect our skin from up to 90 per cent of environmental ageing directly attributed to the sun.

Sunscreen Technology

Sunscreen formulations have become more sophisticated over the years, with a new generation of high-tech broad-spectrum nano-filters covering both UVA and UVB, creating simpler products with fewer irritants that are kinder to the environment – think lightweight lotions and matt-finish gels, rather than the thick creams of old – meaning that protecting our skin is easier than ever.

Broad-spectrum UV protection combines organic filters (that absorb, convert and release harmful UV radiation) with physical filters (containing titanium dioxide or zinc oxide to reflect UV radiation from the skin) which when combined protect against both UVA and UVB rays. SPF protection represents protection against UVB rays – and therefore sunburn – which is why broad-spectrum protection is essential to guard against the dangerous and often invisible signs of UVA damage. Protection is needed even in cold or cloudy weather, as the sun's ultraviolet radiation can still penetrate the clouds.

Sunscreen filters fall into two broad categories: chemical and physical (often marketed as natural).

- **CHEMICAL BARRIERS** (e.g. octinoxate or avobenzone) work by forming a thin, protective film on the skin's surface that absorbs the UV radiation before it penetrates the skin.
- **PHYSICAL BARRIERS** (e.g. micronised zinc oxide and/or titanium oxide) are insoluble particles that reflect UV away from the skin.

No sun-cream can give you 100 per cent protection, even one with a very high SPF. To give your skin – and your body – the best protection possible, choose a broad-spectrum sunscreen with an adequate SPF plus some combination of UVA-screening ingredients (such as stabilised avobenzone, ecamsule (aka Mexoryl), oxybenzone, titanium dioxide and zinc oxide).

What is clear from scientific research is that we need to take more responsibility for ourselves while in the sun by heeding the instructions on sunscreens, avoiding direct midday sun and wearing a wide-brimmed hat, sunglasses and protective clothing, especially when in intense heat.

We now know that almost all active ingredients in sunscreens break apart or react with other chemicals to some extent once in the sun – hence the need to reapply the product every couple of hours (as indicated on the label).

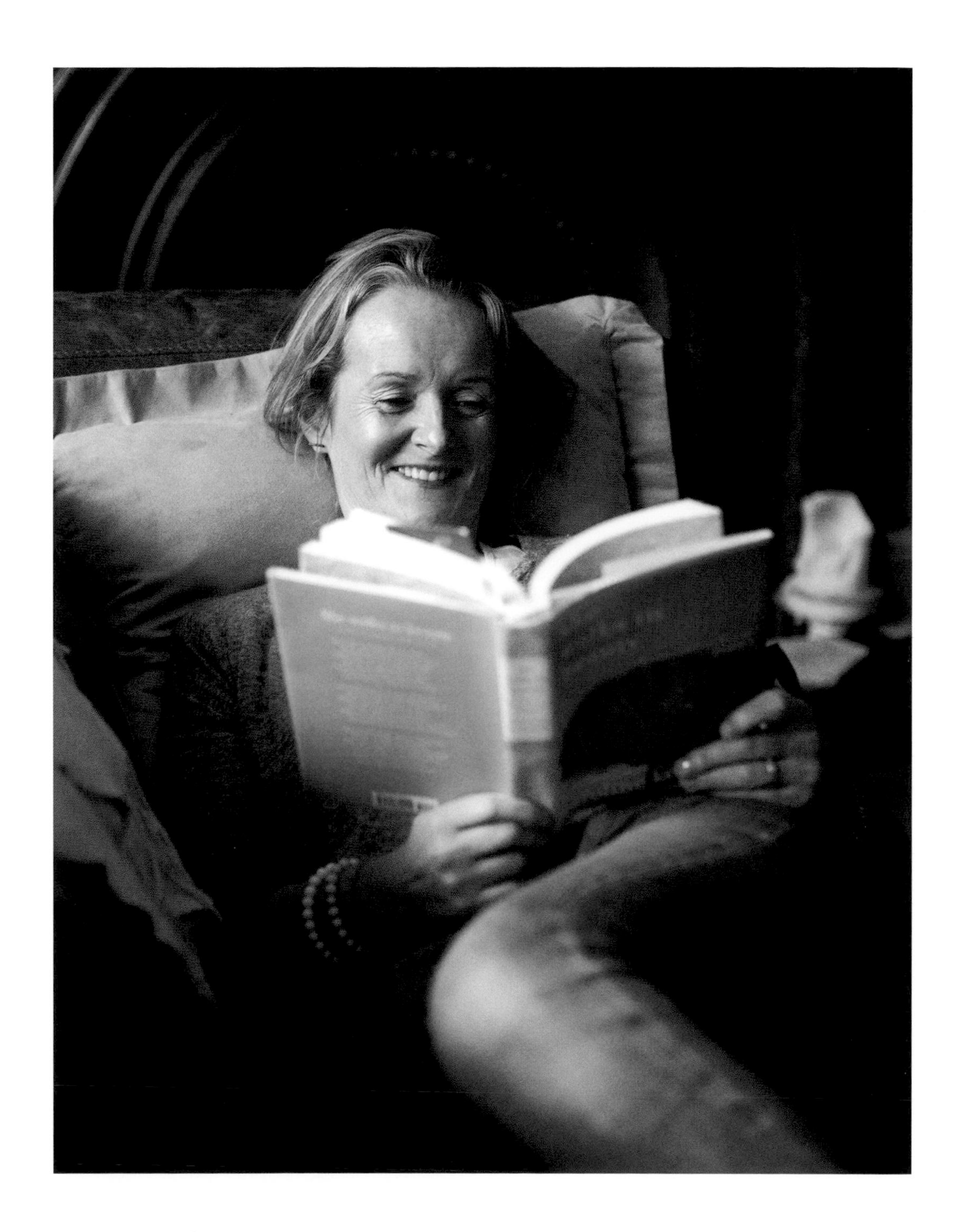

Some of the most commonly asked questions about the use of sunscreen are:

- **WHAT FACTOR TO USE?** Double the SPF doesn't translate into double the time in the sun. SPF30 protects against 97 per cent of UVB rays; SPF50 protects against 98 per cent of UVB rays. Regardless of skin type, use SPF30 or higher broad-spectrum, water-resistant sunscreen, reapplied every two hours when in direct sun.
- **HOW MUCH TO APPLY?** For a lotion, apply one tablespoon-sized dollop to the face and the equivalent of a table-tennis ball over the body (slightly less will suffice for children). One bottle should last no longer than one week or so. The same applies to sprays, although it is not quite so easy to determine the amount applied. After application, wait thirty minutes before going into direct sun.
- **HOW LONG TO KEEP?** Check the open-pot symbol on the back of the packaging to see how long the sunscreen lasts once open – many expire after six months. Keep sunscreen out of direct sunlight and replace every year.

No sunscreen is fully waterproof so always read the label. If a sunscreen says two hours' water resistance, the product needs to be generously reapplied after this time to maintain its water resistance.

Multitasking Skincare

While an increasing number of multitasking moisturisers and make-up products advertise some degree of sun protection, for the vast majority of us it is not enough, especially when facing direct sunlight. SPF is powerful and can compromise the benefits of certain active ingredients in skincare, so it is wise to use a separate broad-spectrum sunscreen, rather than choosing a multitasking serum/moisturiser inclusive of sunscreen protection, especially during the hotter months of the year when the sun's rays are the most damaging. Eyes and lips need protection too, as UV damage can make the lips hard, dry and prone to cold sores, while predisposing the eyes to cataracts, macular degeneration and the possibility of other medical issues. Always wear quality polarised, UV-protecting sunglasses (that block 99.9% of UV rays) when directly exposed to the sun and use broad-spectrum SPF on the lips.

Many make-up products have an SPF rating that users believe offers sufficient protection, but do not assume that make-up products will give adequate protection for your skin. Apply sunscreen before applying make-up.

POLLUTION

With global air pollution at an all-time high, anti-pollution skincare is a current trend. Airborne pollution contains many chemicals identical to cigarette smoke, including sulphur dioxide, nitrogen oxides and particulate matter, that have been shown to penetrate the skin's surface and impact its function at the cellular level.

Some particles, such as soot, dust and smoke, are large and can be seen with the naked eye. Others can be up to twenty times smaller than a human pore, making it easy for them to penetrate and damage the cells. Scientists refer to these as polyaromatic hydrocarbons (PAHs) and they include the sulphur dioxides and nitrogen oxides emitted from coal fires, power plants and automobiles. Experts say that these PAHs are lipophilic, meaning they dissolve in oil, so can easily penetrate the outer layers of the skin where they can damage the protective skin barrier, disrupting the connections between the surface cells, leaving deeper skin layers vulnerable to attack.

Many studies have found that pollution leads to the generation of free radical particles in the skin that significantly contribute to collagen deterioration, irritation, dryness, pigmentation, acne, disrupted moisture balance and chronic inflammation. A study published in the *Journal of Investigative Dermatology* involving groups of Chinese and German women linked exposure to a high level of pollutants to a 25 per cent increase in dark spots on the cheeks.

Remember that, although pollution can be higher in major cities, the countryside is not exempt from damaging PAHs, so it is up to us to protect ourselves through the foods we eat and the products we use on our skin.

THINK ANTIOXIDANTS – Eat Them, Drink Them, Wear Them. Combine an antioxidant-rich diet, overflowing with GLOW skin foods (see page 71) with thorough cleansing (see page 107) and a protective daily skincare routine. With anti-pollution skincare now somewhat of a trend, it's good to know that many of the best pollution-fighting ingredients are already in our food and in superior skincare products on the market.

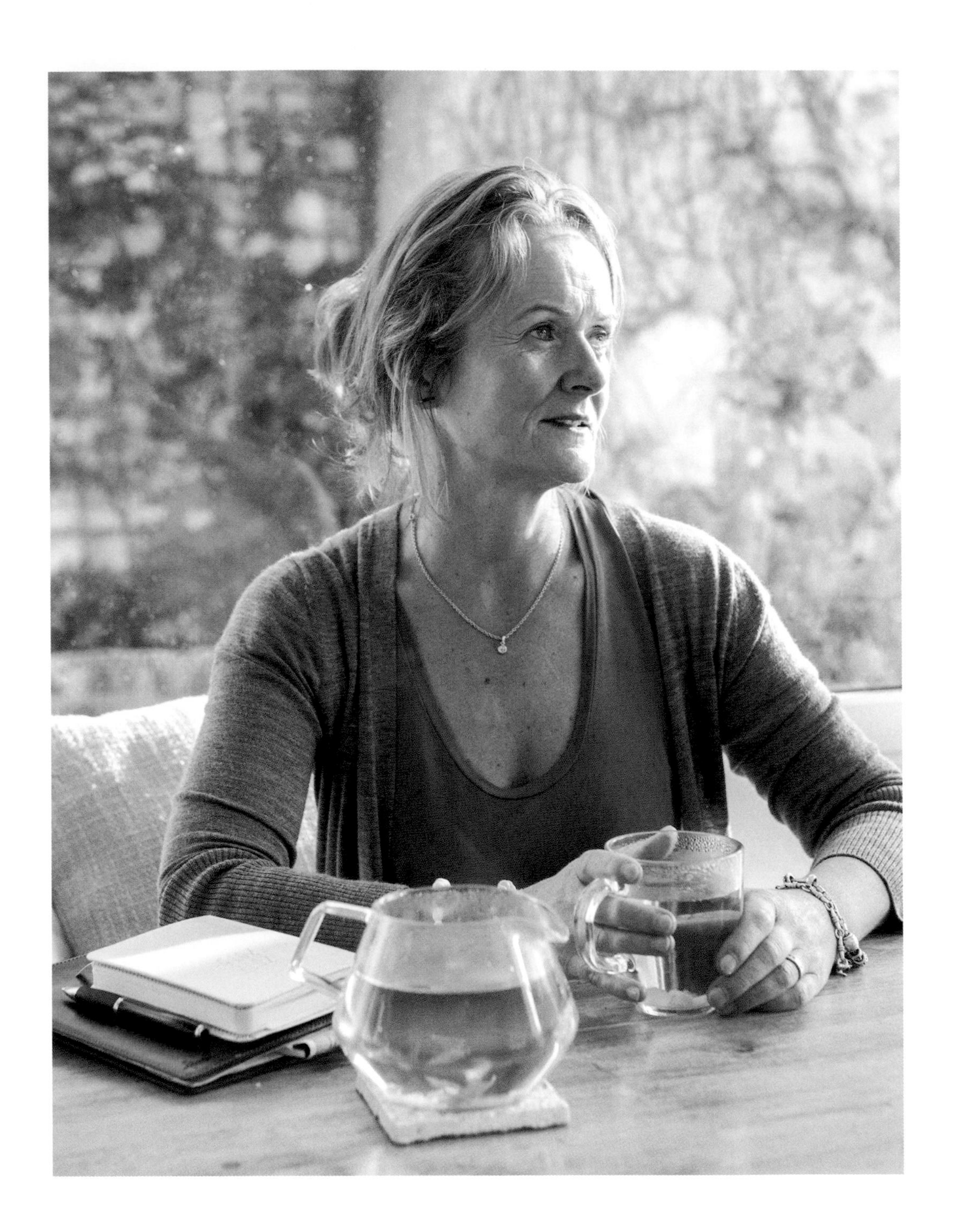

SUGAR AND PROCESSED FOODS

In today's world of excess, sugar and refined carbohydrates are at the root of many diseases and the ill health society is now experiencing. Put simply, if you eat a high-sugar/processed food diet, your body and your skin will suffer the consequences.

All forms of natural sugar (raw sugar, honey, maple syrup, fruit, coconut nectar, date purée and so on) impact blood glucose levels to some extent and lead to the release of the hormone insulin. This directs the body to move glucose from the bloodstream and into the body cells where it is either used for energy or, if not required, converted into fat for storage.

Much skin damage is the end result of a chemical process called glycation. This happens when sugar builds up in the body and the sugar molecules attach themselves to proteins to form advanced glycation end products or AGEs. As the body ages it becomes more susceptible to the formation of AGEs, but a high-sugar and processed food diet exacerbates this. Take the skin, for instance: glycation degrades collagen and elastin proteins in the skin, resulting in the generation of free radicals and inflammation, both of which compromise skin integrity and its capacity to repair and regenerate. Put simply, the more sugar in your body, the more AGEs will be formed and, if your diet is high in sugar and refined foods, your skin will age faster and will be more prone to inflammatory skin conditions like rosacea and acne. With a high processed food diet, AGEs accumulate in other parts of the body too, with joints and muscles especially susceptible and a propensity for pain and inflammation.

While sugar and highly processed foods are the most likely causes of glycation and AGE formation, the manner in which our food is cooked can also have an impact, with fried foods believed to have higher concentrations of AGEs than their boiled or steamed counterparts. Smoking and UV radiation are also believed to accelerate the glycation process.

Science now warns us that it's not just the sugar in coffee that needs to be eliminated – the white breads, breakfast cereals, pastas, cakes, biscuits and other refined foods are equally damaging. Once digested, these break down to form sugar in the intestine. Although fruit is rich in fructose – fruit sugar – that is also degraded in the intestine, it is not as damaging as other types of sugar, as the whole fruit contains many beneficial nutrients and fibres that are essential for skin health.

Studies have shown that the repeated spikes and troughs of glucose and insulin are incredibly stressful on the body, stimulating the release of stress hormones cortisol and adrenaline that, through a cascade of chemical reactions, lead to the breakdown of collagen and other essential skin components. Hence the importance of regular mealtimes and overall balance in how and when we choose to eat.

Reducing both obvious and hidden sugars in the diet is one of the most effective steps we can take for our skin and overall health. Rest assured, once you start to reduce added sugars, your taste buds will adjust and you will begin to appreciate the real flavour of the whole food much more.

STRATEGIC SWAPS

- **SUGARY BREAKFAST CEREALS** *for* porridge in its many guises, sourdough or wholemeal breads, yoghurts with fruit, and smoothies (see Breakfasts and Brunches, page 142)
- **WHITE BREAD** *for* sourdough or wholemeal bread or wraps
- **PASTA AND WHITE RICE** *for* quinoa, couscous, farro, wholewheat pasta, short grain brown/wild rice and other natural grains (see page 77)
- **BISCUITS AND CAKES** *for* oatcakes with nut butters/chopped banana or home-cooked banana breads and other sweeter options (see Snacks and Sweet Things, page 222)
- **MILK CHOCOLATE** *for* a few squares of top-quality dark chocolate (minimum 75 per cent cocoa solids)
- **SWEETENED YOGHURTS** *for* natural unsweetened Greek, sheep's or coconut yoghurt
- **SUGAR IN COOKING** *for* dried fruit and small amounts of maple syrup or honey
- **PACKAGED JUICES** *for* fresh homemade juices and smoothies (see pages 150, 156, 238) or coconut water
- **SUGAR IN TEA/COFFEE:** Wean yourself off sugar by slowly reducing the amount added to drinks. Remember, the plasticity of our brain allows it to change with constant repetition.
- **ARTIFICIAL SWEETENERS** are best avoided as there are concerns about the safety of some brands on the market. What's more, artificial sweeteners do not re-educate taste buds to enjoy the taste of real, unadulterated food.

Many of today's bloggers cite **MAPLE SYRUP** as a healthier alternative to sugar. Maple syrup is the concentrated sap of the Canadian maple tree. It is a natural sugar with a lower fructose content than honey and when used in moderation has some nutritional value – it contains iron, manganese, potassium and zinc. It has a deep caramel flavour and is a useful alternative to sugar in baking and on porridge, pancakes and so on. 'Maple-flavoured syrup' is literally sugar disguised as maple syrup and should be avoided!

ALCOHOL

Studies have shown that a little wine can be good for us. However, we also know that excessive drinking on a regular basis overloads the liver, disrupts sleep patterns and damages the skin, leaving a trail of destruction through the body at large.

The context in which we drink is believed to be important too. Wine (most notably red) is considered an important part of the famed Mediterranean diet, with studies showing the protective effects of moderate consumption of mainly red wine, taken with meals, spread evenly through the week and rarely (if ever) in excess. This said, the overall scientific consensus is that less is most definitely more, and if you don't already drink, there is *no* good evidence to start! If you are pregnant or planning on becoming so, there is *no* safe limit for drinking during pregnancy.

This four-week plan is designed to give skin every possible opportunity to glow and to give our gut a clean break by abstaining completely from alcohol. If, or when, you resume drinking, do try to stick well within the limits recommended by expert advisory boards, and for the sake of your skin and your body as a whole, have at least four alcohol-free days each week. When you do drink, try some of the new varieties of organic and biodynamic wines that can be less damaging on the gut and skin or drink pure spirits – diluted of course!

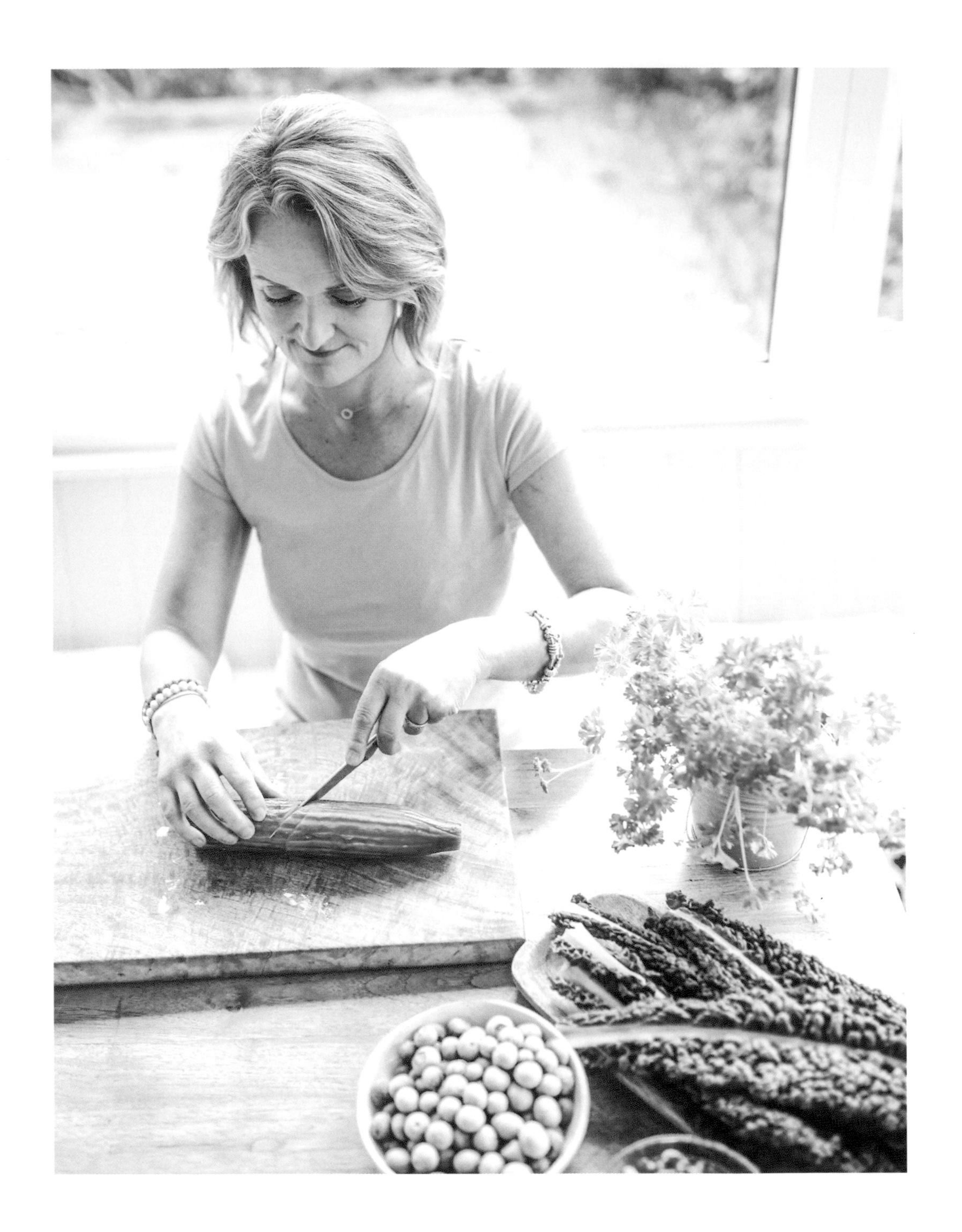

GUT AND SKIN

◊

Hippocrates supposedly believed that all disease begins in the gut and by all accounts, we are on the verge of a new era in medicine, with gut health topping the agenda for almost all healthcare practitioners, from the mainstream medical community to nutritionists, naturopaths, psychotherapists and others. Taking care of our gut is the number one priority in a universal bid to relieve the debilitating effects of chronic stress, obesity and other diseases on our lives – and our skin and brains. In essence, when we invest in our gut, our body at large will begin to thrive.

THE MICROBIOME

Our bodies live in a complex symbiotic relationship with over a hundred trillion bacterial cells (the highest concentration of which is located in the gut) weighing close to two kilograms and considered by many to be the 'forgotten organ' in the human body. This great ecosystem is called the microbiome, an ecological community of microorganisms that literally share our body space.

Since the characterisation of the body's **INTESTINAL FLORA** was made official via the National Institute of Health (NIH) Human Microbiome Project in 2008, there has been an explosion in gut research. While it will be some time before we fully understand the extent of the influence of the microbiome on health at large, experts are beginning to understand the role certain foods play in either supporting or disrupting a well-balanced gut.

Our gut provides these bacteria with indigestible carbohydrates (resistant starch from plant fibres) and a space to flourish, while we, in turn, benefit enormously, as science is now showing us. The bacteria derive energy from the fermentation of otherwise indigestible waste to manufacture key enzymes, nutrients and neurotransmitters, while also secreting anti-microbial proteins that prevent the growth of harmful, or pathogenic, bacteria. In fact, it is now thought that up to 70 per cent of our body's defence system is found in the gut.

SKIN

The skin has a microbiome of its own, being home to millions of microorganisms that act as the body's primary defence from the outside world. This microbiome is affected by many factors, including genetics, the environment and what we eat (or don't eat), and the key to skin health lies in nourishing the good bacteria so they continue to thrive and outnumber those not-so-great varieties.

GUT–BRAIN–SKIN AXIS

There is active two-way communication between the gut and skin and we now know that eating in tune with our gut enhances the resilience of the skin's microbiome, adding a further layer of protective armoury to the body. For this to occur, a healthy balance between the favourable and pathogenic bacteria in the skin is essential, as an overload of the less beneficial varieties can contribute to skin disorders – just as happens in the gut.

The brain and gut are closely connected too through an active two-way system. Even the thought of food can release digestive juices in the stomach, and further research is bringing this communication pathway to life by demonstrating the potential for probiotic foods to impact our mental health. It is now accepted that anxiety and stress lead to intestinal permeability and gut dysbiosis, which, in turn, can result in skin irritation and inflammation. What's more, certain skin disorders are more common in people suffering from gut issues, and a strong association between gut dysbiosis and acne has also been demonstrated.

PROBIOTICS

Probiotics are active live microorganisms naturally present in foods like organic fermented dairy products (milk drinks, live yoghurt, aged cheese), sourdough breads, kefir, kombucha, miso, sauerkraut and tempeh, with different products containing different microbial species, each with unique benefits (hence the importance of variety in what we eat). They are also widely available as over-the-counter supplements in tablet and powder form.

Most probiotic foods or supplements contain strains of either lactobacillus or bifidobacterium bacteria that must pass intact through the acidic environment of the stomach and cope with the various digestive juices and enzymes on their route to the gut where they begin to act. The biggest challenge is maintaining sufficient quantities of these bacteria in the gut, as many are destroyed by the typical acidic stomach environment.

We now know that what we eat has a critical impact on the microbiome, so the potential for probiotic food products is enormous. Certain probiotics are being used to treat irritable bowel syndrome while others help prevent lactose intolerance. When it comes to skin health, studies have shown the benefits of key probiotics in reinforcing the skin barrier function, while also reducing skin sensitivity.

PROBIOTIC SKINCARE

As the popularity of probiotics in food rises, the concept of probiotics in skincare is fast gaining credence too. Just as our stomachs need to be repopulated with good bacteria to function smoothly, so does our skin, and this new wave of probiotic and fermented ingredient-enriched skincare claims to stabilise the skin's natural microflora and generally rebalance the bacterial ecosystem of the skin.

Studies suggest that probiotic ingredients can help strengthen the skin's microbiome and have an overall calming effect, making them especially beneficial for sensitive and acne-prone skin. However, to be truly effective, ingredients need to penetrate the skin barrier and must be concentrated enough to be useful in the first place. While research is encouraging, it is by no means conclusive, and whether topical beauty products are as potent and beneficial for the skin as probiotic supplements and foods remains to be seen. So whether you choose the probiotic skincare route or not, always ensure that the products you ultimately buy are packed with at least some of the essential active ingredients outlined on pages 34–5).

PREBIOTICS

Prebiotics are non-digestible, fermentable carbohydrates that pass through the upper part of the gut to stimulate the growth of friendly bacteria and prevent the propagation of harmful strains. Prebiotic foods include chicory, onions, globe and Jerusalem artichokes, savoy cabbage, mangetout, leeks, beetroot, pomegranates, peaches, garlic, watermelon and barley, amongst others. Although beneficial to the gut, some people with irritable bowel syndrome (IBS) may not be able to tolerate them so, in that case, it's best to first seek advice from a healthcare professional.

FERMENTED FOODS

Hand in hand with the explosion in gut research is the upsurge in interest in fermented foods (think kefir, sauerkraut and kombucha). Fermenting is nothing new – it was the preservation method used for thousands of years before refrigeration and canning. Fresh foods (primarily vegetables) were packed into large wooden containers, salted and left for months or even years to ferment, generating B vitamins, probiotics, omega-3 fatty acids, beneficial enzymes and more, and thereby enhancing the nutritional value of the foods. Kefir, sauerkraut and kombucha are now widely available, as is the know-how on how to ferment. (See page 257 for guidelines on making kombucha.)

CREATING A HEALTHY MICROBIOME

- Improving the diversity of gut bacteria brings an endless list of benefits for skin and body, so nourish your gut with a colourful, varied diet. The colourful fresh fruits and vegetables, oily fish, nuts, seeds, unrefined grains and fermented foods discussed in these pages will help reduce inflammation through the body and maintain a healthy gut.

- Eat more prebiotic and fermented foods and take a daily probiotic (get advice from a healthcare practitioner).
- Eat more polyphenol-rich foods, including berries, flaxseeds, plums, hazelnuts, green tea, raw cacao and red wine (in moderation and organic and preservative-free), as research has shown that they can further support the gut microbiome.
- If you drink, have at least four alcohol-free days every week. Alcohol irritates the gut.
- Exercise regularly.
- Rest and digest – the body will digest food more efficiently and effectively when the mind is calmer, so even simple steps like taking a few minutes to breathe deeply before eating and eating more slowly – chewing food more thoroughly – can have a large impact on the health of our skin and body.
- Manage stress levels (see page 39).
- Get adequate sleep (see page 59).

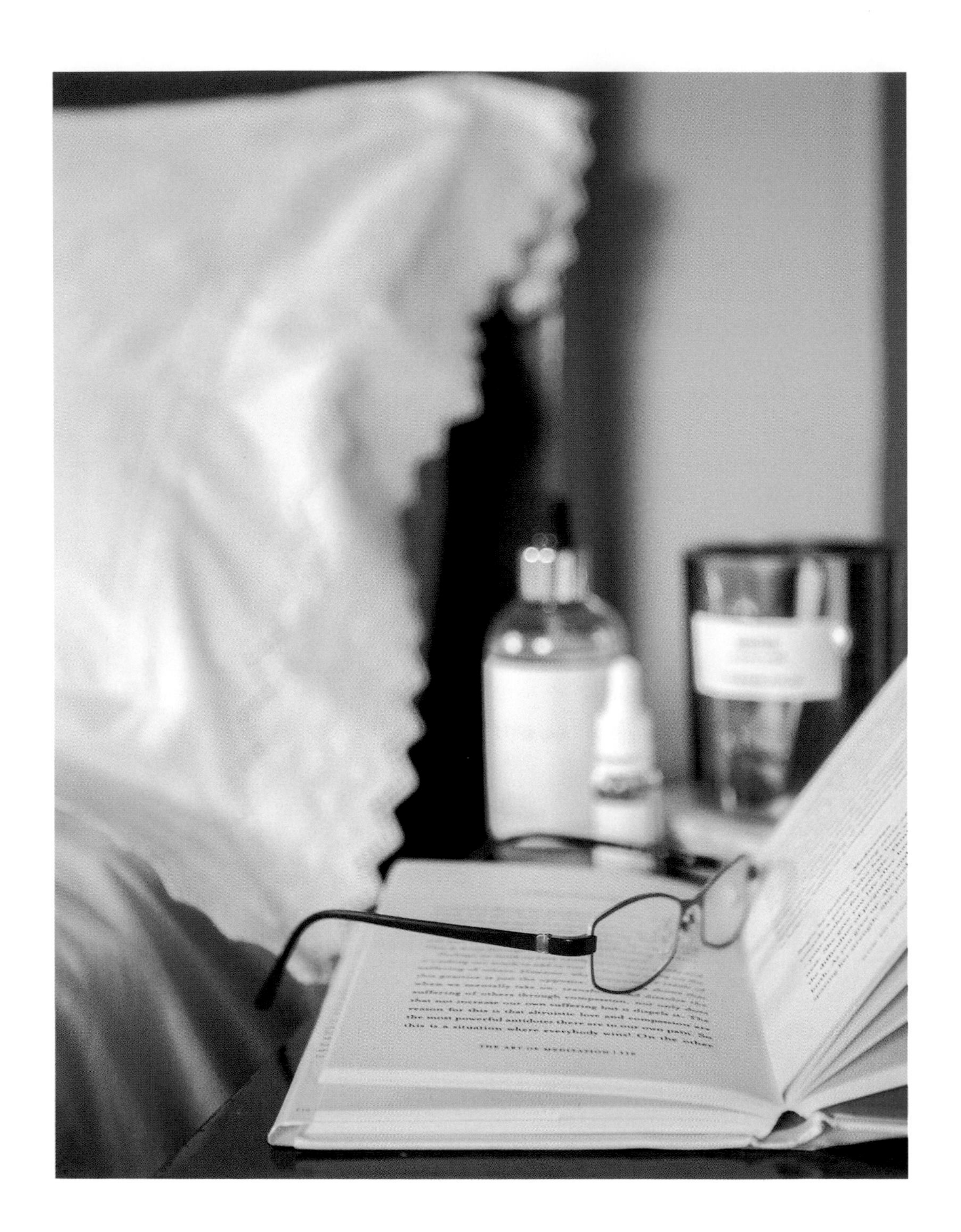
the most powerful antidotes there are to our own pain. So
this is a situation where everybody wins! On the other

SLEEP AND SKIN

◊

With sufficient sleep now scientifically recognised as a key part of our fight against premature skin ageing, tuning in to our skin's natural rhythms and harnessing the benefits of the night's calm has become the holy grail for healing and nurturing from within. Life in the fast lane has taken its toll and now, more than ever before, we need to slow down and sleep longer and deeper.

It has been estimated that up to 30 per cent of the population worldwide is having trouble sleeping at any given time. But sleep is widely considered to be our body's most important recovery mechanism. It is a biological imperative that does far more than rest the body – it heightens the senses, sharpens the mind and mellows the spirit. It's hardly surprising, then, that beauty experts consistently rate sleep among their top essentials because, when sufficient and deep, a good night's sleep can transform our appearance. As we grow older, even a couple of late or relatively sleepless nights can leave our minds overwhelmed and inefficient. What's more, when we don't sleep well, our bodies begin to feel more strained, releasing more of the stress hormone cortisol, with potential knock-on effects on weight, on collagen production in the skin and on other body systems.

With the toxic load from our unrelenting environment at an all-time high, our skin is in overdrive through the day in an unyielding attempt to protect itself, which is why we need sufficient time to regenerate when we sleep. During these precious hours, our body's innate healing capacity kicks into full gear, as toxic build-up is cleared, growth hormone is produced, our immune systems are revitalised, breathing and heart rate slow, cells are repaired and our systems are rebalanced. However, as most of us just don't get enough sleep time to complete these (and other) tasks, our skin suffers and signs of premature ageing and other skin concerns have become the norm.

HOW MUCH IS ENOUGH SLEEP? While needs vary considerably, experts recommend an average of six to eight hours' sleep a night to keep the body working efficiently. According to the US National Sleep Foundation (NSF), women are more likely to suffer sleep problems like insomnia and to experience excessive sleepiness than men. And while we know that that a few nights of broken sleep won't kill us, lack of sleep long term accelerates the ageing process in the brain, leaving us slow, exhausted and hugely compromised in both body and mind.

SKIN REPAIR

Research has shown that our skin synchronises with both the sleep–wake cycle and the dark–light rhythms, and that essential evening skin healing begins as early as dusk, when the sun goes down, and the skin slowly starts to move into repair mode. So, as outlined below, to maximise skin repair, it makes sense to remove the day's grime and thoroughly cleanse the skin as early as possible in the evening.

The skin's fibroblast cells start producing collagen once the skin is completely clean, with output believed to peak around midnight. Overnight cell renewal and collagen production pinnacles about 2 a.m., triggered by a peak in growth hormone activity and enhanced blood flow to the skin. As the new day dawns, rejuvenated skin switches from repair to protection mode once again and the cycle recommences.

AS THE DELICATE skin barrier thins overnight, this can lead to increased water evaporation and skin feeling parched on rising. Hence the benefits of using a night cream or nourishing face oil that locks moisture into the skin.

Prior to the digital age, our bodies were more balanced and in sync with these natural rhythms, but scientists now believe that we have not evolved fast enough to adapt to the alien environment we now call home, with pollution, blue light and our always-on lifestyles, reducing growth hormone production, weakening skin repair and increasing inflammation through the body.

A joint 2013 study carried out by Estée Lauder and University Hospitals Case Medical Center in Cleveland, Ohio, recounted the long-term effects of poor sleep (five hours or less per night for one month) on the skin's barrier function. After lifting off the skin's protective barrier, the study found that those who slept well (seven hours or more per night) had fully repaired their skin barrier within twenty-four hours. However, with the poor sleepers a water loss of over 30 per cent was noted over a three-day period, as the skin barrier continued to deteriorate. In all areas considered, from the levels of elasticity and sensitivity to the skin's ability to repair itself after a controlled sunburn, the poor sleepers scored only half as well as the good sleepers, with increased signs of skin ageing and significantly slower recovery from environmental stressors.

NON-NEGOTIABLE NIGHTLY SKIN REGIME

Regardless of your age, if you want better skin, not just for now but for always, the following evening routine is non-negotiable. Remember, even small changes like prepping skin for sleep two hours earlier will pay dividends in the long term.

- Prep skin as early in the evening as possible
- Thoroughly cleanse/double cleanse (see page 107)
- Layer up for active skin repair with a targeted serum rich in active ingredients to speed up cell turnover (see The Skin We're In, page 7)
- As skin grows older, use a more occlusive cream or oil to lock in the goodness and prevent moisture loss through the weakened skin barrier
- Use nourishing vitamin-rich natural oils targeted to specific skin concerns. Combine these with moisturiser or apply them directly to the skin after moisturiser to enhance absorption.
- Use one of the advanced generation of deeply nourishing masks formulated to remain in place overnight one to two times per week (depending on needs)

CIRCADIAN RHYTHMS

Our sleep–wake pattern is partially controlled by our circadian rhythms and understanding our unique rhythm will help ensure more restful sleep. The lives of the ancient Chinese revolved around the natural order of day into night, with *Qi* (the vital energy that sustains life) being dominant during the working daylight hours and the body entering its calm, resting phase after dark. Today, working in tune with these rhythms is as important for health and well-being as it was centuries ago.

The master timekeeper of our internal twenty-four-hour clock is located in the hypothalamus region of the brain, and the rhythms generated govern the timing of many behavioural, physiological and metabolic functions in the body including sleep, temperature regulation, the production of hormones like melatonin and cortisol, heart and lung function, glucose and insulin levels and much more.

The sleep-inducing hormone melatonin is produced by the brain's pineal gland and is regarded as the most powerful reset button for our biological clocks. Melatonin is present in the body at low levels during the day, slowly increasing a couple of hours before bedtime and peaking in the middle of the night. The appearance of light at dawn suppresses its production and this becomes our signal to wake up and be active.

Our bodies evolved in harmony with these light signals but sleep experts warn that one of the most fundamental stresses on our bodies today is that we are living completely out of sync with these natural fluctuations. That said, we are also told that under the right conditions our internal clocks can be reset – the key rests in listening to our bodies and working with them.

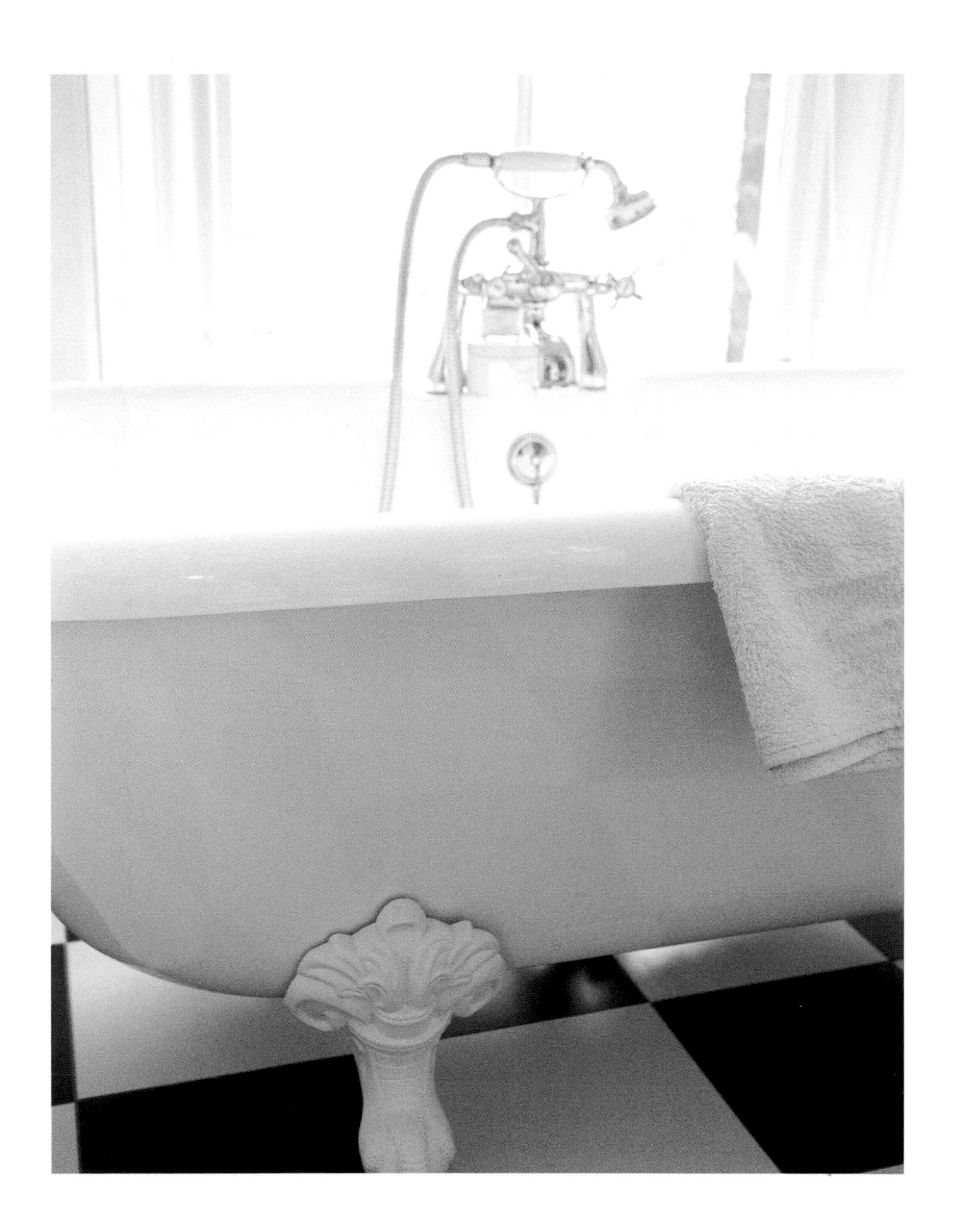

SOUNDER SLEEP STRATEGIES

Being permanently exhausted does not mean we are super busy or super important – it just means we are not prioritising. Following the well-documented advice below will help us keep more in sync with our bodies, so we can sleep sounder at night and wake up feeling – and looking – refreshed and ready to tackle what lies ahead.

1. GET SOME NATURAL SUNLIGHT

Sunlight entering our eyes helps regulate and reset our body clocks. So work with your body's unique rhythms by letting in as much early morning light as possible: open the curtains and let the daylight in or go out for a short walk or run – whatever exercise works for you.

2. EXERCISE

Regular exercise encourages deeper sleep cycles. While fitness experts believe that the best time to exercise is a time that works well for you, it has been shown that people are more likely to stick to a routine if they exercise first thing in the morning. Strenuous exercise before going to bed can stimulate the body, making it more difficult to fall asleep.

3. CREATE A ROUTINE

We are hardwired to rise at dawn and go to sleep at sunset and our body's ability to regulate healthy sleep patterns depends on this consistency. The production of melatonin drops rapidly in the morning light and this sets the pace for the next twenty-four-hour cycle, so using the weekend to make up for lost sleep can disrupt this rhythm. Try to rise at a similar time every morning (occasionally allowing up to one hour's variation if needed). If you must catch up on lost sleep during the day, have a nap for about forty-five minutes – no more.

4. SWITCH OFF

Our body doesn't go from full speed to stop without slowing down. So take time to wind down. Switch off electronic devices – leave them charging in the kitchen, not the bedroom. Backlit screens and devices such as smartphones, tablets and laptops have blue light, which can suppress melatonin production and disrupt sleep quality. Turn off the TV at least one hour before sleep and don't bring devices to bed (if you must read on an e-reader or tablet, reduce the light to a minimum). Power off social media: you can catch up in the morning – and you won't have missed much!

5. CUT OUT STIMULANTS

Caffeine and alcohol are stimulants with effects that can last many hours. If you are a coffee drinker, enjoy it – in moderation – in the morning. If you are experiencing problems getting to sleep, cut out all caffeinated beverages, including soft drinks, many teas (check ingredient listing), chocolate and certain medications after midday.

When taken in excess alcohol can induce sleep, but it's not deep sleep and it doesn't last. Drinking alcohol just before bed reduces overall sleep quality while also waking the body during the night. It is scientifically proven that alcohol at all dosages causes a reduction in sleep onset latency, meaning a more consolidated first half of sleep and a disrupted second half of sleep.

SLEEP-INDUCING FOODS

Foods naturally high in melatonin such as cherries, bananas, oranges, pineapples and oats can help improve sleep.

Tryptophan is another key sleep helper. This essential amino acid is a prerequisite for serotonin and melatonin, with studies showing that eating foods high in tryptophan (nuts, sesame seeds, tofu, turkey and pumpkin seeds) can reduce the time taken to fall asleep.

Instead of sleeping pills or alcohol, try herbal teas that help induce an inner calm, like chamomile, valerian root, lemon balm or the many mixed blends widely available.

6. SLEEP MEDITATIONS

Numerous studies support the benefits of mindfulness meditations, including self-guided meditation and guided sleep apps, in improving sleep quality and quantity. These are widely available online or via app stores.

- **SELF-GUIDED MEDITATION:** Progressive muscle relaxation (PMR), or the 'Body Scan', helps prepare the body for sleep. As you lie in bed, tense and relax your muscles in groups from the toes up to the forehead. Squeeze each muscle group for a few seconds, then release, before moving on to the next. Alternatively, mentally talk yourself through relaxing each part of the body: 'I am relaxing my toes. My toes are relaxed. I am relaxing my knees. My knees are relaxed.' And so on. This can be especially effective for those who struggle to stop the relentless mental chatter, as the brain is focused on the body scan, not the mental activity.
- **SLEEP APPS:** A whole range of sleep apps using a plethora of musical arrangements, guided meditations and other effects to help soothe the senses and induce sleep

are available. Many of these come with sound scientific support. This said, some experts are cautious about having any form of technology at hand when trying to sleep for the reasons outlined above.

7. LETTING GO

Most of us think in terms of 'going to sleep' at bedtime. We forget that sleep is not a place. You cannot will yourself to sleep and worrying about it makes anxiety worse. Sleep is about letting go and should be something that comes naturally. Experts tell us that often it is our anxiety about not falling asleep quickly that is keeping us awake, rather than there being an actual problem with our sleep routine or rhythms. For many people, getting to sleep means detaching themselves from the myriad thoughts running through their heads. If your brain is still working overtime as you lie in bed, practise the meditation and breathing techniques outlined or try jotting down ideas that come to mind or jobs that need to be done in a notepad kept by your bed, instead of mulling them over and hoping they won't be forgotten. Most important, don't worry about not sleeping. Sleep will come.

8. THE QUARTER-OF-AN-HOUR RULE

If you spend a lot of time lying in bed awake, your bed may become connected with being awake, rather than asleep. So to encourage a healthier bed–sleep connection, follow the quarter-of-an-hour rule recommended by the Sleep and Circadian Neuroscience Institute at Oxford University: if you are not asleep within around fifteen minutes of going to bed, get up, go to a different room and relax until you are feeling really tired and ready to sleep. But just estimate that quarter of an hour – don't add stress by checking the time. *https://www.ndcn.ox.ac.uk/*

9. SETTING THE SCENE

- **COOL AND DARK:** Darkness is a prerequisite for melatonin production. Close curtains and blinds and minimise or remove glowing indicator lights from alarm clocks and charging indicators on cordless phones, etc.
- **TEMPERATURE:** An ambient temperature of 65–70 degrees Fahrenheit (18–21 Celsius) is believed to suit most people, even during cooler months. During hot weather use a fan or air-conditioner, if available.
- **BEDDING:** Invest in a comfortable mattress and pillows made from natural rather than synthetic fibres, designed for breathability. Your mattress should be firm enough to support the spine in correct alignment (but not too hard). Replace pillows that are uncomfortable or out of shape.
- **ESSENTIAL OILS:** Aromatherapy stimulates the limbic system in the brain and can affect how we feel and experience

emotions. Essential oils like lavender, chamomile, bergamot and ylang-ylang create a sense of calm, making it easier to drift off. These can be added to a burner or diffuser, applied to the pulse points before going to bed, added to a bath or used as pillow sprays. Many sleep-inducing essential oil blends are available, but always choose reputable brands and check the labels for quality.

10. SOOTHING SOUNDS

Certain types of music have been shown to affect internal biometrics, including heart rate, brain activity and sleep patterns. While the genres of music can vary, a tempo between 60 and 80 BPM, a regular rhythm, low pitches and tranquil melodies have been found to be most conducive to sleep. Researchers also found that the positive effects of listening to music accumulated over time, meaning that the more nights you listen to music, the more beneficial it will be to overall sleep quality.

11. BE THANKFUL

While this may sound somewhat New Agey, thinking of one or two things you can be thankful for from your day (regardless of how difficult your life may be at the time) helps focus the mind on the positive, rather than that wakeful tossing and turning associated with negative thoughts.

QUICK SLEEP FIX: BREATHING

In Indian and Tibetan yoga philosophy, our thoughts and breath are inextricably linked. Try the following when lying on your back in bed. Focus both your mind and body on taking slow and very deep breaths. With lips lightly touching, breathe in deeply through your nose for a count of four, hold for four seconds, breathe out through your nose for a count of six, and hold for four. Repeat this four times without letting the mind wander. Work slowly up to eight repetitions. If the mind wanders, gently bring it back to the breath. If it continues to do so, then begin the exercise again. With slow breathing, the rib cage expands allowing the lungs to fill completely, before emptying naturally on the exhale. By training your mind to focus on the breath, the rest will come naturally.

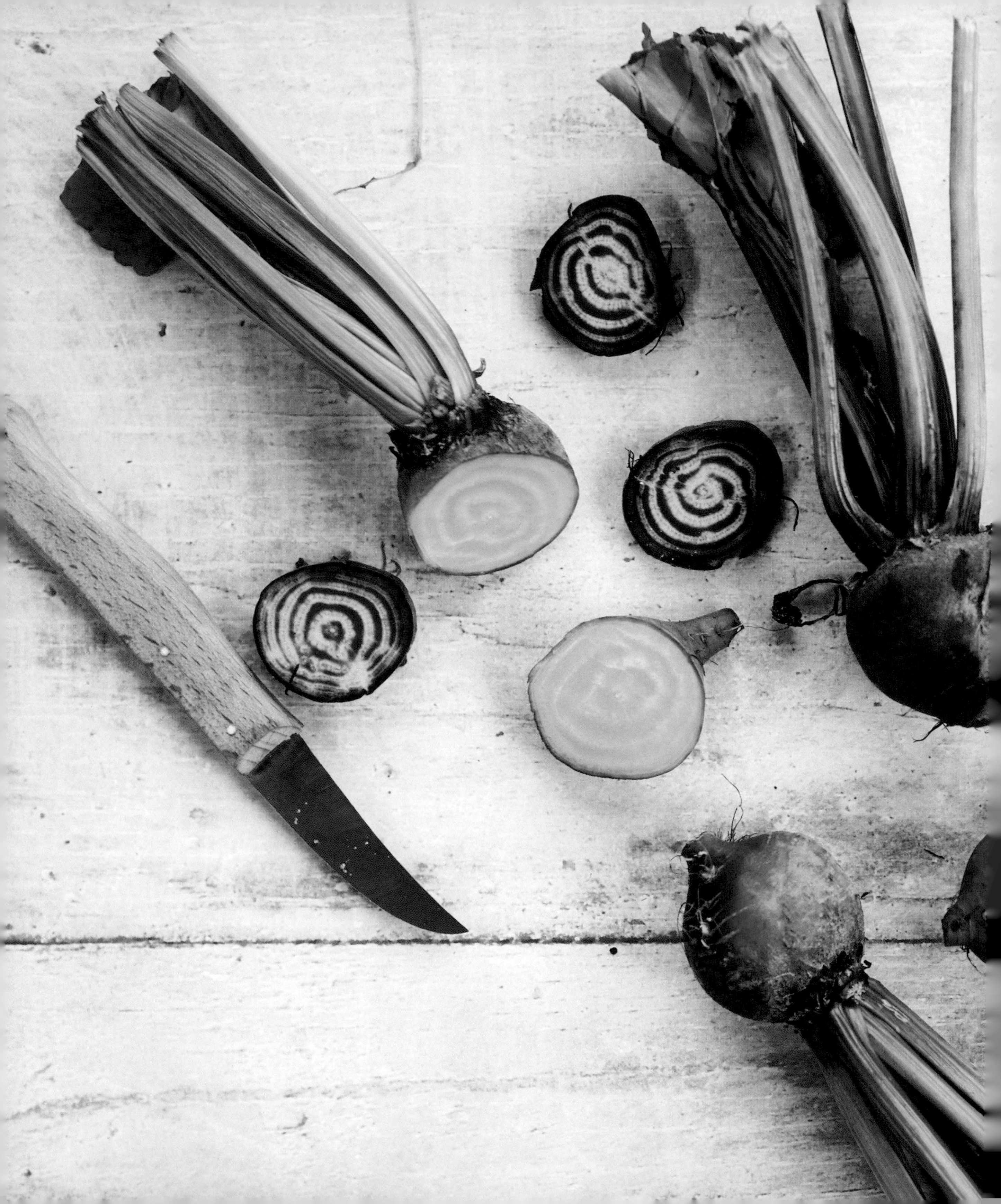

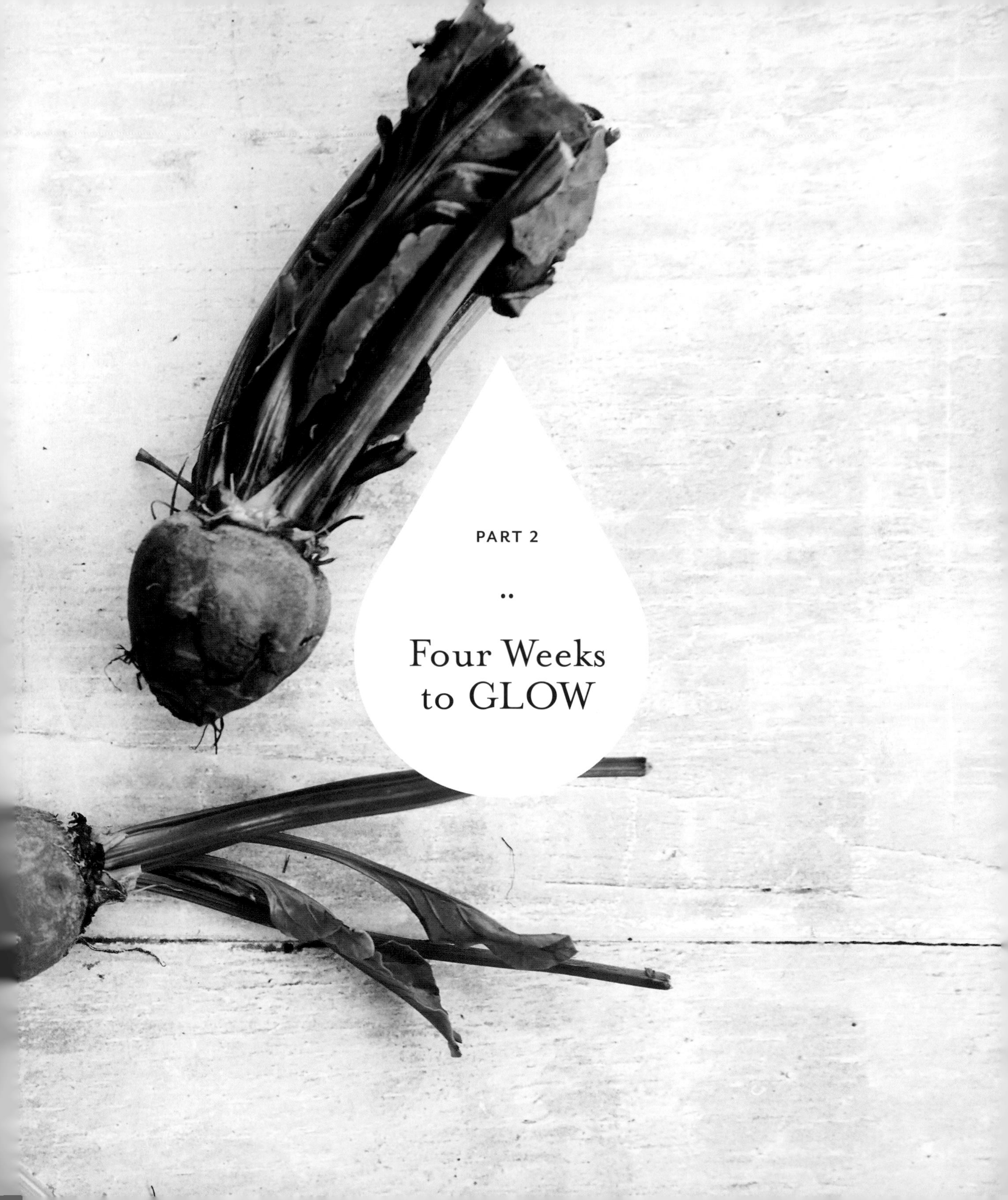

PART 2

Four Weeks to GLOW

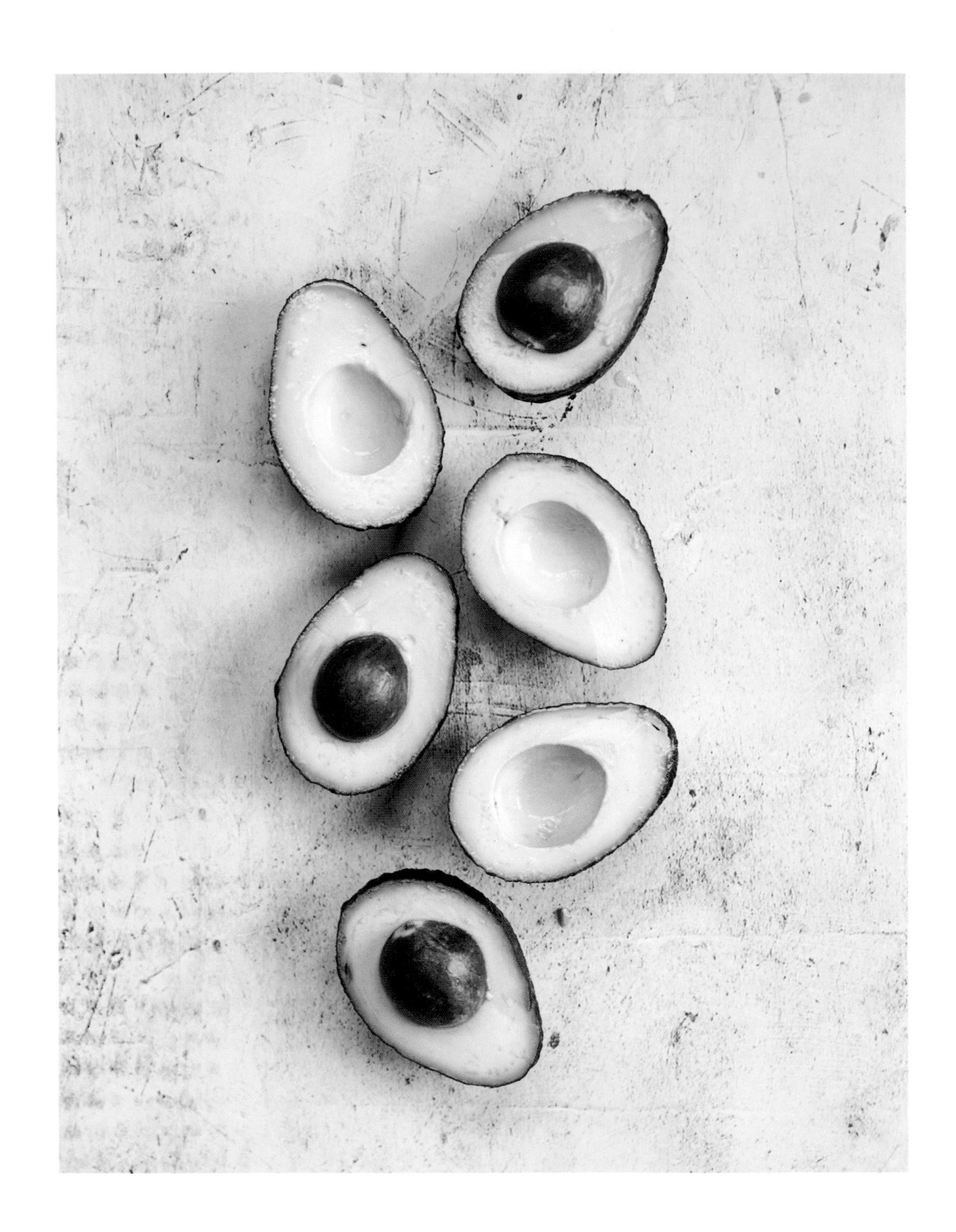

GLOW FOODS

◊

Top of every great skin care plan is fresh, seasonal, colourful, skin-loving food – just as Mother Nature intended. Basically, feed your face with what it needs and it will glow and radiate vitality – always. The good news is that this is not difficult to do, as the best skin foods are deliciously tasty and easy to prepare – think rich pink salmon, grains, nuts, seeds and the massive variety of seasonal fruits and vegetables now on hand and all radiating energy and goodness.

There are so many skin-loving choices on offer that it is impossible to outline them all here, but if we eat most of the following foods, almost daily, both our bodies and minds will thrive.

Certain foods are grouped together, like seeds and nuts – they are all great, although some are marginally more nutritious than others, but all should be a cupboard staple to be enjoyed.

One of the **COMMONEST CAUSES** of dehydrated skin is lack of water. 1.5–2 litres of fluid is recommended each day, taken primarily as water, with green tea and other caffeine-free teas also included in this mix.

APPLE CIDER VINEGAR (ACV)

All vinegar, regardless of brand, contains an active ingredient called acetic acid. ACV is made from freshly crushed apples fermented in wooden barrels, and it's this fermentation process that results in a natural brown colour and some floating particles. These particle bits (or 'mother') comprise strands of protein, enzymes and gut-friendly bacteria that give the vinegar a slightly dense, murky appearance. As the vinegar ages, more of this mother accumulates. ACV is especially potent if the fermentation process is left untouched (filtering and pasteurisation can lead to poorer nutrient content).

The benefits of vinegar have been recognised from as far back as 5000 BC, when the Babylonians used it as a tonic and pickling agent, and for the ancient Chinese it was the go-to remedy for everything from flu to stomach upsets and warts, not to forget its use through the ages as a household cleaning agent. Other reported benefits of ACV include its role in maintaining healthy cholesterol levels in the body (the high pectin content is thought to help reduce cholesterol), more evenly controlled blood sugar and maintaining a healthier gut. Used as a hair rinse, ACV washes away the residue of styling products, leaving hair clean and super shiny.

When choosing ACV make sure to buy the organic, unfiltered variety. You can take it daily – start with 1 tablespoon mixed into a glass of warm(ish) water and increase slowly to 2 tablespoons if you tolerate it well. Add some honey or lemon if desired. If drinking it isn't your thing, use ACV in a salad dressing (see recipe pages 165).

Skin-Loving Nutrients

- **DIETARY FIBRE** (from pectin)
- **FATTY ACIDS:** monounsaturated (oleic acid) and omega-3
- **PHYTOCHEMICALS:** carotenoids (alpha- and beta-carotene, lutein)
- **VITAMINS:** A (as beta-carotene), B2, B6, B7, C, E, K
- **MINERALS:** calcium, magnesium, potassium, phosphorus

AVOCADOS

Not so long ago, avocados were bottom of the pile, perceived as being fat-laden and highly calorific. How times have changed, as these nutritious fruits are now top of every skin-essential list. Avocados are loaded with monounsaturated fatty acids that work to keep the skin moist and protect it from UV damage, among numerous other benefits. Used as a skin mask or an oil applied directly to the skin, avocados help soothe sensitivity and curb skin inflammation (see Nourishing Avocado Mess, page 128). Just imagine how nourished your skin would feel after a slathering of mashed avocado – just like we eat on sourdough toast (see page 158).

Avocados and avocado oil contain antioxidants, fibre, potassium, magnesium and folate, while also providing a source of linoleic acid to help strengthen skin membranes. Avocado oil is one of the best plant oils for soothing dry skin.

Skin-Loving Nutrients

- **DIETARY FIBRE**
- **FATTY ACIDS:** polyunsaturated (linoleic acid), monounsaturated (oleic acid) and omega-3
- **PHYTOCHEMICALS:** carotenoids (alpha- and beta-carotene, lutein)
- **VITAMINS:** A (as beta-carotene), B2, B6, B7, C, E, K
- **MINERALS:** copper, magnesium, potassium

BEETROOT

Our skin can become a dumping ground for toxins that the body is unable to eliminate through the usual pathways of the liver and kidneys, and beetroot has long been used for its liver-cleansing and detoxification benefits (thanks to its antioxidant and anti-inflammatory phytochemical betalin). So it is especially beneficial during the first week of this four-week plan, as it digs deep to cleanse the system. Beetroot also contains pectin, a form of soluble fibre that further flushes the system. It is also rich in vitamins and minerals to help support the production of collagen in the skin.

Skin-Loving Nutrients

- **DIETARY FIBRE:** pectin
- **PHYTOCHEMICALS:** betalin, carotenoids (beta-carotene, lycopene)
- **VITAMINS:** C, K
- **MINERALS:** iron, manganese, potassium

BLUEBERRIES

Blueberries are overflowing with antioxidant-rich flavonoids and vitamin C to protect the skin and support connective tissue, keeping it supple and taut. Just a handful of blueberries on their own or with breakfast will make your skin smile.

Skin-Loving Nutrients

- **DIETARY FIBRE**
- **PHYTOCHEMICALS:** flavonoids (anthocyanin); carotenoids (lutein)
- **VITAMINS:** C, K
- **MINERALS:** manganese

CARROTS

Carrots are one of the richest sources of the antioxidant beta-carotene, a precursor to vitamin A in the body. They are also rich in fibre and vitamin C and help enhance the production of collagen and elastin in the skin, while also protecting and supporting the skin against environmental hazards.

Skin-Loving Nutrients

- **DIETARY FIBRE**
- **PHYTOCHEMICALS:** carotenoids (beta-carotene)
- **VITAMINS** A, B6, B9, C, E
- **MINERALS:** copper, iron, manganese, potassium

DARK CHOCOLATE

Chocolate, or rather the low sugar, unsweetened dark variety with at least 75 per cent cocoa solids, is packed with antioxidant-rich flavonoids to repair and protect the skin. With most other lower-grade chocolate any potential health benefits are far outweighed by the sugar and fat content.

It is also widely accepted that chocolate makes us happy – and why wouldn't it, as it tastes delicious! Research has shown that eating quality dark chocolate increases the production of mood-enhancing neurotransmitters, thereby reducing stress hormones like cortisol that are linked to collagen breakdown – so a real win-win on all counts, and when you feel good, you look even better.

Skin-Loving Nutrients

- **FATTY ACIDS:** monounsaturated (oleic acid)
- **PHYTOCHEMICALS:** flavonoids, polyphenols
- **VITAMINS:** A, B1, B2, B3, B5
- **MINERALS:** calcium, copper, iron, magnesium, potassium, sulphur, zinc

EDAMAME BEANS

These nutritious young soya beans have enjoyed a long history in Japanese cuisine, eaten on their own as a tasty snack or added to main meals and dips, but they have only recently made their appearance in supermarkets in this part of the world. Edamames can be bought shelled (much like frozen peas) or as the whole bean in its shell, ready to be shucked. They are an excellent source of protein, choline, complex carbohydrates and fibre, releasing energy slowly to nourish the skin and fuel both body and mind.

Skin-Loving Nutrients

- **DIETARY FIBRE**
- **PROTEIN:** amino acids
- **PHYTOCHEMICALS**
- **CHOLINE**
- **VITAMINS:** K, B1, folate
- **MINERALS:** copper, iron, magnesium, molybdenum, phosphorous

EGGS

Eggs are a nutritional powerhouse – a complete protein source packed with the necessary essential amino acids, essential fats, lecithin and much more. Both the yellow and white parts of the egg are naturally loaded with nutrients. The lecithin and fat-soluble vitamins A and D in the yolk help regulate cell turnover in the skin, while also keeping it soft and supple. The whites contain the bulk of the protein (an estimated 4 g per egg white) as well as certain nourishing vitamins and minerals. Contrary to previous belief, it is now accepted that moderate consumption of eggs does not have a negative impact on cholesterol levels. In fact, studies have shown that regular consumption of two eggs per day does not adversely affect lipid profiles and may, in fact, improve them.

Choose organic or free range where possible, as these tend to have a superior nutritional profile. Eggs from ethically reared chickens taste far better too, with a richer, more vibrant yolk.

Skin-Loving Nutrients

- **FATTY ACIDS:** omega-3
- **LECITHIN**
- **PROTEIN:** all essential amino acids (mostly in the white)
- **VITAMINS:** B2, B6, B12, folate, A, D, E, K
- **MINERALS:** copper, iron, magnesium, phosphorus, potassium, selenium, zinc

FERMENTED FOODS

Fermented foods, including kombucha, sauerkraut and kefir amongst others, provide a wealth of beneficial probiotic bacteria, organic acids, active enzymes, amino acids and antioxidants that are particularly supportive for the gut. These bacteria enhance digestion, immunity, neurological health and overall health, while also enhancing skin elasticity and helping to keep it clear and fresh. See pages 257–62 for kombucha recipes.

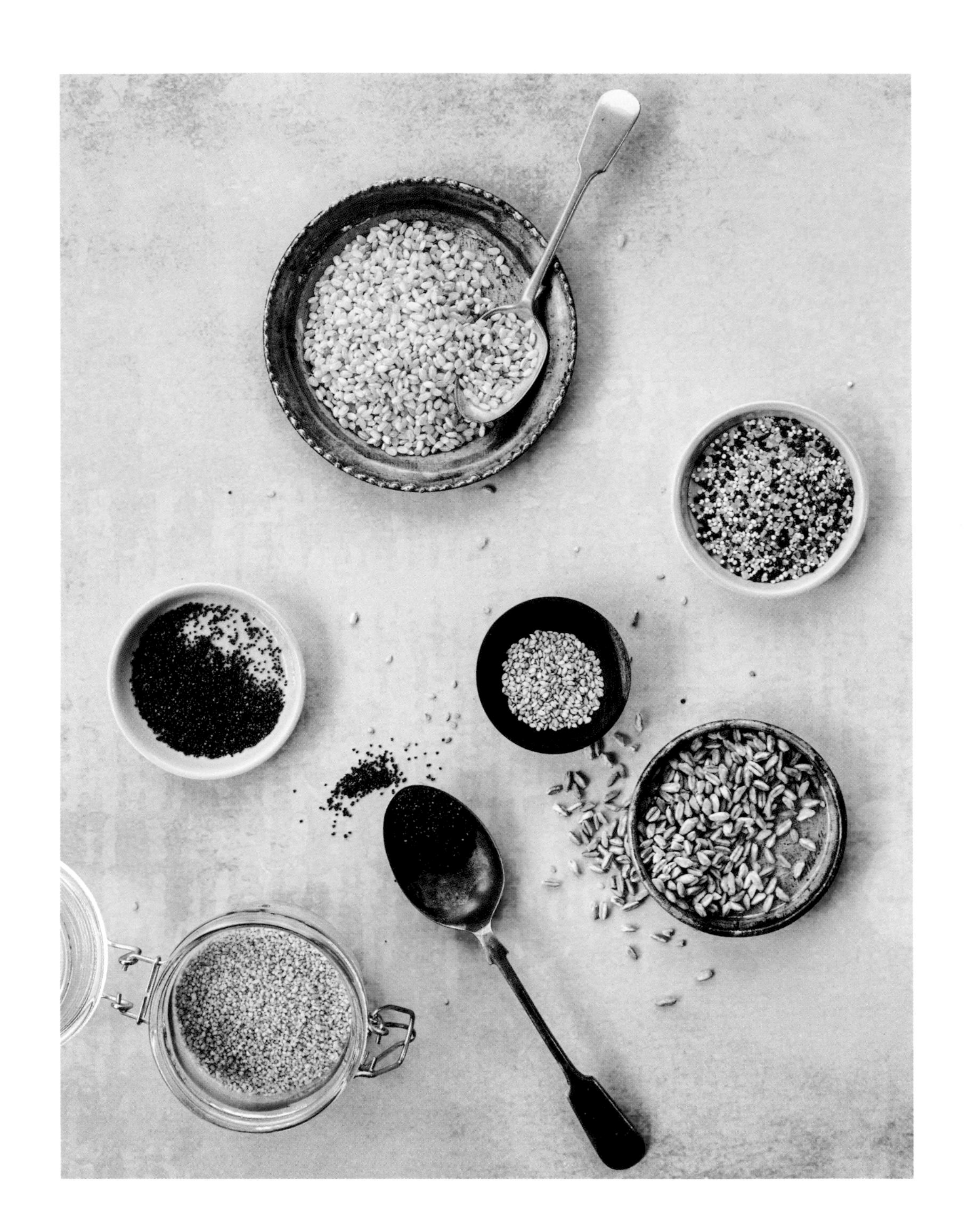

GRAINS

For meals that positively sing of goodness, you cannot beat grains. These nutritional powerhouses are readily available, easy to prepare and, when herbs and spices are woven in, packed with flavour.

While numerous grains line supermarket shelves now, only certain ones, most notably the natural, unrefined versions, are included in this plan. The processed or white versions of the more commonly eaten grains have gone through a chemical process to bleach them that naturally removes much of their goodness.

Quinoa and buckwheat are 'pseudo-grains' – they look and cook like grains but are in fact seeds. They have been used in a multitude of ways for centuries and are now enjoying a revival, thanks to an increased focus on more nutritious grains.

When buying grains, choose the least processed varieties that have been altered little since their original cultivation and have kept their goodness intact.

This is the perfect time to experiment with some of the less familiar grains, like farro and buckwheat and many others. Increasing your range of foods means that you are getting the complete spectrum of essential minerals and vitamins – you might even surprise yourself with what you can create with just a little effort!

Pre-cooked grains are popular now too and are great to have on standby when time is tight. A quick read of the ingredients is advised to see what else has been added – choose the pack with the shortest ingredient list!

While all grains can be cooked in plain water, adding a little mint or other herbs intensifies their flavour. Alternatively, cook in vegetable stock (see recipe on page 173). The grains listed here are included in the four-week plan, along with guidelines on how best to cook them. Please also refer to packet instructions, as cooking recommendations can vary.

GLUTEN FREE OR WHEAT FREE? While this book is not a manifesto on the pros or cons of gluten, the following scientifically grounded facts are important.

Gluten is created when two molecules, glutenin and gliadin, form a bond. When bakers knead dough, this bond creates an elastic membrane, which is what gives bread its chewy texture and elasticity. Gluten also traps carbon dioxide, which adds volume to the loaf as it ferments.

For people with coeliac disease, the briefest exposure to gluten can trigger an immune reaction that can damage the lining of the small intestine. However, for the vast majority of us who do not have an intolerance to this protein-rich ingredient, gluten is perfectly fine to eat.

Many experts believe that the perceived problem with gluten – and wheat, for that matter – in society today is more to do with the mass production of bread and the quality of ingredients in that bread.

The only scientifically proven way to decipher if you are sensitive or intolerant to wheat, gluten or any food is by doing a blood test with a qualified health practitioner. If the results are positive then you should work with a qualified dietitian or registered nutritional therapist to ensure you are making healthy substitutes and not comprising your health in any way.

BUCKWHEAT

Despite its name, buckwheat is not part of the wheat family. It is a gluten-free seed bearing the scientific name *Fagopyrum esculentum*. Buckwheat generally comes in two forms – kasha, meaning toasted, and buckwheat groats, the untoasted version. It is grown mostly in central and eastern Europe, Russia and China. The groats can have a slightly bitter taste so it's best to rinse the grain well ahead of cooking. When ground into flour, buckwheat is becoming an increasingly popular alternative to wheat flour for breads, for pancakes and in baking.

Buckwheat is a complete protein, containing all essential amino acids and minerals including zinc, copper, magnesium and manganese. Being a seed, it is rich in flavonoids. It is also high in soluble fibre so can help balance blood sugar levels.

Skin-Loving Nutrients

- **DIETARY FIBRE**
- **PROTEIN:** complete
- **PHYTONUTRIENTS:** flavonoids, quercetin
- **VITAMINS:** trace amounts only
- **MINERALS:** copper, iron, magnesium, manganese, phosphorus, zinc

How to Cook

Rinse groats under cold water until the water

runs clear. Use 2 cups of liquid per cup of buckwheat. Bring to the boil and simmer for 20–30 minutes (15–20 mins for toasted buckwheat) or follow directions on label.

COUSCOUS

Couscous is small pasta made of durum wheat or semolina, a form of wheat native to North Africa. It has a mild flavour and is extremely versatile. While it lacks the range of nutrients found in whole grains, it is an excellent base for tasty salads and a great accompaniment to main meals.

Skin-Loving Nutrients

- **DIETARY FIBRE**
- **PROTEIN:** small amounts only
- **PHYTONUTRIENTS:** ferulic and phytic acid
- **VITAMINS:** B3, folate with trace amounts of others
- **MINERALS:** magnesium, phosphorus, selenium

How to Cook

The general rule is to use 1 cup of dry couscous to approximately 1½ cups boiling water. Cover and allow to sit for about 5 minutes. Fluff up with a fork.

FARRO

Farro is an ancient wheat grain, believed to have originated in Mesopotamia, with a nutty flavour and chewy texture. It is higher in protein (similar to quinoa, and a great protein source for vegetarians) and significantly lower in gluten than typical wheat.

Skin-Loving Nutrients

- **DIETARY FIBRE**
- **PROTEIN:** most essential amino acids
- **PHYTONUTRIENTS:** polyphenols, carotenoids
- **VITAMINS:** B3 and E with trace amounts of others
- **MINERALS:** iron, magnesium, selenium, zinc

How to Cook

Use about 2 cups of water per cup of farro. Add a handful of fresh mint for added flavour. Bring to the boil and simmer for 20–30 minutes or until tender.

OATS

Oats are a wholegrain cereal known scientifically as *Avena sativa*. They are mainly grown in North America and Europe. The whole oat with the outer hull of the grain removed is called a groat. Oat groats are most commonly rolled or crushed into flat flakes and lightly toasted to produce oatmeal. Typical instant porridge oats are made of more thinly rolled or cut oats that absorb water more easily and cook faster. The fibre-rich outer layer of the grain is the bran, which is used in cereals or in baking where it is becoming an increasingly popular alternative to wheat flour.

Oats are one of the richest sources of the essential mineral silica, which helps the skin (and hair) retain moisture. They are a good source of protein and fibre (almost 11 per cent), much of this in the form of the soluble fibre beta-glucan, released when the oats are soaked and adding creaminess while also helping to reduce blood cholesterol levels and balance blood sugar.

Colloidal oatmeal, produced by finely grinding oats and boiling them to extract the colloidal material, is found in many skincare products from shampoos to face creams. It is incredibly gentle on skin and is deemed safe for use even on the most sensitive skin types. It is believed to help normalise skin pH levels and can help soothe and calm irritations and soreness. To use this way, simply grind the oatmeal into a fine powder. It can then be used as part of a gentle healing face mask (see page 109) or put into a muslin bag and added to a running bath with a few drops of lavender essential oil to calm and soothe the body.

Skin-Loving Nutrients

- **DIETARY FIBRE:** beta-glucan
- **PROTEIN:** essential amino acids
- **PHYTONUTRIENTS:** avenathramides, ferulic acid, phytic acid, silica
- **VITAMINS:** B1 with trace amounts of other B vitamins
- **MINERALS:** copper, iron, magnesium, manganese, selenium, zinc
- **TRACE ELEMENTS:** silica

How to Cook

Use about 1 cup of oats to 2 cups of liquid (water, milk or non-dairy alternative). Combine in a pot over a medium heat. Bring slowly to the boil, then reduce heat to a simmer, stirring frequently. Once the oats soften and the liquid starts to thicken, remove from the heat and add your chosen fruits, nuts and seeds.

QUINOA

Quinoa is a member of the grass family and comes in three forms – red, black and white. It was first harvested in the Andes Mountains of South America where it is called the 'mother grain'. It has a higher protein content than most other grains (approximately 16 per cent by dry weight) and is rich in iron, fibre and magnesium (among other nutrients). It has a crunchy texture and nutty flavour and is extremely versatile, albeit somewhat bland on its own, but is easily spiced up for flavour. If using for porridge, use quinoa flakes.

Skin-Loving Nutrients

- **DIETARY FIBRE**
- **PROTEIN:** all essential amino acids

- **PHYTONUTRIENTS:** quercetin and others
- **VITAMINS:** B2, folate, B6
- **MINERALS:** copper, iron, potassium, magnesium, manganese, zinc

How to Cook

While cooking recommendations vary, the general guideline is 2 cups of water per cup of quinoa. Some chefs suggest toasting the uncooked grain on a dry pan for a few minutes before cooking, as this adds a deeper nutty flavour. Bring to the boil and cook for 10–15 minutes until all the water has been absorbed. Red and black quinoa can take slightly longer to cook than white.

RICE

Rice is the most versatile grain on the planet, grown on almost every continent. The main varieties of rice are white, brown, red, black and purple. White rice is highly refined and stripped of its seed coat (bran) and germ, while brown rice is an intact whole grain and a superior source of fibre, vitamins, minerals and other healthy components, which are mostly concentrated in the bran and germ of the grain.

- **LONG GRAIN** rice maintains its texture and shape through cooking and is the most widely used rice.
- **MEDIUM GRAIN** rice contains slightly more starch so is a little stickier and generally used in paella and risotto.
- **SHORT GRAIN** brown rice adds a deliciously nutty flavour to meals, while the white variety works well in puddings.

Skin-Loving Nutrients

- **DIETARY FIBRE**
- **PROTEIN:** small amounts only
- **PHYTONUTRIENTS:** ferulic and phytic acid
- **VITAMINS:** B1, B3
- **MINERALS:** copper, manganese, magnesium, selenium

How to Cook

For brown rice, rinse under running water to remove excess starch. Use 1¼ cups of water per cup of long grain brown rice (a little more water if using short grain). Bring to the boil and simmer for 25–30 minutes until the rice is tender. Drain and leave in the pot for a few minutes before serving.

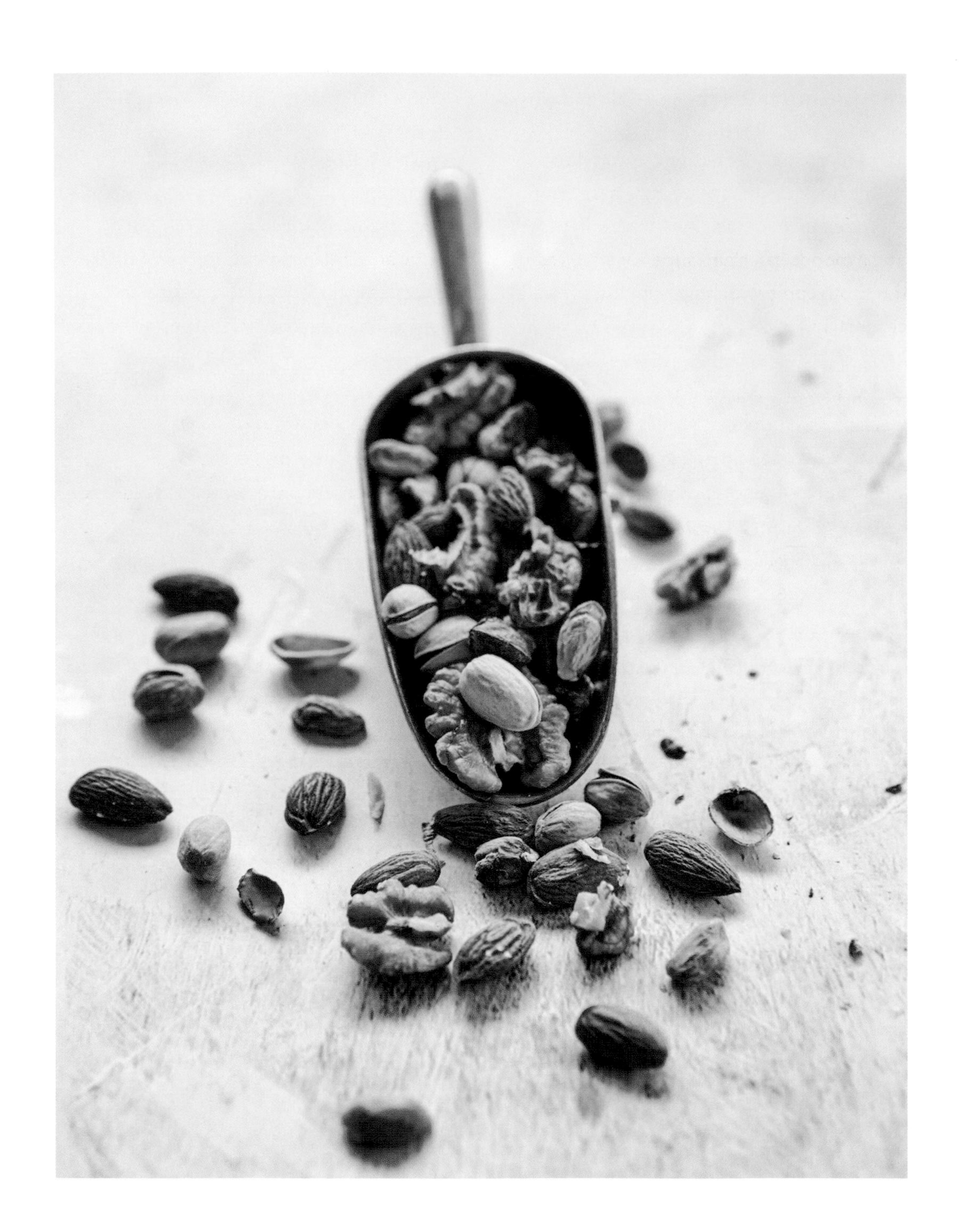

NUTS

Most nuts are beneficial to the skin due to their high content of healthy fats, vitamins and minerals. This said, walnuts and almonds can claim superior status as they both come with hugely impressive credentials.

Skin-Loving Nutrients

- **DIETARY FIBRE**
- **FATTY ACIDS:** omega-3
- **PROTEIN:** amino acids
- **PHYTOCHEMICALS:** flavonoids
- **VITAMINS:** B1, B2, B3, B5, B6, B9, E, K
- **MINERALS:** calcium, copper, iron, magnesium, manganese, phosphorus, potassium, selenium, zinc

WALNUTS

Walnuts are one of richest plant sources of omega-3 fatty acids, crucial for brain health and protection against the risk of depression and associated disorders. The fatty acids profile of walnuts works alongside their high vitamin E content to keep skin moist, soft and plump. Walnuts are anti-inflammatory and excellent for treating acne and other issues related to the skin's sebaceous gland. They also protect hair from UV damage and keep it lustrous and shiny. Just a ¼ cup of walnuts as a snack or added to a breakfast bowl gives almost 95 per cent of daily omega-3 requirements.

ALMONDS

Almonds are overflowing with fibre, protein, vitamin E and essential fatty acids, all of which help promote a healthy heart and maintain plump, glowing skin. They are a natural anti-inflammatory and can help treat skin issues including acne, psoriasis and eczema. They are also rich in the hair-loving minerals manganese and selenium.

A handful of almonds eaten as a snack, chopped into smoothies or salads, or enjoyed as almond butter spread helps keep your skin glowing.

OILY FISH

Cold water oily fish, notably salmon, trout and tuna, are packed with omega-3 fatty acids to strengthen blood cells and plump the skin, boosting the production of the essential proteins collagen and elastin.

Books have been written exclusively dedicated to the powers of oily fish – and for good reason too as, simply put, the more you eat, the more your skin (not to forget your brain, heart and the rest of your body too) will benefit. Studies have shown that eating more omega-3 fatty acids may result in smoother, younger-looking skin with a reduction in inflammatory skin conditions, including acne and psoriasis.

As with many other foods, quality is key and it's important to check where your fish has come from before buying. Where possible, choose organic line-caught fish.

Skin-Loving Nutrients

- **FATTY ACIDS:** omega-3
- **PROTEIN:** all essential amino acids
- **CHOLINE**
- **VITAMINS:** B5, B7, B12, D
- **MINERALS:** iodine, phosphorus, selenium

ORANGES

Sunshine in a skin, oranges are the embodiment of vitamin C. This essential vitamin helps the body absorb iron from food and is needed for the production of collagen. The high fibre content in the orange flesh helps keep the digestive system in motion, eliminating waste for a cleaner colon and skin.

Skin-Loving Nutrients

- **DIETARY FIBRE:** pectin
- **PHYTOCHEMICALS:** flavonoids, polyphenols
- **VITAMINS:** B1, B6, B9, C
- **MINERALS:** calcium, potassium

POMEGRANATES

Pomegranate seeds have been used for centuries in the Middle East. They are overflowing with vitamin C to stimulate collagen production and boost elasticity in the skin. They also help protect and repair damaged skin and combat inflammation, making them especially beneficial when tackling acne and other skin conditions.

Pomegranate seeds are extremely versatile and readily available. Use on their own or in everything from smoothies to salads, tagines, couscous, farro, quinoa or rice.

Skin-Loving Nutrients

- **DIETARY FIBRE**
- **PHYTOCHEMICALS:** flavonoids (ellagic acid), polyphenols
- **CHOLINE**
- **VITAMINS:** B1, B2, B3, B5, B6, B9, C, E, K
- **MINERALS:** calcium, copper, iron, magnesium, manganese, phosphorus, potassium, selenium, zinc

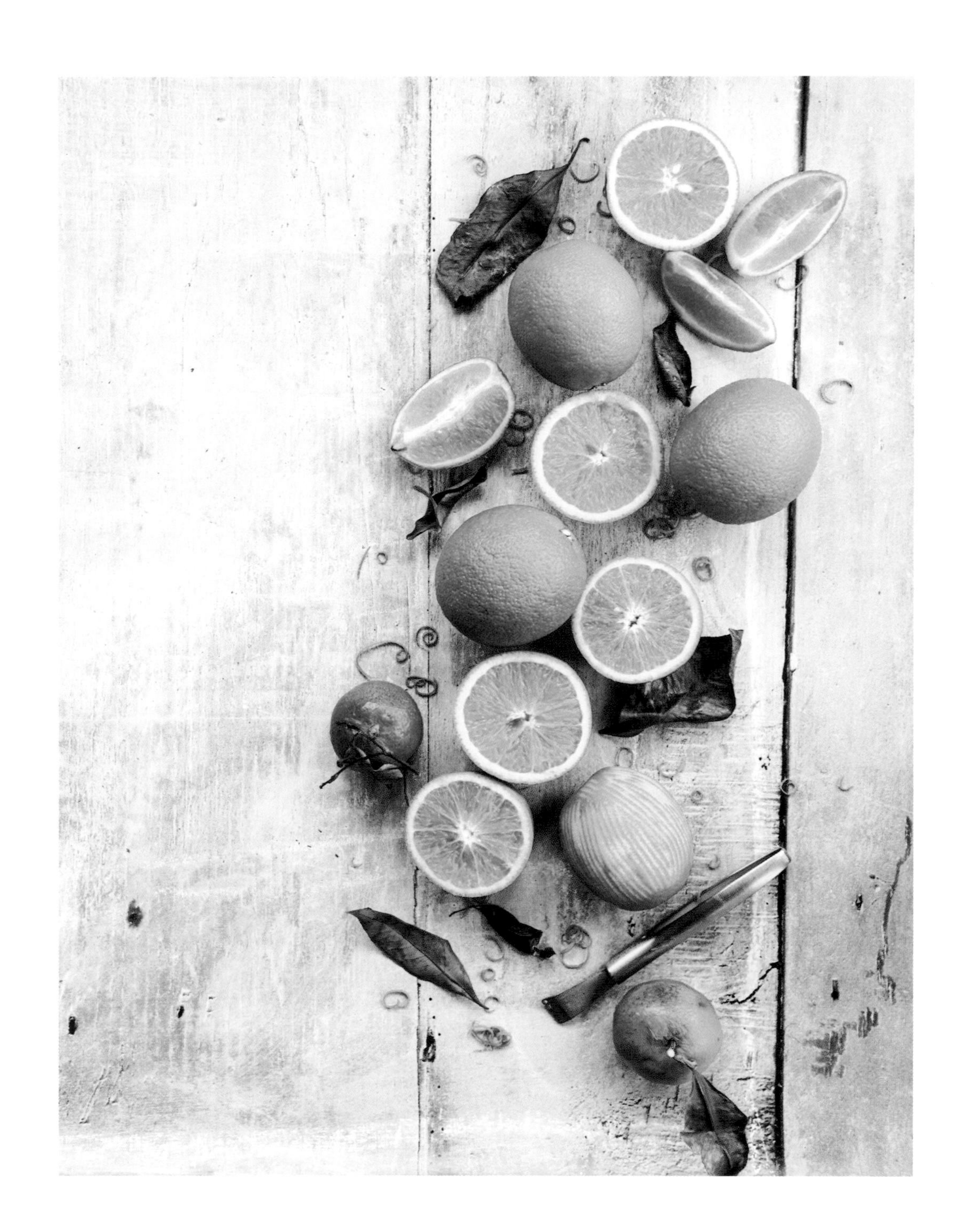

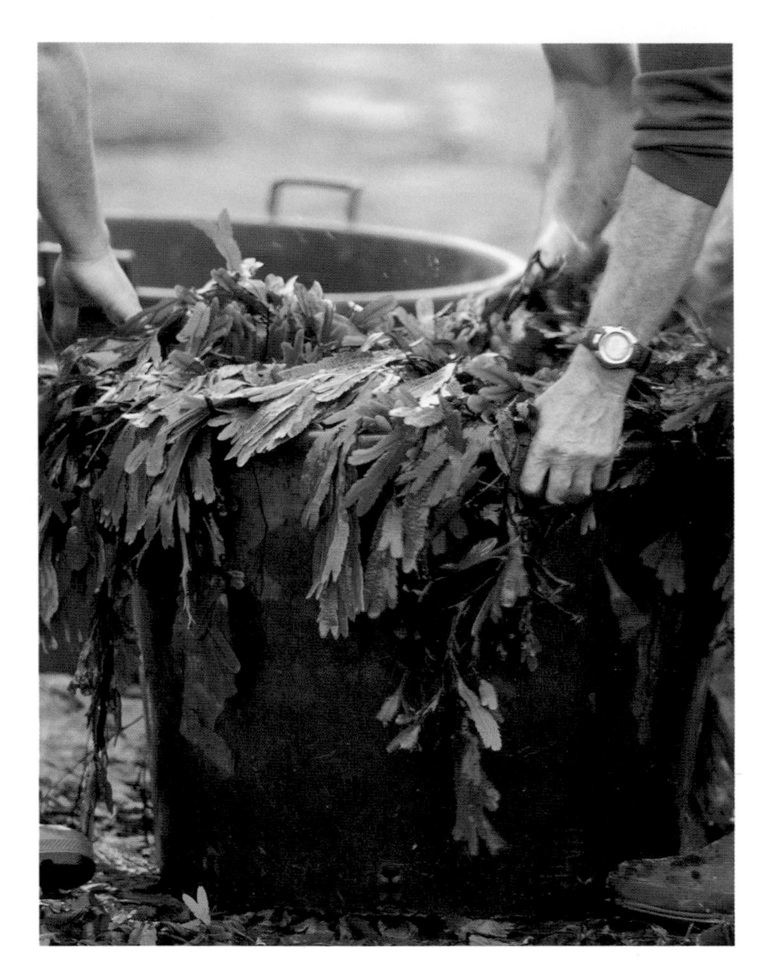

Courtesy of Voya

SEA VEGETABLES

'In the internal environment of our human system, and only there, do we find the same mineral make-up and the same physiognomy as that of seawater' – René Quinton, French scientist, c. 1897

Seaweed is the oldest form of life on the planet and one of today's hottest superfoods. Hardly surprising, really, as the Ancient Polynesians availed of the curative properties of seaweed to treat wounds, bruises and swellings, while the Japanese have sworn by it for over 2,000 years, and Ireland, being cocooned in it, is only now appreciating the extent of its goodness.

There are an estimated 30,000 algae varieties in the world, many not yet identified (and most not yet extensively researched). And whether you drink its extract, bathe in it or rub it into your skin, seaweed is the tonic of the moment and a great all-rounder for balancing and boosting the body both inside and out. It is also appearing as a key ingredient in results-driven skincare from some of the world's leading skincare brands.

SEAWEED CLASSIFICATION

Seaweeds come in three colour categories, depending on their level of chlorophyll and the amount of light they have been exposed to. The more readily available types include:

- **GREEN ALGAE (CHLOROPHYTA):** sea lettuce, *Chlorella/Codium*
- **RED ALGAE (RHODOPHYTA):** *Lithothamnium/Corallina*, nori, agar, dulse, Irish moss
- **BROWN ALGAE (PHAEOPHYTA):** *Fucus/Laminaria*, kelp, kombu, arame, hijiki, wakame

Seaweeds draw a wealth of minerals, vitamins and trace elements from the sea that can account for well over half of seaweed's dry mass. These include sodium, calcium, magnesium, potassium, chlorine, sulphur, iodine, iron, zinc, copper, selenium and fluoride, among countless others. Nutritionally, they are as good as any land vegetable and often superior in their vitamin, mineral, trace element and protein content. Most varieties are particularly high in iron and vitamin C (to facilitate the absorption of iron in the body). They rate among the few sources of vitamin B12-enriched plant foods, so are especially beneficial for plant-based foodies and vegans. Fresh and dried seaweeds are now widely available in supermarkets and, like other vegetables, they differ in their uses and cooking methods. A snack of dried wakame, for instance, is a source of numerous essential nutrients including vitamin C and zinc, iodine, iron, magnesium, calcium and vitamin B12, while nori and kelp are loaded with iron, essential fatty acids and phytonutrients that suffuse the skin, hair and nails with moisture and nourishment. Toss some wakame into your miso soup, or wrap some vegetables in nori sheets to make nori rolls. Dulse is a natural flavour enhancer, with a rich savoury taste that works well in risottos and casseroles, and sea spaghetti is nature's pasta and can be cooked in a similar fashion.

When steamed, seaweed produces amazingly luxurious oils that detoxify and nourish the body. Put simply, the algae act as a large poultice, quickly removing toxins while transferring nutrients to the body. Sea buckthorn oil is a well-recognised cleanser and skin soother that is also beneficial in the treatment of acne and rosacea.

Seaweed is enriched with proven antioxidants, algal polyphenols and carotenoids that protect the skin against environmental damage, while the vast store of EFAs helps maintain skin's suppleness and elasticity. It has long been used in products designed to treat conditions like psoriasis, eczema, dermatitis and acne.

Seaweed extracts also have a pronounced moisturising effect on the hair, increasing lustre and softness while decreasing its electrostatic charge.

Algae soaks are now extensively used for bathing in the home. To maximise benefits, the body must soak in the cleansing oils twice a week (at about 36° C). Be warned, however: the higher the grade of seaweed soak the more pungent it can be. If yours is at the upper end, then add a few drops of lavender oil to soften the aroma.

SEAWEED BATHS

Seaweed baths have long been used as a way of relaxing and relieving pain, and in more modern times as a way to unwind and destress. This is largely due to the detoxifying benefits of the seaweed and the recuperative effects of its high mineral content. When seaweed is steamed, the polymers act as a carrier for minerals, vitamins, proteins and polysaccharides, creating a natural alkaline poultice that gently clears toxins. The oils are naturally suspended in the water and as the heat opens the pores in the skin, the oils are readily absorbed.

Skin-Loving Nutrients

- **DIETARY FIBRE**
- **VITAMINS:** C, B12, Copper
- **MINERALS:** calcium, iodine, iron, magnesium, phosphorous, potassium, sodium

SEEDS

A handful of seeds will boost the nutritional content of every meal. Top of the skin-loving list are chia, flaxseeds, pumpkin and sunflower. They can be sprinkled over salads and yoghurts, added to breads and in other baking or just eaten on their own by the handful.

Skin-Loving Nutrients

- **DIETARY FIBRE**
- **PROTEIN**
- **PHYTOCHEMICALS:** carotenoids (beta-carotene)
- **VITAMINS:** A, folate, C, E, K
- **MINERALS:** iron, magnesium, zinc

CHIA

Chia seeds are packed with protein, fibre, and omega-3s – all great for your skin and hair. As they absorb close to twelve times their weight in water, they keep you feeling fuller longer, which is a benefit if trying to lose weight. They are a handy replacement for eggs in vegan baking.

FLAXSEEDS

Flaxseeds provide a huge boost of omega-3 fatty acids to help prevent and treat skin conditions like acne and eczema. Their anti-inflammatory properties also help skin repair and cell renewal.

PUMPKIN

Pumpkin seeds (or pepitas) are overflowing with protein, vitamin E, zinc and magnesium to promote regeneration of skin cells and fight off acne-inducing bacteria. Their high vitamin-E content is an added bonus to help keep skin supple and strong

SUNFLOWER

Sunflower seeds are high in protein and magnesium, both important to keep skin nourished and strong. Magnesium helps to calm and relax nerves and muscles.

- Nuts and seeds are best eaten raw and unsalted.
- Store nuts and seeds in the refrigerator or freezer to preserve freshness.
- If you cannot eat nuts and seeds without salt, buy them raw, roast them and sprinkle with a pinch of sea salt.

SPINACH

A symbol of strength and vitality, spinach is as nourishing as its powerful image portrays. It is a rich source of iron, an essential component of the blood's haemoglobin, and its vitamin K

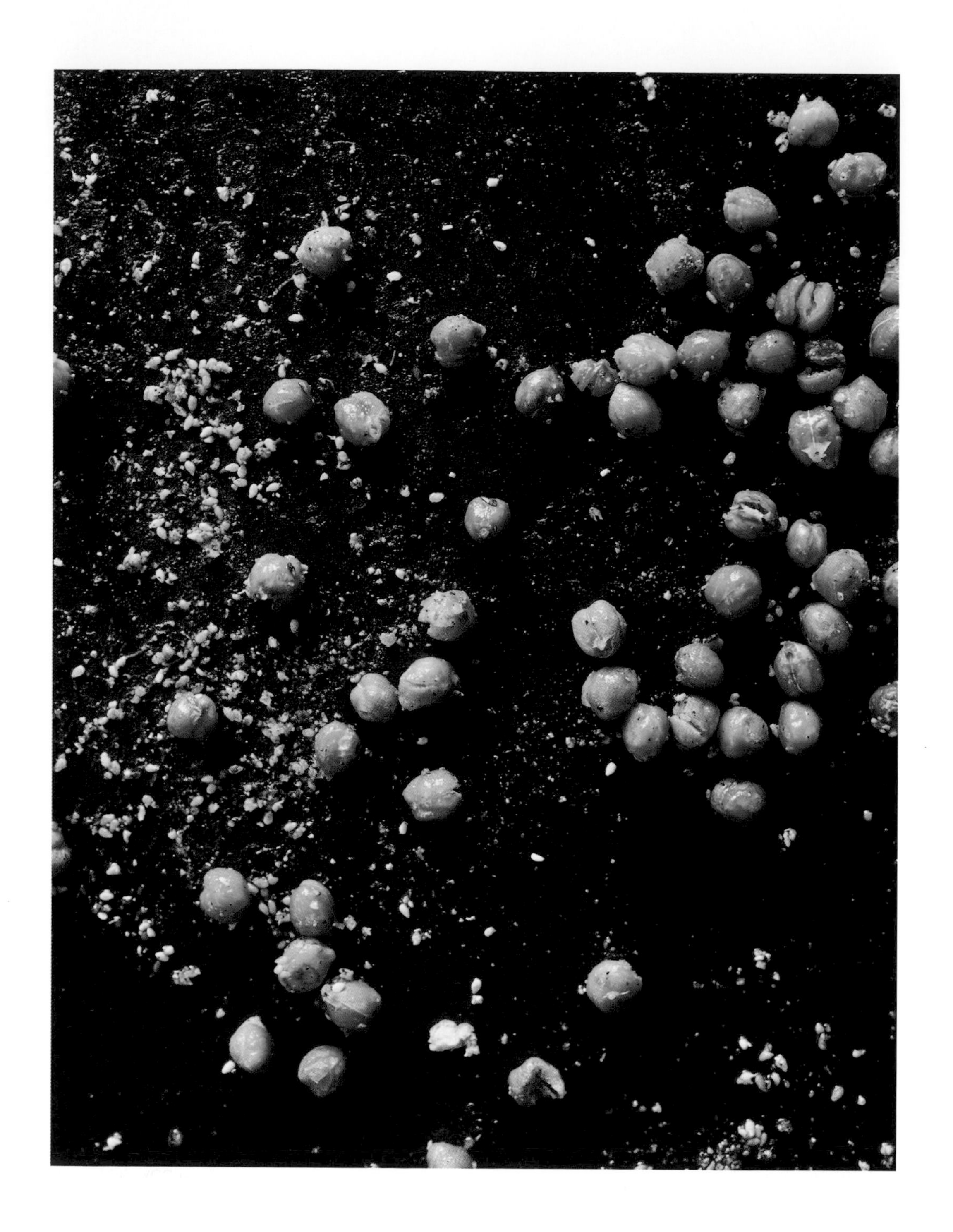

content enhances blood circulation. As with other leafy green vegetables, spinach is an excellent source of skin-protecting and collagen-boosting antioxidant vitamins A, C and E and beta-carotene and can be enjoyed in salads, in smoothies or lightly sautéed with olive oil, garlic and a dash of sea salt.

Skin-Loving Nutrients

- **DIETARY FIBRE**
- **PROTEIN**
- **PHYTOCHEMICALS:** carotenoids (beta-carotene)
- **VITAMINS:** folate, A, C, E, K
- **MINERALS:** iron, magnesium

TOMATOES

Few foods can beat the deliciously sweet taste of juicy, ripe tomatoes in summer, eaten on their own with a pinch of black pepper or sliced with fresh mozzarella, a dash of olive oil and torn basil leaves. Tomatoes ooze skin-glowing goodness and are best known for their high content of the antioxidant lycopene that gives them their rich red colour. They are also excellent sources of vitamins A, K and the B-complex group, which all play key roles in in keeping skin fresh supple and glowing.

Skin-Loving Nutrients

- **DIETARY FIBRE**
- **PHYTOCHEMICALS:** carotenoids (lycopene)
- **VITAMINS:** B1, B3, B5, B6, A, C, E, K
- **MINERALS:** iron, magnesium, phosphorus, potassium

TURMERIC

Long revered by both Chinese medicine and Ayurvedic experts for its far-reaching medicinal benefits, this colourful, fragrant spice is now weaving its magic in the West.

In Ayurvedic medicine, turmeric is referred to as 'Indian solid gold' and used to help curb inflammation and treat an array of ailments from infections to stomach upsets and arthritis. Mixed with honey to form a thick paste, it can be taken orally for sore throats and colds and can also be applied directly to the skin to relieve infections and certain inflammatory conditions like acne and rosacea (see page 121).

Recent scientific studies support the time-tested belief that turmeric is indeed a potent antioxidant and anti-inflammatory. The spice's active ingredient is a group of polyphenol plant pigments called curcumin that give the distinctive saffron/orange colour. Studies have confirmed how powerful curcumin is in protecting against arthritis-related joint pain and swelling, inflammation, high cholesterol and so much more.

The fresh root is preferred, but dried works too, especially in cooking. The dried variety is made by peeling, boiling and drying the turmeric root, before grinding and bottling (1 inch/2.5cm fresh turmeric root = approx. 1 tsp ground turmeric).

Skin-Loving Nutrients

- **CURCUMIN**
- **DIETARY FIBRE**
- **PHYTOCHEMICALS:** carotenoids (beta-carotene)
- **VITAMIN C**
- **MINERALS:** calcium, iron, magnesium, potassium, zinc

SKIN BARRIER-STRENGTHENING FOODS

The GLOW plan is structured to fuel our bodies with the building blocks for stronger, healthier skin that is better able to withstand the toxic assaults of daily life. Lecithin, otherwise known as phosphatidylcholine, is a phospholipid molecule and an essential component of the body's cellular membranes. Lecithin helps maintain a healthy active skin barrier that helps lock water into the cells to hydrate the deeper layers of the skin.

The majority of nutrients found in lecithin are stored in the form of choline (a softening and soothing agent), which the body can only produce in limited quantities so must be topped up through our diet. Choline is often added to products designed for mature, dry or overworked skin but is best used by the body when taken through food.

Egg yolk is among the best sources of lecithin, while edamame beans and pomegranate seeds are rich in choline. Other foods that protect this essential skin barrier include blueberries, nuts (especially walnuts and almonds) and dark green leafy vegetables.

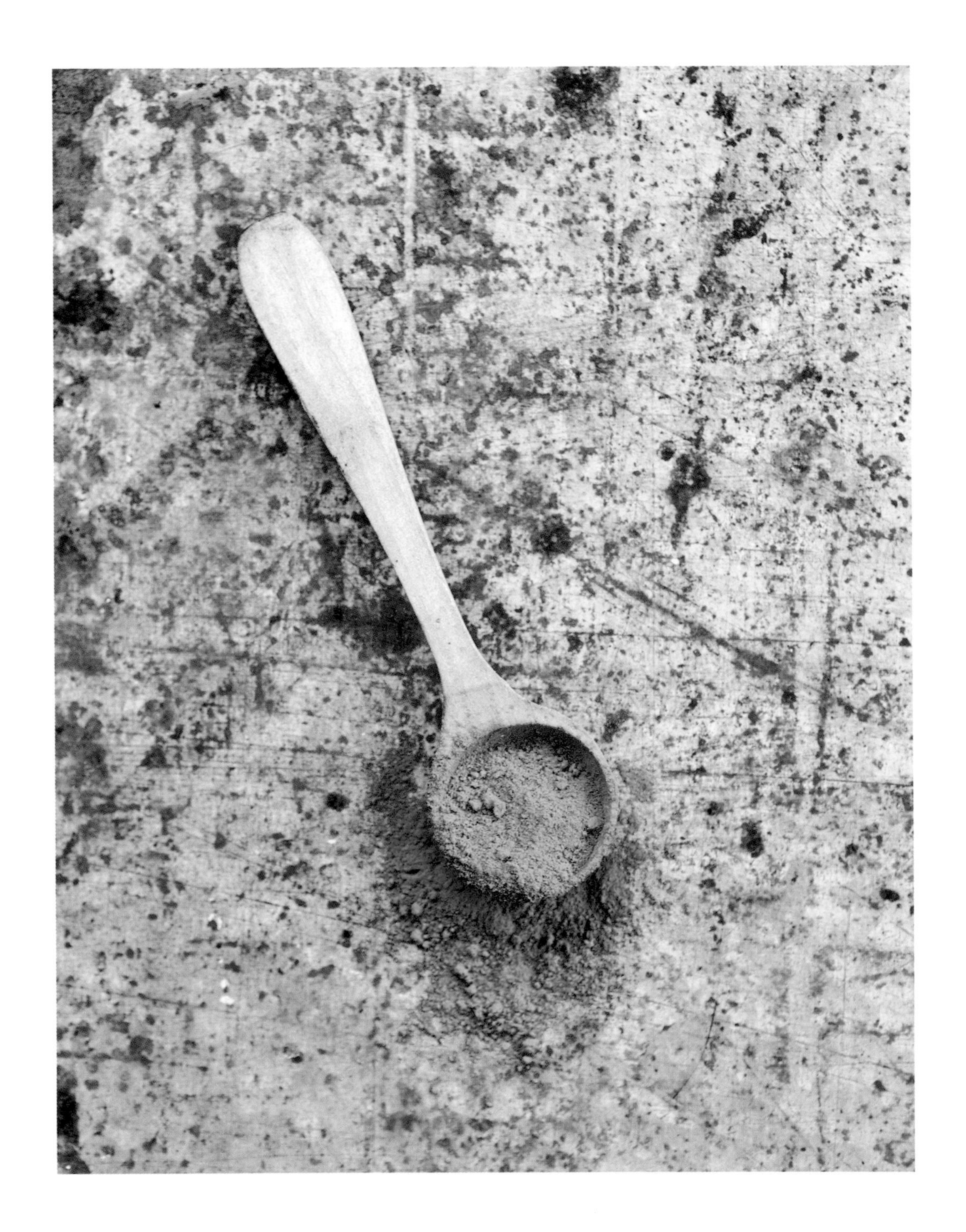

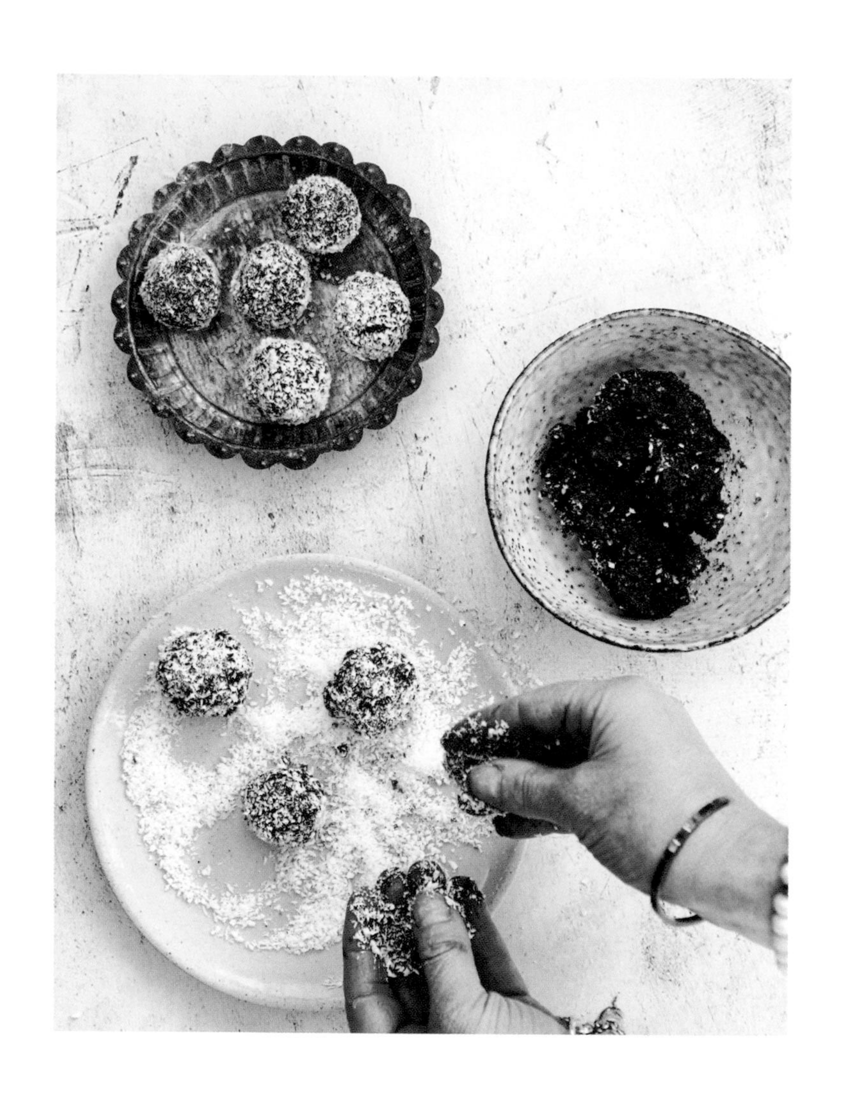

KITCHEN ESSENTIALS

◊

With this GLOW plan, time, or lack of, is no excuse for not eating deliciously healthy skin-loving foods every day. Just a little effort and organisation is required and it pays off big time. You won't need to buy lots of expensive equipment – you'll just need some kitchen basics and to focus on buying top quality, fresh ingredients, the majority of which should be vegetables and fish.

Personally, I relish quick and easy foods – if the ingredient list is too long, I move on. And although I am less impatient than I was pre-children, I still struggle with long preparation times. Thus, almost all of the recipes in this book are quick and easy to prepare – some might take time to prove or breathe, but other than that they are good to go.

The following skin-loving foods are included in many of the GLOW recipes and useful to have on hand when preparing meals during the four-week plan.

FRIDGE

FRUIT AND VEGETABLES

- Bananas
- Oranges
- Limes and lemons
- Apples
- Pomegranates
- Berries – blueberries, strawberries, etc. (when in season)
- Avocados
- Tomatoes
- Red peppers
- Seasonal root vegetables (beetroot, carrots, parsnips, etc.)
- Spinach and other leafy greens
- Rocket
- Fresh mint, parsley and coriander

DAIRY AND DAIRY ALTERNATIVES

- Natural unsweetened or Greek yoghurt; sheep's or coconut milk yoghurt
- Coconut milk or almond milk (unsweetened)
- Feta cheese

FISH

- Salmon, tuna or other oily fish

FREEZER

- Mixed berries (if fresh are not in season)
- Chopped bananas
- Edamame beans
- Peas
- Salmon – in reserve for when no time to shop

CUPBOARD

VEGETABLES

- Sweet potatoes
- Squash
- Potatoes
- Seasonal root vegetables

OILS, HERBS, CONDIMENTS AND SPICES

- Apple cider vinegar (ACV)
- Balsamic vinegar
- Extra virgin olive oil – for dressings
- Olive oil or coconut oil – for cooking
- Vegetable stock cubes
- Black pepper
- Pink or sea salt
- Ground chilli
- Ground cinnamon
- Ground cumin
- Dried mixed herbs
- Fresh root ginger
- Fresh or dried turmeric

- Smoked paprika
- Bay leaves
- Tamari or soy sauce
- Maple syrup
- Miso paste
- Honey

NUTS AND SEEDS

- Almonds
- Walnuts
- Chia seeds
- Flaxseeds, ground
- Sunflower seeds
- Pumpkin seeds
- Almond butter
- Tahini

GRAINS AND FLOURS

- Oats
- Quinoa
- Farro
- Short grain brown rice
- Buckwheat flour
- Spelt flour
- Couscous
- Puy lentils
- Pitta breads and/or wholewheat wraps
- Sourdough bread from a reputable bakery

TINS AND EXTRAS

- Chickpeas
- Kidney beans
- Tinned tomatoes
- Eggs
- Seaweed
- Dark chocolate (more than 70 per cent cocoa solids)
- Herbal teas (berry, mint, rooibos)
- Dates

COOKING WITH OILS

To get the most from plant oils look for the words 'natural', 'unrefined' and 'cold-pressed' on the label. Cold-pressed simply means that the nuts or seeds are first ground, then pressed to release the oil (think olive oil). And while they can be more expensive, they are well worth it. Many everyday cooking oils are treated with chemical solvents to enhance the oil – however, this can destroy some of the goodness. Oils are at their best when unheated, but some (including rapeseed and camelina oils) have a high smoking point and are safe to cook with.

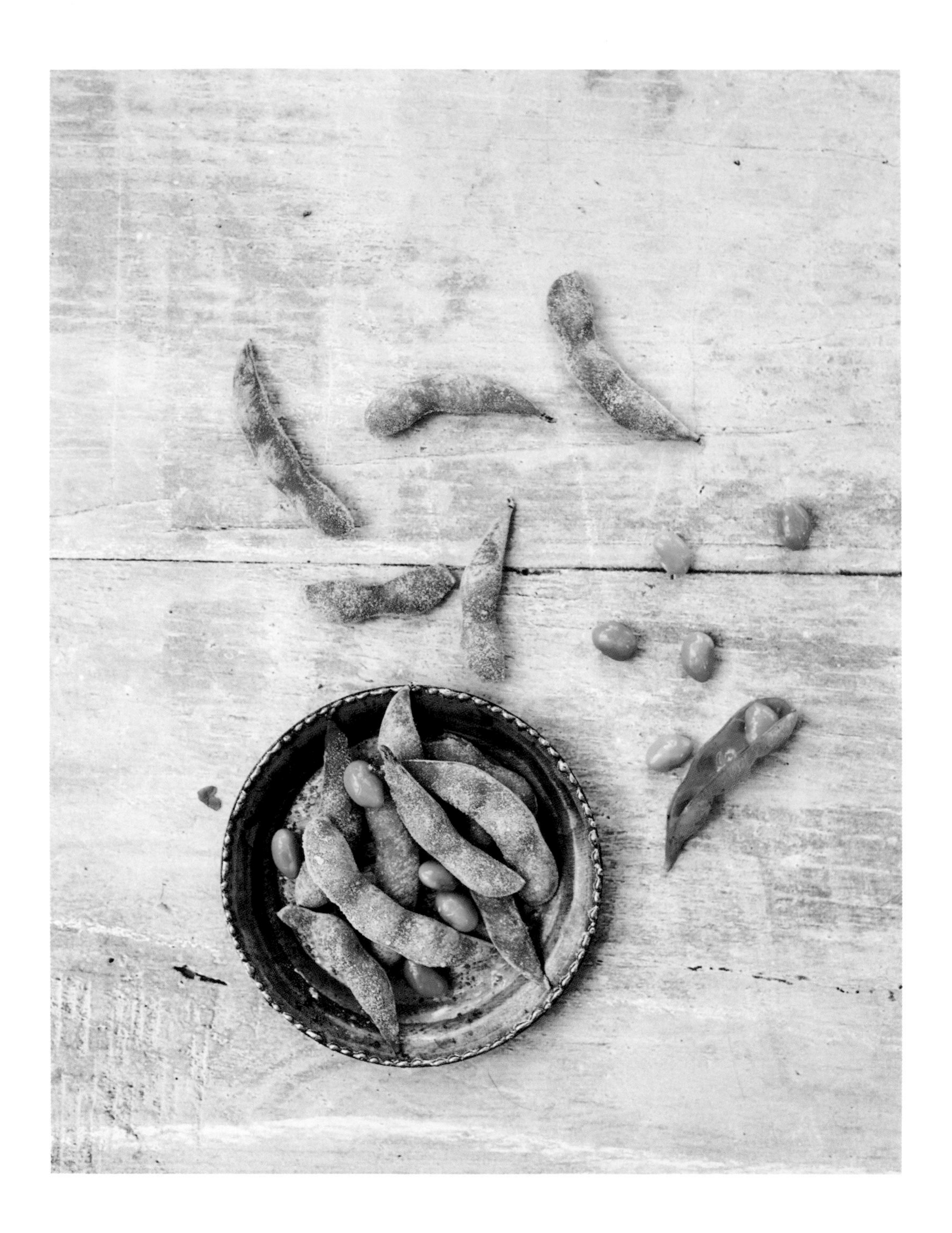

BETTER SKIN TIPS

◊

Applying the following tips to your daily life will keep your skin vibrant and healthy all year long, while also benefiting your general health. Trust me – your body will thank you!

EAT MOSTLY PLANTS

This idea is nothing new, but what *is* new is that research is now proving just how beneficial a plant-based diet is for your skin and your body. The majority of the recipes included here are plant-based, so get experimenting! The more plants you eat the happier and brighter you will feel.

MAKE YOUR MEALS AS COLOURFUL AS POSSIBLE

If your plate looks bland and boring, then it probably is! Spice it up with colour: think leafy green veggies and fruits; and spices like turmeric and cinnamon, for instance, will add colour, taste and a multitude of health benefits.

TUNE IN TO THE SEASONS

Nothing compares to the freshest seasonal foods eaten when they are at their most colourful and nutritious – and their tastiest. So follow the time-tested principles of Ayurveda by tuning in to the best time of year to eat your fruits (generally summer – keep frozen fruits in the freezer for winter time) and root vegetables. Once your body becomes attuned to the seasons, you will automatically reach for fresh, colourful, seasonal foods every time.

DON'T SKIP MEALS

Many people believe that missing meals will hasten weight loss, but numerous studies have shown that regularly missing meals can in fact be detrimental to health and does not promote weight loss. Eating regular meals ensures blood sugar levels are better controlled and can help keep hunger at bay. Lack of time is no excuse for missing meals. Many of the recipes included in this plan are quick and easy to prepare. If time is tight, then cook in bulk and freeze.

CHEW FOOD WELL

Food needs to be thoroughly chewed to stimulate digestive enzymes. Experts recommend thirty to forty chews per mouthful – yes, that sounds a lot, but by eating more mindfully and consciously, you will start to enjoy food more.

EAT MORE GOOD FATS

Think avocados, oily fish and nuts – overflowing with nourishment. The more of them you eat, the more your skin will glow. (If weight loss is your main objective, just eat slightly less of them.)

READ LABELS

Be more label savvy when food shopping – avoid packets with long, complex lists of ingredients and products containing suspect chemicals or sugar in its various guises (glucose, maltose, sucrose, fructose, corn syrup and so on) near the top of the ingredient list. You will soon learn to recognise what you should buy and what is best left on the shelf, thereby reducing the amount of processed, sugar-laden foods you are eating.

MEAT

Meat is one of the best sources of protein and iron we can eat. However, it is not included in this plan – primarily to give the liver a break. The focus of the plan is oily fish, eggs and generally plant-based foods.

If you are a regular meat eater then by all means enjoy it after the four weeks. But bear in mind that the quality and quantity of meat we buy and eat is important. Many studies highlight the dangers of regularly eating processed and cured meats, like bacon, sausages and ham. What's more, dietary recommendations for meat suggest limiting overall meat intake to about 70g a day – roughly one small steak or lamb chop. Most of us eat far more than this at a typical meal.

Choose the best quality organic, grass-fed meat you can afford and enjoy it every so often, rather than every day or every other day. Always buy from a trusted butcher. Cheap, mass-produced meat doesn't support animal welfare, nor does it taste as good. We should also consider the impact of greenhouse gas emissions from livestock on the environment.

Meat, while sometimes delicious, is not essential to our health. We can live equally well, and in many cases more healthily, on fish and the pure plant goodness outlined in this four-week plan.

CAFFEINE

Most of us enjoy the hit that our morning cup of freshly brewed coffee or caffeine-rich tea brings. However, if that hit becomes a necessity every couple of hours, then it needs to be reduced for the sake of your skin and health in general. Caffeine is a diuretic and dehydrates the body. It increases the load on the liver, which when over-burdened can result in a toxic build-up on the skin. The end result of this caffeine chain is a lacklustre, dehydrated and worn look.

Coffee or caffeine-rich tea are not included in this four-week plan so should be avoided for the duration. However, if the consequent withdrawal symptoms prove debilitating to the mind and body, then the occasional coffee that you truly look forward to can be relished; top up with herbal teas and water in between.

Start each day with a morning tonic of hot water, turmeric and lime (see page 107). This helps cleanse and prep the liver for the day ahead, while also kickstarting the brain into activity. For the remainder of the day drink teas, such as the GLOW teas and other caffeine-free herbal options (see recipes page 246).

EXERCISE

It is now pretty much a given that regular exercise can make an enormous difference to how you look and feel in and about yourself at every stage of life. With regular exercise everything improves – our skin, our hair, our heart, our brain and our memory. The hardest part is getting started. Whether it's running, yoga, walking, swimming or dancing, once exercise becomes a part of your life you will quickly feel the benefits. So find something that works for you and move yourself – every day.

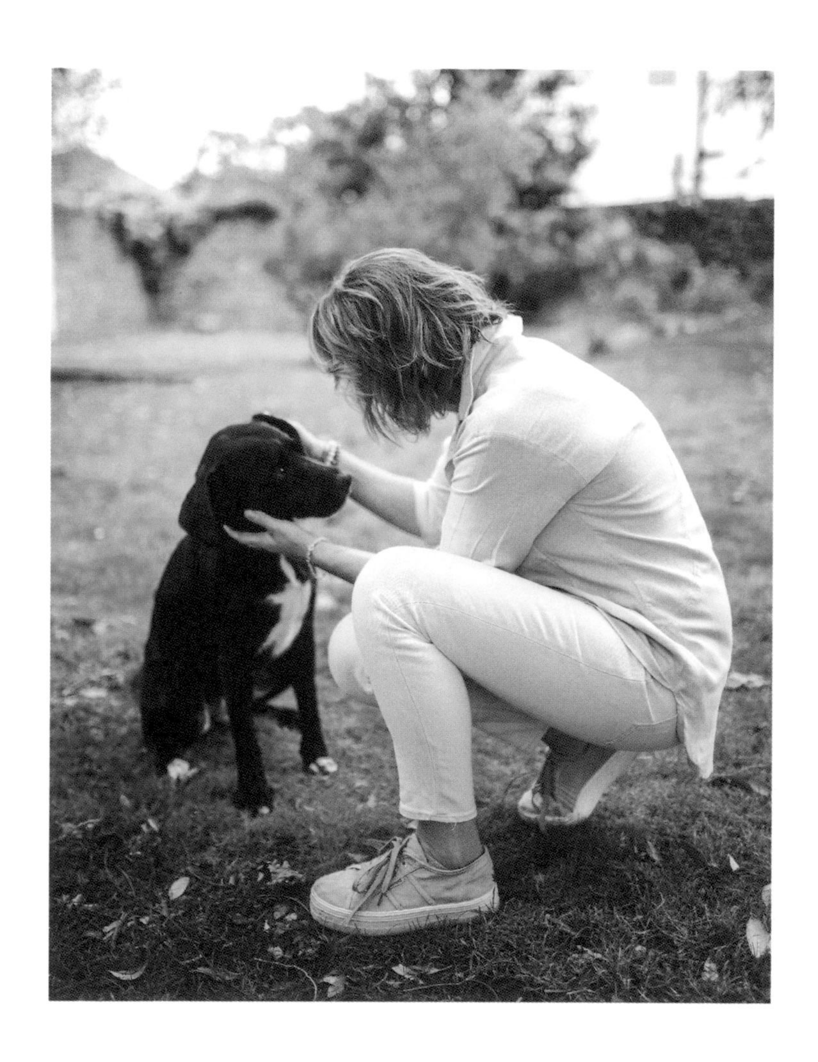

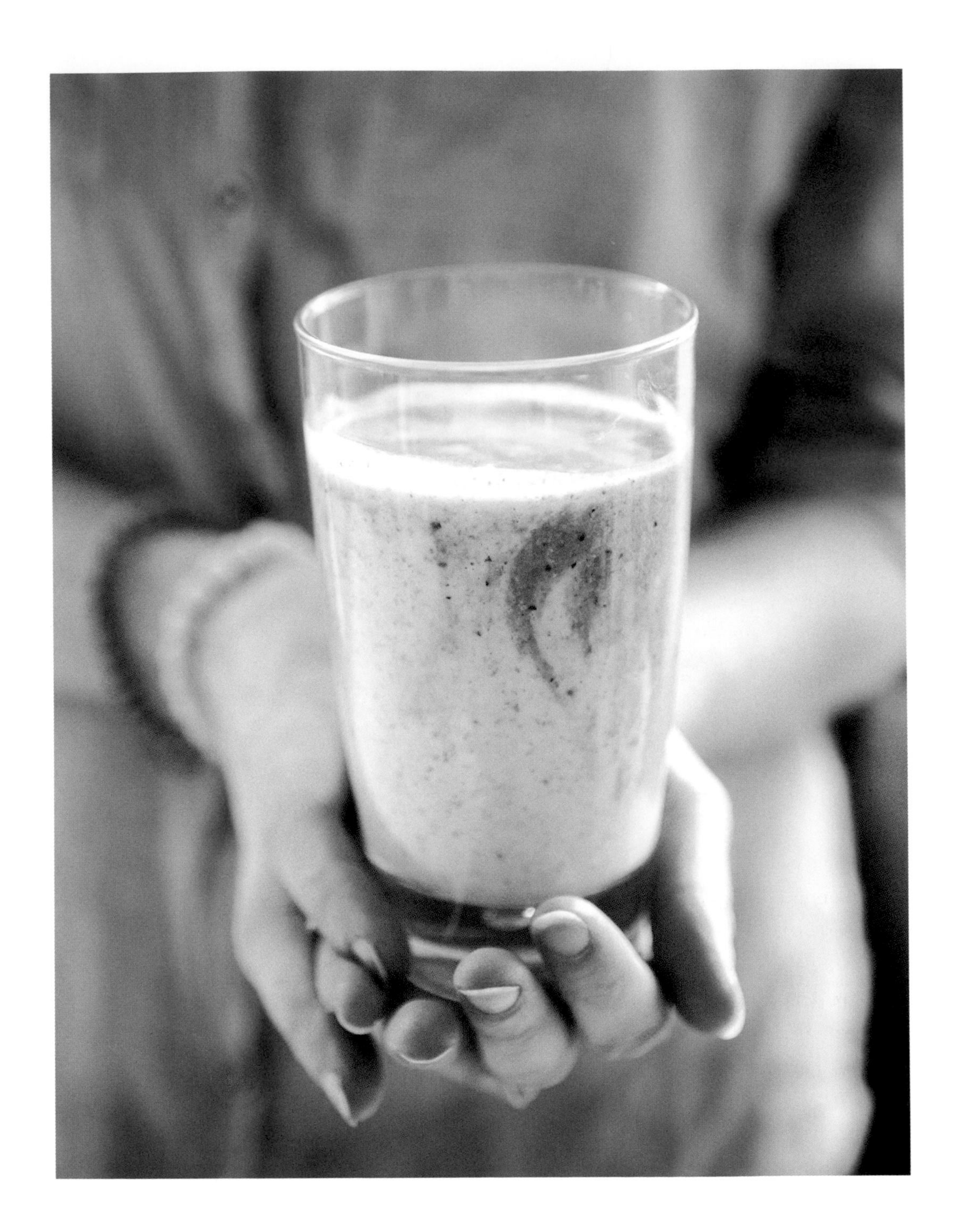

THE PLAN

◊

This four-week plan to better skin combines the best of skin-enhancing skincare with the tastiest, most nurturing recipes imaginable. Each week focuses on a different aspect of skincare, from cleansing and exfoliating to healing, nourishing/balancing and, ultimately, the GLOW, and combines simple tried and tested recipes for skin masks, scrubs and oils appropriate for the task in hand and designed to affect skin on the outside, with the extensive menu of GLOW foods, drinks, teas and other tips to cleanse, heal and nourish from within.

Most of the recipes are straightforward and easy to prepare, as for the majority of us time is tight. However, a couple require a little forward planning, so when time is limited during the week, use the weekend to stock up on essentials and prepare meals for the days to come. Most can be kept in the freezer. Remember, all GLOW foods and recipes will help repair and nourish the skin, so if you don't like, or don't have the ingredients for, a recommended recipe, there are suggested alternatives, or you can cook something else from the list. That said, certain foods are deliberately included during specific weeks as they work particularly well for that week's target – be it cleansing, healing or nourishing the skin. Seasons are considered too to make the most of the superior nutritional value and taste of foods when they are at their best, with choices of soups, salads and so on.

Encouraging variety is one of the main reasons I have included a detailed meal plan, as the more varied your food choices are, the more likely you are to get the complete spectrum of nutrients for your skin. It also lessens the risk of boredom!

If you are not normally a breakfast person, then you can try one of the quick, light and skin-nourishing smoothies, all topped with a handful of the super-nourishing GLOW Trail Mix, but breaking the fast (which is what breakfast literally means) is essential for both the skin and body as a whole, so it should not be missed. When time allows, make the most of the Shakshuka, Herby Edamame Omelette and Buckwheat Pancakes with Caramelised Banana Bites – they take longer to prepare but are worth the effort!

The Sweet Things are all deliciously sweet and satisfying. They can be eaten as snacks or made for special occasions. As many of them are quite filling, a small amount should be enough. If, however, you are doing a lot of exercise, your body may require extra fuel. A selection of dips and spreads are also included to encourage variety and for when healthy snacks are needed. For example, avocados are full of skin-nurturing goodness, so the Guacamole recipe on page 167 will be an added bonus at snack times – it tastes delicious too! The comprehensive menu of herbal teas will ensure there is something for every taste and time of year. They can be enjoyed whenever you choose during the plan and for always.

The recipes for facemasks and scrubs are relevant to specific weeks. These only take a few minutes to prepare, as long as the necessary ingredients are on hand. There is no obligation to make these, however, as there are plenty of great products on the market. But do ensure that the products you buy are packed with essential skin ingredients – think hyaluronic acid, vitamin C and so on (see What Skin Needs, pages 19–36) – and only buy a trusted brand.

All the foods and recipes included here are among the healthiest you will eat, but bear in mind that four weeks to better skin is *not* a guide to weight loss. For this reason, recipes have no calorie counts attached. This is deliberate, as when calorie counts are included focus immediately shifts to weight and often unnecessary guilt about the number of calories in a particular food or meal. Take avocados: they are among the most nourishing foods for our skin, as they are so rich in essential fats – but these same fats move the calorie counter up a gear! One of the key intentions of the plan is that the best of fresh, seasonal and local (where possible) produce will be savoured and enjoyed and that skin will thrive with the best fuel possible.

If you *are* trying to lose weight, four weeks to better skin is a great resource too, but pay attention to portion sizes, limit the amount of sweet things and, most important, move your body more. You will soon feel the benefits.

Remember, the more colourful your meals are the greater the chances that they are nurturing your skin, so eat plenty of berries, pomegranates, leafy green vegetables, vibrant pink oily fish and the rich yolks of fresh free-range eggs.

MORNING MANTRA

Take one minute every morning before rising to set your intentions for the day ahead – or to be grateful, even if times are quite stressful. Make your intentions positive, affirming and nourishing for the soul. Even if you think this is not for you, just try it – you might surprise yourself with how much better you feel when you do this daily.

TURMERIC TONIC

Mix half a fingernail-sized slice of grated fresh turmeric (or less than ½ tsp turmeric powder) with a pinch of black pepper and a slice fresh lime in a glass of warm water. Drink it first thing every morning. You will grow to love it, as I did!

WEEK ONE: CLEANSE

Cleanse and **exfoliate** are the key words for this week. Beauty experts are adamant that cleansing is the most important step in every effective skincare routine. It makes sense, too, as you wouldn't lather luxurious body oil over sweaty, grubby skin!

This is the week to dig deep and thoroughly remove all traces of our stress-inducing lifestyles. By combining simple and effective cleansing techniques with key foods that work to detoxify the liver and remove stagnant energy, your skin will once again be a blank canvas to be renewed and nourished.

ON THE OUTSIDE

CLEANSING OILS: lemon, lime, bitter orange, peppermint, tea tree, eucalyptus
USE WHENEVER YOU CAN: burn them as you work or read, mix with water and spritz onto your skin through the day or use in a bath in the evening.

THE FACE

Healthy skin sheds thousands of dead cells every day that are replaced by fresh, plump newbies. As the new cells move towards the surface of the skin they flatten and develop protective qualities that give them a two-way barrier function: they seal moisture into the skin and keep germs and toxins out. As healthy skin ages, the speed at which cells shed and renew starts to slow. Cell turnover allows the body to exfoliate naturally, and a slowing down of this process causes a build-up of dead skin cells on the surface, clogging pores and giving a dull, lacklustre texture to the skin – hence the need to deeply exfoliate to remove these cells and freshen the complexion. However, we now know that one of the main causes of dehydrated and damaged skin is over-zealous exfoliation, where skin is left thin and fragile with the outer protective skin barrier scrubbed to nothing. So the rule of thumb is to be gentle when scrubbing and to avoid harsh ingredients.

This is the week for a deep, deep cleanse – use the scrub detailed below and enjoy a deep exfoliating facial with a trusted expert. Choose a product that works for you and is not too aggressive. For example, if your skin is hormonally aggravated choose a creamy or oily product that is gentler on the skin, and if you experience redness or severe dryness stop immediately.

Herbal Steam

Steaming is great way of opening skin pores and loosening impacted dead cells and blackheads. It is especially effective on oily skin and great before applying a scrub or mask. Eucalyptus or tea tree oil both help decongest the lungs and chest area too. All you need is a bowl, essential oils, a towel and hot water.

Tie your hair back from your face or wear a shower cap. Double cleanse the skin using a cotton cloth and cleansing products. Fill a large(ish) bowl with hot water. Add a few drops of essential oil – lavender with chamomile and one drop of tea tree (normal skin), or lavender with mint (oily/combination skin), or lavender with rose (sensitive skin) – and stir quickly. Put a towel over your head, close your eyes and lean your head over the bowl so the steam can permeate – but not too close to the steam, as your face may burn. Breathe deeply through the mouth and move your head until the whole face is exposed to the steam. Keep breathing for up to two minutes or for as long as you can tolerate it. Lift head and remove towel. Spritz your face with cooling toner or flower water.

BODY STEAMING

If you have access to a steam room in a local gym or club, now is the time to reap the benefits. Each session in a steam room should be quickly followed by a cold shower or a plunge in cold water to close the skin pores.

Quick Skin Fix: Oatmeal Mask for Oily Skin

For a simple brightening and moisturising mask, just mix one heaped tablespoon of thick organic natural yoghurt with one tablespoon of finely ground oatmeal. Add a few drops of warmed honey (warm spoon under hot water and add honey to warmed spoon) and stir well. If the mask is too runny, add a little extra oatmeal to thicken. Cleanse and tone the face. Deeply massage the mask over the face and leave in place for up to twenty minutes. Rinse off with warm water and apply pure natural face oil or moisturiser to hydrate. Apply this mask about three times this week, then one to two times per week, or as required, to balance oiliness.

EXPERT INPUT

Alexandra Soveral

Alexandra Soveral has been my go-to facialist in London for many years now. I trust her implicitly and both her therapies and her products are wonderful.

'I have been using honey in my facials in a rather unique way for many years. I blend honey with vitamins and plant extracts to enhance its anti-inflammatory benefits, but at home plain honey works too! When removing the honey, I developed a technique that helps lift the underlying facial tissues to improve detoxification and move stagnant lymph. We must protect our acid mantle from being destroyed – it's our first line of defence against pollution and pathogens. Honey is wonderful, as when lifted off the skin, it only removes what is ready to be removed, while also calming and nourishing the skin.'

Alexandra Soveral's Honey Cleanse

- Apply a thin layer of thick honey all over a damp face, as you would a mask. Leave it on for ten minutes to nourish the skin.
- With four fingers together, press onto the skin and lift off by lifting from the index to the little finger. Continue to do these quick movements all over the face. Use a stronger lifting technique around the T-Zone and be gentler over the rest of the face where the skin is more fragile.
- If it gets too sticky and starts to hurt while lifting, wet a finger to add a little water. Work through the whole face including the glands behind the ears to ensure the lymph is being drained. Once you practise you will get to grips with the technique.
- When the skin feels alive and stimulated the mask can be removed by placing a damp, hot face cloth over the face to create a little steam that will efficiently remove all the honey and dead skin cells.
- Skin should feel squeaky clean, but if you want to go one step further now is the perfect time for a deep pore cleanse, as the pores are open and the outer layer of dead cells is removed.
- Simply massage Soveral Angel Balm (or other natural balm) onto the skin and the fats in the balm will blend with the sebum in the pores and the geranium in the balm will help balance the skin's sebaceous glands. Once the balm is removed with another hot, damp flannel, the skin will be even cleaner.
- This treatment should be performed weekly for those with dry, flaky or congested skin, and every two weeks for normal skin types.

TIP: Alexandra Soveral uses organic rose water made from the steam distillation of rose petals as a cleanser, toner, eye wash (diluted) and compress to reduce thread veins and to cool inflammation in the body.

Face Massage

Those who appreciate the benefits of massage will know how powerful the technique can be for relieving tension and easing both body and mind. This centuries-old panacea remains as popular as ever, but it is only recently that the Western world is waking up to its benefits in

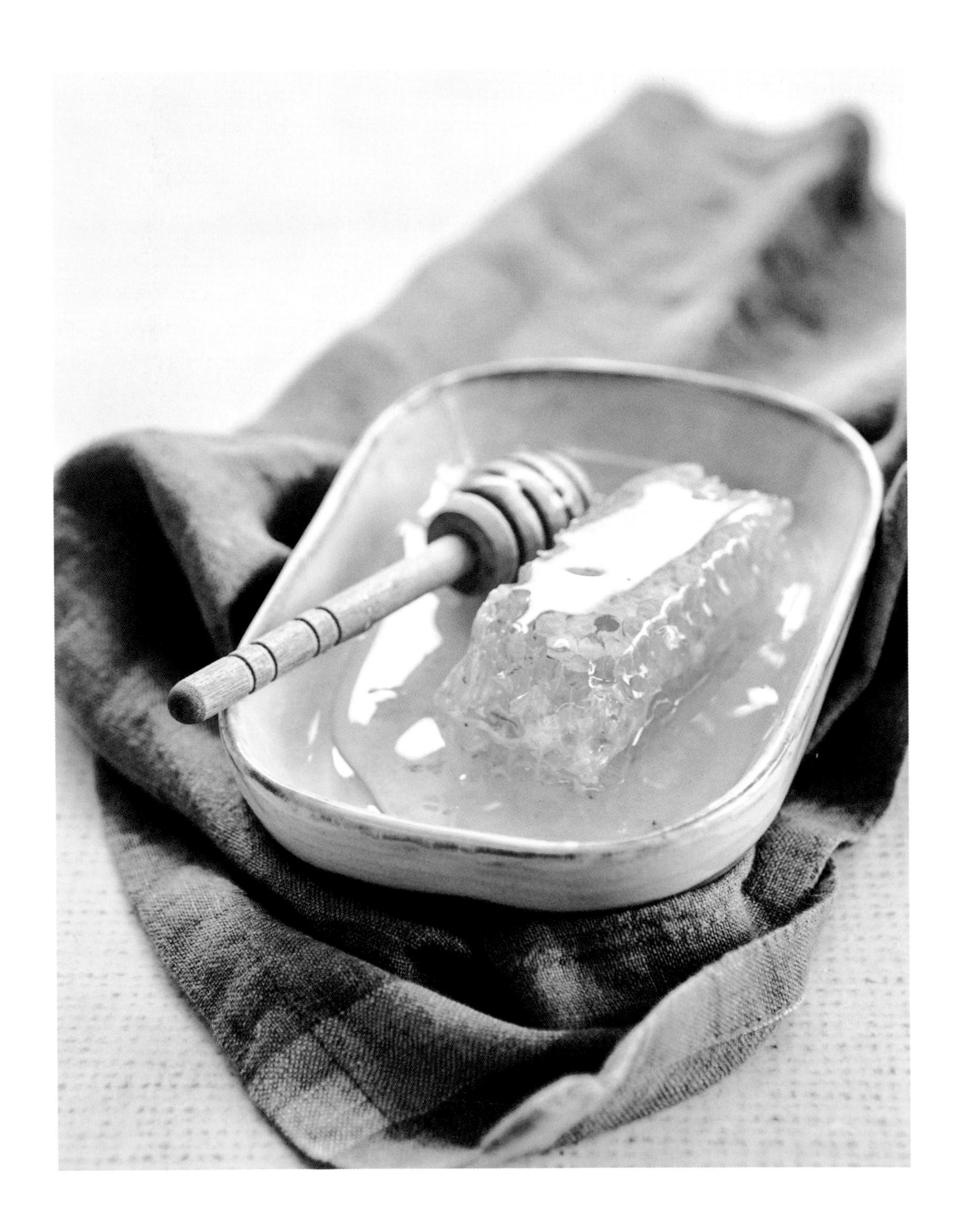

tightening, toning and rejuvenating the face and neck. Just as an active, fit body looks healthy and invigorated, a skilled facialist will use massage to stimulate blood circulation and bring facial muscles to life.

What's more, massaging products into the skin helps work them deeper, while a more gentle massage around the delicate eye area helps drain lymph and de-puff the eye contour. As well as seeking out a skilled therapist, why not become your own facialist? Try the GLOW Face Blend (page 135), massaging the blend deep into the skin around the face and neck, with more gentle movement around the eye area. And remember, as with every effective gym workout, the more you put in, the more you gain and the more vibrant your skin will be.

THE BODY

Body Brushing

Body brushing is an easy and effective way to remove waste products built up on the skin. It's a perfect cleansing tool that exfoliates the skin, boosts blood and lymphatic flow through the body and helps manage the appearance of cellulite. It is best done first thing in the morning before stepping into the shower. All you need is a body brush and a few minutes. The most effective body brushes are those made from cactus bristle: firm enough to create friction, yet gentle enough not to scratch skin. Long-handled brushes can reach all body parts.

Brush dry skin (before showering) in an upward direction towards the heart – from feet (including soles) to knees (behind knees too, where there is a density of lymph), over thighs, hips and buttocks, to the arms, underarms and shoulders. Do not scrub skin with the brush, but maintain steady, long, swift strokes of the bristles. The benefits are immediate and lasting.

Exfoliating Scrubs

When applied correctly (as per the body brushing technique above) exfoliating body scrubs help remove dead skin cells to leave the skin smooth and soft. The best scrubs are those containing natural granules like sea salt that cleanse and invigorate the system. There are many on the market, but always choose natural. And they can be homemade too!

Quick Skin Fix: Cleansing Body Scrub

For a simple and effective body scrub, all you need are a few spoons of an organic carrier oil (e.g. sweet almond, pure olive or coconut oil), a few drops of a trusted essential oil and an abrasive ingredient (e.g. sea salt or sugar). The following recipe can be used as a guide to experiment with until you find what works best for you and your skin. Remember, this is a body scrub and too harsh for the sensitive skin on the face.

- 3 tbsp sea salt
- 1 tbsp sweet almond or pure olive oil
- 4–5 drops lemon, lime, lavender or sweet apricot essential oil – or a blend

Mix ingredients in a bowl. Massage gently into skin using a slow circular motion. Rinse thoroughly in warm water.

You can adjust this basic recipe as desired. It will last a few weeks, so it can be prepared in a larger quantity, stored in a glass jar with secure lid and kept in a dark place to protect the precious essential oils.

Cellulite

Cellulite is essentially congestion in the fat cells in certain parts of the body, including the buttocks, thighs, back of the arms and upper and lower back. Although much medical uncertainty exists about its actual cause, it is widely accepted that poor circulation, inadequate diet, lack of exercise and genetics all play a role. It is thought to be less of a problem in men, due to their more muscular build and body fat distribution. Other factors including weight change, stress and smoking, and age-related tissue weakening can exacerbate the problem.

Unfortunately most topical cosmetic creams will rarely, if ever, show long-term benefits in helping relieve the appearance of cellulite as, despite what manufacturers say, they just don't penetrate deeply enough. More invasive treatments carried out by a medical doctor or skilled therapist can temporarily improve the appearance of cellulite, but only in a fraction of people treated.

Realistically, cellulite bumps are rarely noticed by others, and by taking a few minutes to body brush every day, by moving more and paying more attention to when and what you eat, cellulite can be kept under control.

ON THE INSIDE

This meal plan has been formulated to help cleanse and flush the body from within. If, however, you don't like a particular food or find it hard to get, then feel free to swap for another recipe or meal, as every recipe in this plan is skin friendly. However, some foods are richer in particular nutrients and more suited to specific weeks of the plan.

LIVER CLEANSE

The liver is the body's ultimate detox organ and works incessantly to cleanse the body of waste matter. Now is the time to give your liver the break it so desperately needs. The foods, juices and cleansing teas outlined this week will help to repair and support the liver, leaving it ripe for some deep nourishment later in the plan.

Liver-Supporting Herbs

MILK THISTLE

Also known as silymarin, milk thistle hails from Europe and North America. It has a great affinity for the liver and has been used for many years by herbalists. The leaves exude a milky sap when crushed or broken – hence the name. It is available dried and in tincture and capsule form. It is a widely used hangover remedy.

ARTICHOKE

Artichokes are a natural liver support and can be eaten as a food or as an extract of the leaves, stems and roots. They are part of the daisy family (Asteraceae), and are rich in antioxidants and vitamins.

NETTLE

The analgesic and anti-inflammatory properties of the stinging nettle (*Urtica dioica*) can help relieve symptoms of acne and skin irritation. They are widely available to pick in many parts of the world – but beware of the stings (see page 247).

DANDELION

A powerful healer, dandelion is available as a dried herb, a tincture and in capsule form. When gathering dandelions, choose tender young leaves and avoid busy roads and other polluted areas.

KEY FOODS

Every GLOW food is good but the following work a little harder and deeper to cleanse from within and so are especially helpful this week:

- Apple cider vinegar (ACV)
- Beetroot
- Celery
- Oats
- Oranges, lemons and limes
- Pomegranate
- Seaweed
- Seeds
- Spinach and all dark green leafy vegetables

CLEANSING JUICES

Earthy Goodness *or* Zesty Cleanser (see page 242)

CLEANSING TEAS

Lemongrass, Ginger and Mint *and* Nettle and Ginger (see page 247); Kombucha (see page 257)

WEEKLY CLEANSE PLAN

EVERY DAY

- Cleansing teas
- Cleansing juice
- Turmeric Tonic (see page 107)
- 1 tbsp ACV on its own or mixed in warm water
- GLOW Trail Mix

MONDAY

BREAKFAST

Oaty Breakfast Bars (page 149) **OR** Oaty Banana Smoothie (page 150)

LUNCH/LIGHT MEAL

Spinach and Broccoli Soup with Flaked Almonds (page 181) **OR** Quinoa, Pomegranate and Feta Salad (page 184)

MAIN MEAL

Shepherdless Pie (page 202) **OR** salmon/oily fish – one of three ways (pages 205-8)

TUESDAY

BREAKFAST

Maya's Granola (page 145) **OR** Shakshuka (page 163)

LUNCH/LIGHT MEAL

Quick Miso Broth with Edamame (page 178) **OR** Orange, Walnut and Quinoa Salad (page 186)

MAIN MEAL

Cannellini Bean Salad with Marinated Alaria (page 192) **OR** Sweet Potato, Pea and Courgette Cakes (page 197) with Mango, Pomegranate and Cucumber Salsa (page 171)

WEDNESDAY

BREAKFAST

GLOW Banana Bread (page 152) **OR** Oaty Breakfast Bars (page 149)

LUNCH/LIGHT MEAL

Spinach and Broccoli Soup with Flaked Almonds (page 181) **OR** Beetroot, Edamame and Orange Salad (page 188)

MAIN MEAL

Salmon – one of three ways (page 205–8) **OR** Cannellini Bean Salad with Marinated Alaria (page 192)

THURSDAY

BREAKFAST

Overnight Oats with Seasonal Berries (page 146) **OR** Salted Caramel Smoothie Bowl (page 155)

LUNCH/LIGHT MEAL

Quick Miso Broth with Edamame (page 178) **OR** Avocado on Toast – one of three ways (page 158)

MAIN MEAL

Salmon/oily fish – one of three ways (pages 205-8) **OR** Warming Squash, Red Pepper and Chickpea Curry Bowl (page 218) **OR** other seasonal bowl of choice

FRIDAY

BREAKFAST

Oaty Breakfast Bars (page 149) **OR** Herby Edamame Omelette (page 143)

LUNCH/LIGHT MEAL

Beetroot, Edamame and Orange Salad (page 188) **OR** GLOW Frittata (page 195)

MAIN MEAL

Root Veggie Bowl (page 217) **OR** seasonal bowl of choice **OR** Cannellini Bean Salad with Marinated Alaria (page 192)

SATURDAY

BREAKFAST

Shakshuka (page 163) **OR** Avocado on Toast – one of three ways (page 158)

LUNCH/LIGHT MEAL

Orange, Walnut and Quinoa Salad (page 186) **OR** GLOW Frittata (page 195)

MAIN MEAL

Salmon/oily fish – one of three ways (pages 205-8) **OR** Sweet Potato, Pea and Courgette Cakes (page 197)

SUNDAY

BREAKFAST

Overnight Oats with Seasonal Berries (page 146) **OR** GLOW Banana Bread (page 152)

LUNCH/LIGHT MEAL

Quick Miso Broth with Edamame (page 178) **OR** Orange, Walnut and Quinoa Salad (page 186)

MAIN MEAL

Broccolini Risotto (page 198) **OR** Salmon/oily fish – one of three ways (pages 205-8)

KEY POINTS WEEK 1: CLEANSE ACTION

- Morning mantra
- ACV shot
- Cleanse oils
- Daily body brush before showering
- Daily body scrub while showering
- Facial steaming
- Facial cleansing mask
- Cleanse body steam
- Cleanse foods, teas and juices
- Turmeric Tonic
- GLOW Trail Mix

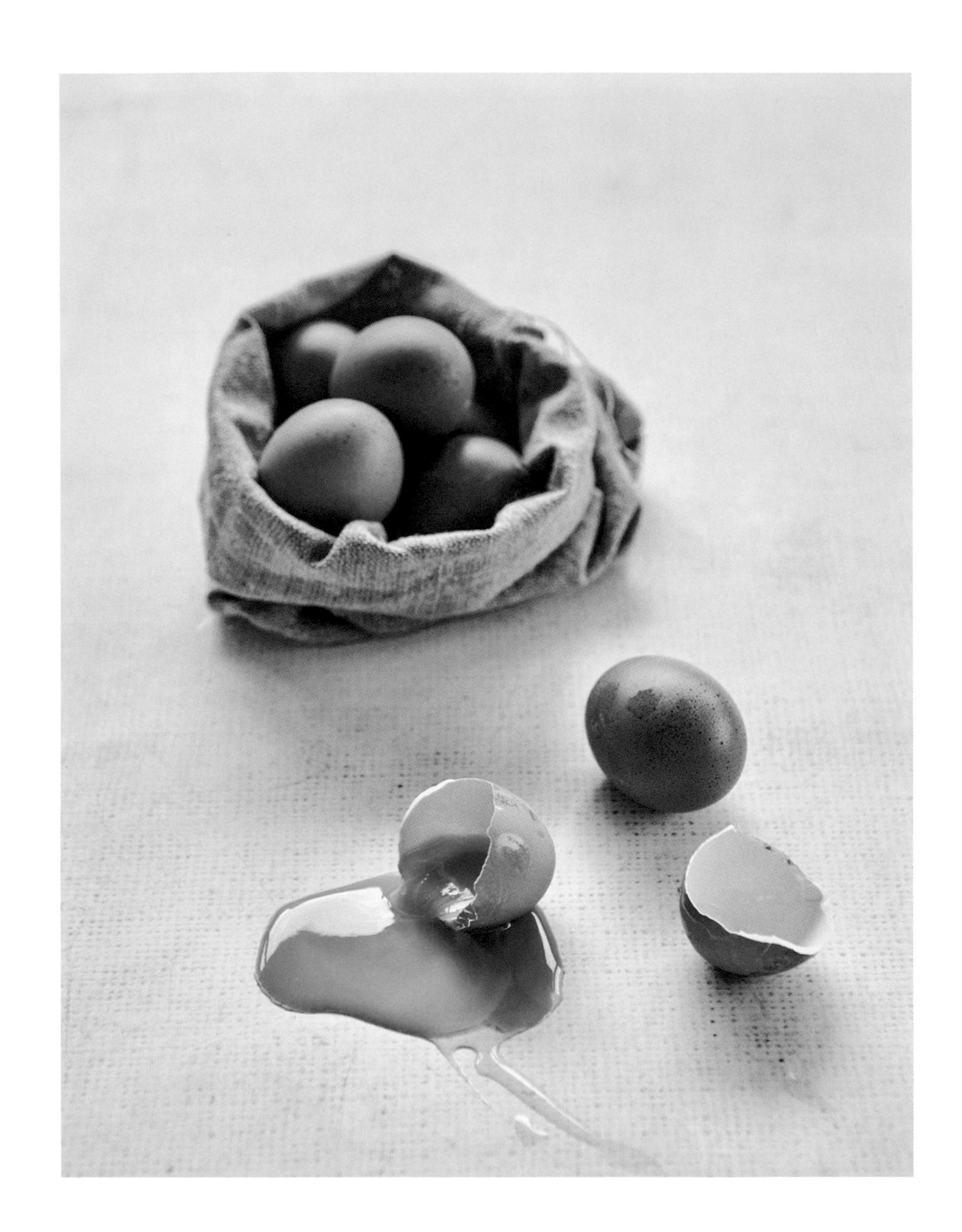

WEEK TWO: HEAL

Heal and **balance** are the key words this week, with the aim of soothing and repairing troubled skin, calming inflammation and rebalancing to leave skin ripe and ready for intense nourishment. With that in mind, this week combines fresh, colourful anti-inflammatory fruits and vegetables, unrefined grains, nuts, seeds and fermented foods with herbal healers and proven skin remedies designed to soothe and rebalance from within.

Skin can flare up at any time but most especially during the hormonal fluctuations of teenage and middle years and during periods of stress. We now know that what we eat largely dictates how well our body feels, looks and operates, so our skin, being the visible us to the greater world, really tells it all – and it can also be the first to heal when given the best healing ingredients.

Balance is key when treating sensitive and inflamed skin, both in terms of what we eat and what we apply to it. If your skin is acting up then treat it kindly – don't over-exfoliate in the belief that the harder you work the quicker the aggravation will disappear. It will get worse! Instead use a gentle foaming or pure, natural oil-based cleanser (remembering that less is more).

Be very careful with the products you use, as they may be too harsh during this very sensitive time. Avoid highly fragranced skincare and any products packed with a list of added extras, most especially sodium lauryl/laureth sulphate (SLS), as these can exacerbate eczema and other irritations. In other words, the purer and simpler the better.

Keep your hands away from your face (except when applying skincare, obviously!) and don't spray perfume directly onto your skin – spray through your hair or on your clothes or, even better, through your scarf if you wear one.

If you are concerned about the health of your skin, it is advisable to speak with a dermatologist or other skin specialist with experience in this area.

ON THE OUTSIDE

HEALING OILS: Argan, borage seed (starflower), chamomile, evening primrose, geranium, lavender, tea tree, ylang-ylang
USE WHENEVER YOU CAN: burn them as you work or read, mix with water and spritz onto your skin through the day or use in a bath in the evening.

THE FACE

Skin Quick Fix: Calming Lavender Mist

- 150ml water
- 5–6 drops lavender essential oil (preferably organic)
- 1 drop witch hazel (if handy)

Combine ingredients in a bottle with a spray head. Mist after cleansing and whenever skin needs a little love. Keep in a cool(ish) place for up to three months.

Skin Quick Fix: Healing Turmeric Face Mask

This mask taps into turmeric's anti-bacterial and anti-inflammatory powers to relieve skin inflammation and irritation. Oatmeal is an excellent exfoliant so this mask is great for treating acne, as it absorbs excess oils and prevents clogging.

- ½ tsp ground turmeric
- 1 tbsp oatmeal (oats can also be used but it's best to grind them into a flour as it's easier to apply)
- 2–3 drops healing oils (see above)
- 1 tbsp milk

Blend ingredients together and apply all over the face. Massage into the skin and leave in place for twenty minutes or longer before washing off with warm water and a muslin cloth or flannel. If skin feels dry, some evening primrose or starflower oil applied to damp skin (use capsules if easier – simply pierce them and apply contents) will instantly hydrate and nourish.

Rosacea

Rosacea is an aggravating skin condition that causes the face to flush and turn red in patches. While the exact cause remains unknown, key triggers are believed to include hot sun, alcohol (especially wine), spicy foods, stress and strenuous exercise. Try to identify triggers and where possible:

- Use a broad-spectrum, mineral-based sunscreen (SPF 30+)
- Avoid saunas and steam rooms
- Don't exfoliate if skin is already irritated, as this may exacerbate the condition
- Eat plenty of calming anti-inflammatory foods and juices – as outlined in this week's healing plan
- Drink plenty of water (1.5 litres per day)
- Try green tea and probiotic supplements
- If the condition persists, consult your dermatologist

THE EYES

The eyes are the most delicate and expressive part of the face and the skin around the eyes is thin and needs to be treated extra carefully. Our always-on lifestyle of computers, lack of sleep, sun exposure, smoke and environmental aggressors can leave the eyes tired, dull and lifeless.

There is an extensive range of specially formulated eye creams and gels on the market, but they can be expensive and many of them are not worthwhile. Often all that is needed is a natural, gentle and nourishing facial or targeted eye oil, applied gently, to bring some fresh vitality to the eyes. If you are buying eye creams or gels shop around to find a product that works for you – one that isn't too heavy (as this can lead to puffy bags) and one that works well under make-up, without pilling.

Always tread lightly by using a gentle circular motion (using the third finger of each hand), starting at the outer eye socket, working under the eye towards the nose (following the line of the socket) and then over the lid (at the base of the eyebrow). Rest the eyes whenever possible too – all the more reason to sleep longer and deeper!

Skin-nourishing foods will also help keep the eye area hydrated and clear, while protective sunglasses will block damaging UV light – even on cloudy days.

Eye Quick Fixes

- To refresh and reduce puffiness: splash iced water over the eyes as many times as possible before patting dry.
- To calm and soothe tired eyes: place cold used tea bags (chamomile is great) over the eyes and leave in place for up to ten minutes.
- To refresh and brighten the eyes: put some very finely chopped cucumber into two muslin cloths and place one over each eye. Relax for at least ten minutes (the longer the better) to let the goodness penetrate.

THE BODY

Seaweed scrubs are renowned for soothing and calming irritated skin. There are many products on the market at various price points, but always choose a more natural, organic brand from a reputable company. You can also add seaweed from a trusted source to a warm bath and feel the oils infuse into thirsty, irritated skin.

A warm bath infused with a few drops of healing essential oils will also instantly soothe and calm the skin while also promoting restful sleep.

Other healing bathing options include:

- **EPSOM SALTS:** rich in magnesium to help relieve body aches and soothe irritated skin. For best results use at least 2 cups of Epsom salts per bath and soak for up to twenty minutes.
- **OATMEAL:** Whizz a cup of oats to a fine powder and put into a small muslin bag. Add to a running bath with a few drops of healing essential oils. Soak for fifteen minutes or more.

ON THE INSIDE

The focus this week is on the healing benefits of a healthy balance of oily fish, eggs, plant proteins, vegetables, fruits, nuts, spices, seeds and fermented foods. As with every week of the plan, refined sugars and processed foods should be avoided.

KEY FOODS

- Apple cider vinegar (ACV)
- Avocados
- Blueberries
- Dark chocolate
- Edamame beans
- Eggs
- Fermented foods (e.g kombucha)
- Oily fish
- Pomegranates
- Seaweed
- Seeds
- Tomatoes
- Turmeric

HEALING JUICES

Skin Soother *or* Intense C (page 243); Kombucha (page 257)

HEALING TEAS

Lavender and Rosemary *and* Fennel and Mint (pages 248)

WEEKLY HEAL PLAN

EVERY DAY

- Healing teas
- Healing juice
- Turmeric Tonic
- 1 tbsp ACV on its own or mixed in warm water
- GLOW Trail Mix

MONDAY

BREAKFAST

Buckwheat Pancakes with Caramelised Banana Bites (page 160) **OR** Oaty Banana Smoothie (page 150)

LUNCH/LIGHT MEAL

Courgette and Almond Soup (page 177) **OR** Orange, Walnut and Quinoa Salad (page 186)

MAIN MEAL

Sautéed Spinach with Edamame served with short grain brown rice (page 189) **OR** Shepheardless Pie (page 202)

TUESDAY

BREAKFAST

Avocado on toast – one of three ways (page 158) **OR** GLOW Banana Bread (page 152)

LUNCH/LIGHT MEAL

Creamy Squash and Red Pepper Soup (page 174) **OR** Minted Farro and Three Bean Salad with Goat's Cheese (page 191)

MAIN MEAL

Salmon/oily fish – one of three ways (pages 205-8) **OR** Shepherdless Pie (page 202)

WEDNESDAY

BREAKFAST

Buckwheat Pancakes with Caramelised Banana Bites (page 160) **OR** Summer Surprise Smoothie (page 156)

LUNCH/LIGHT MEAL

Spinach and Broccoli Soup with Flaked Almonds (page 181) **OR** Avocado on Toast – one of three ways (page 158)

MAIN MEAL

Salmon – one of three ways (pages 205-8) **OR** Broccolini Risotto (page 198)

THURSDAY

BREAKFAST

Avocado on Toast – one of three ways (page 158) **OR** GLOW Banana Bread (page 152)

LUNCH/LIGHT MEAL

Quinoa, Pomegranate and Feta Salad (page 184) **OR** GLOW Frittata (page 195) with Beetroot, Edamame and Orange Salad (page 188)

MAIN MEAL

Cannellini Bean Salad with Marinated Alaria (page 192) **OR** Seasonal Bowl of choice (pages 210-19)

FRIDAY

BREAKFAST

Overnight Oats with Seasonal Berries (page 146) **OR** Maya's Granola (page 145)

LUNCH/LIGHT MEAL

Quick Miso Broth with Edamame (page 178) **OR** Orange, Walnut and Quinoa Salad (page 186)

MAIN MEAL

Salmon/oily fish – one of three ways (pages 205-8) **OR** Broccolini Risotto (page 198)

SATURDAY

BREAKFAST

Shakshuka (page 163) **OR** Salted Caramel Smoothie Bowl (page 155)

LUNCH/LIGHT MEAL

Quinoa, Pomegranate and Feta Salad (page 184) **OR** Spinach and Broccoli Soup with Flaked Almonds (page 181)

MAIN MEAL

Nachos with a Twist (page 200) **OR** Sweet Potato, Pea and Courgette Cakes (page 197) with salad or grain of your choice

SUNDAY

BREAKFAST

Herby Edamame Omelette (page 143) **OR** Avocado on Toast – one of three ways (page 158)

LUNCH/LIGHT MEAL

Nachos with a Twist (page 200) **OR** Minted Farro and Three Bean Salad with Goat's Cheese (page 191)

MAIN MEAL

Warming Squash, Red Pepper and Chickpea Curry Bowl (page 218) **OR** other Seasonal Bowl of choice

KEY POINTS WEEK 2: HEAL ACTION

- Morning mantra
- ACV shot
- Heal oils
- Body brush before shower
- Calming Lavender Mist
- Healing turmeric face mask 2–3 times
- Healing foods, teas and juices
- Turmeric Tonic
- GLOW Trail Mix
- Fermented foods

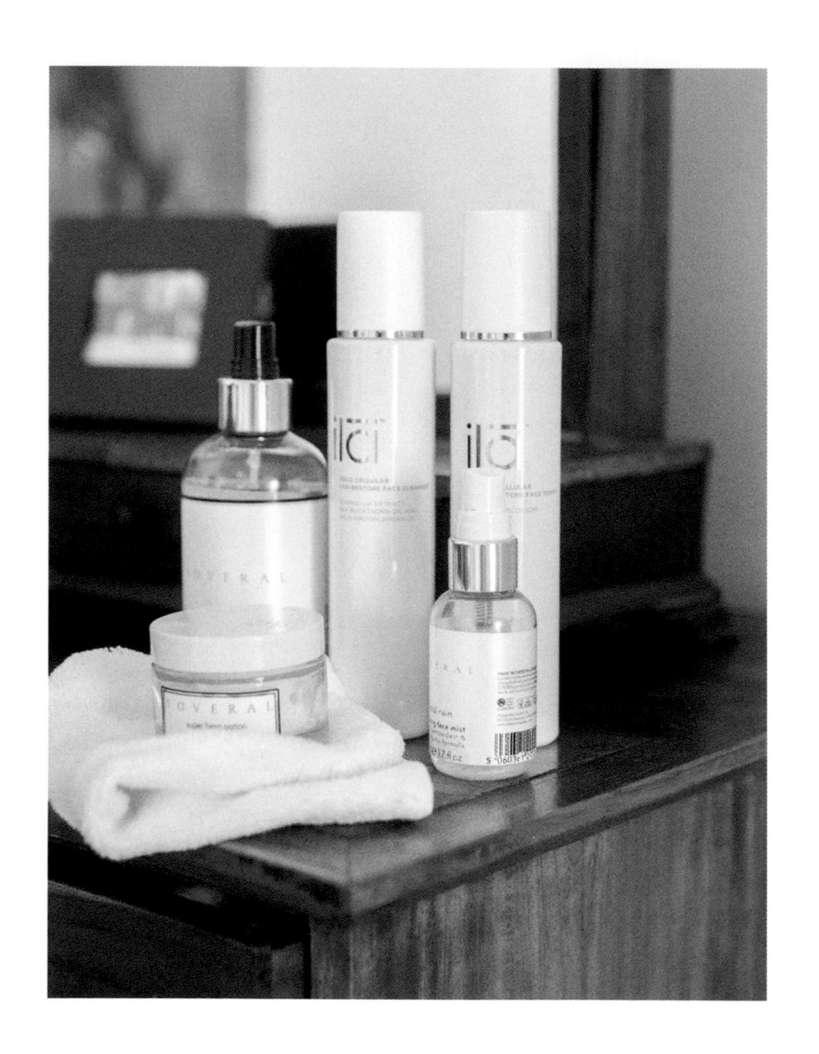

WEEK THREE: NOURISH

Nourish and **protect** are this week's key words, with the objective being to feed the skin from within with a nurturing combination of richly wholesome foods (think oily fish, nuts, seeds, avocados, vegetables and natural grains), skin oils and facial therapies that guarantee the optimum fuel inside and out.

ON THE OUTSIDE

NOURISHING OILS

Argan, avocado, borage seed, evening primrose, rose, rosehip

USE WHENEVER YOU CAN: burn them as you work or read, mix with water and spritz onto your skin through the day or use in a bath in the evening.

THE FACE

Ensuring the skin gets adequate moisture through the day and night is essential to stop the drying effects of sun, wind, central heating, air conditioning and so on taking their toll.

Skin Quick Fix: Nourishing Facial Scrub

- 3 tbsp (45g) approx. carrier oil (sweet almond or pure olive)
- 2–3 drops rose and/or rosehip essential oil
- 1 tbsp sea salt

Mix ingredients together. Massage gently over the skin, avoiding the eye area, for up to five minutes. Leave in place for another ten minutes, or as long as possible, before rinsing off with warm water and a flannel or muslin. Follow this with a generous smothering of nourishing facial oil that will work overnight to deeply restore the skin.

Skin Quick Fix: Nourishing Avocado Mess

- 1 ripe avocado, mashed
- 1 tsp natural yoghurt
- 1 tsp olive oil
- 1 tsp honey (the more natural the better)
- 2 drops rose or rosehip essential oil

Mix ingredients together and massage gently over the face, avoiding the eye area, for two to three minutes (or longer). Leave in place for another fifteen minutes, or as long as possible, before rinsing off with warm water and a muslin or flannel.

HAIR

Our hair is delicate and should be treated gently by avoiding harsh chemicals and by not brushing or pulling too hard. As the body ages hair starts to become finer and more brittle. Hair loss is an added problem too – often the result of years of dieting, prolonged periods of stress, reduced iron levels or certain diseases and medications.

There are numerous hair-restoring products and therapies on the market, but to ensure hair follicles are sufficiently nourished, the best advice is to surround them with a rich supply of blood through a nutritious, protein-rich diet.

Hair Loss

Healthy hair follicles typically go through a lifecycle with three different phases every six years or thereabouts: the growing (anagen) phase, the resting (catagen) phase and the shedding (telogen) phase.

While the average person typically sheds about fifty to a hundred hairs per day, research is showing that an increasing number of women are experiencing hair thinning by their early forties, primarily due to stress and fluctuating hormones. Androgenetic alopecia, more commonly termed 'female pattern hair loss', is often the result of changes in hormone levels, primarily the male androgen hormones. It can be triggered by a range of factors including pregnancy, menopause and ageing. Telogen effluvium is the term used to describe stress-

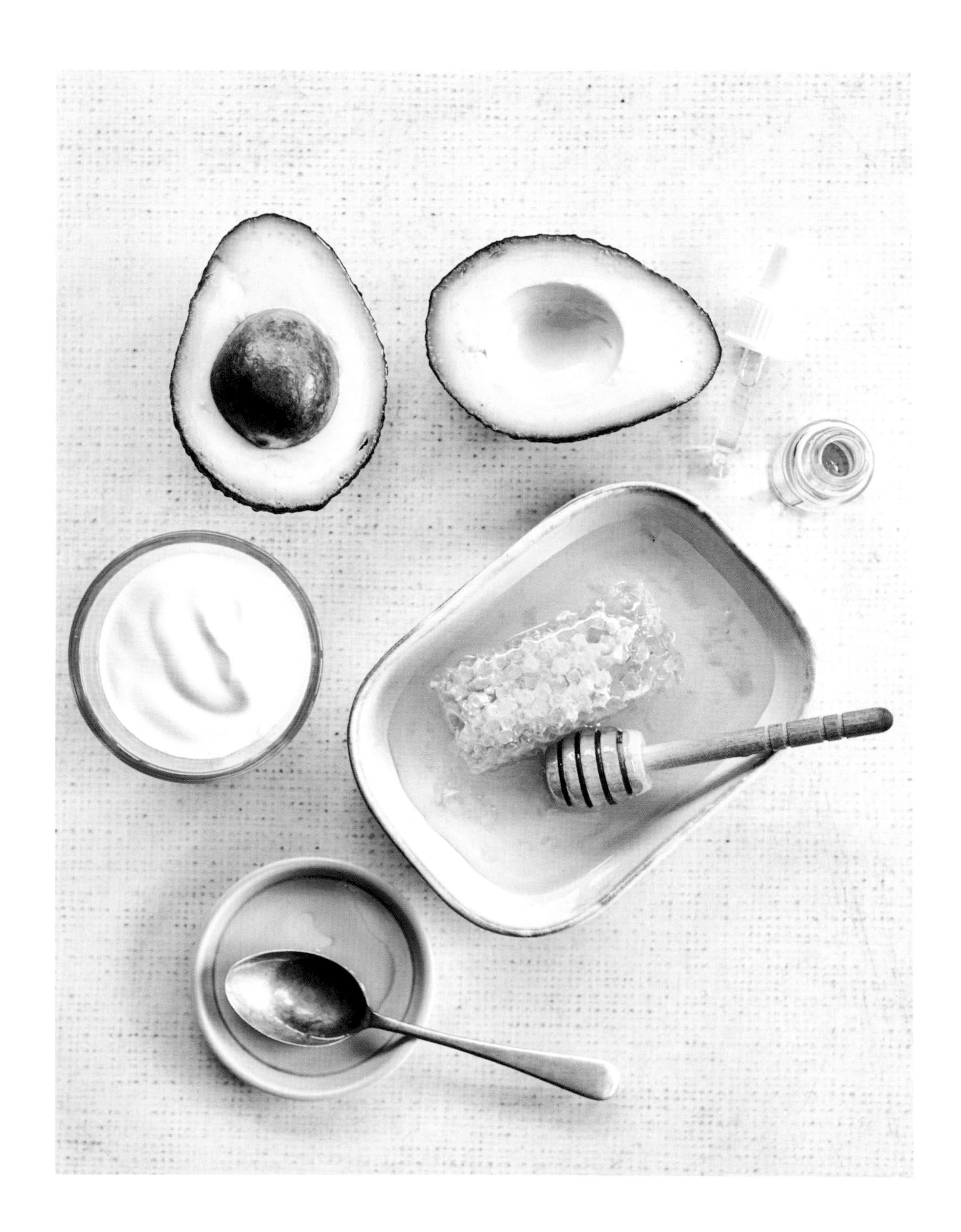

related hair loss that can happen after the body goes through a major trauma such as illness, childbirth or another stressful event and the hair reacts by shedding in clumps. With the right advice and treatment hair will regrow and complete recovery is possible in this case.

Hair Quick Fixes

Try one of the following hair treats at least once a week to keep hair deeply nourished and healthy.

- **COCONUT OIL RINSE:** Warm about ¼ cup of coconut oil and massage into wet or dry hair. This is best done in the bath or shower where the steam will encourage absorption of the oils into the hair and scalp. Leave in for at least one hour.
- **RESTORATIVE HAIR MASK:** Mix ½ an avocado with 2 egg yolks. Apply to wet or dry hair and leave for twenty minutes before rinsing off and washing hair as normal.
- **DAMAGED HAIR MASK:** Mix 1 tbsp honey with 2 parts unrefined coconut oil (the exact quantity depends on hair length – more will be required for longer hair) and 1 part natural argan oil in a small bowl. Massage into brushed, tangle-free hair, focusing on the ends and midsection (avoid applying to the scalp). Wrap hair in a bun, cover with a warm towel or shower cap and leave on for at least thirty minutes, depending on the degree of hair damage (if badly damaged, leave in place as long as possible). Alternatively enjoy a bath with your hair in a bun so the steam can penetrate. Rinse off and shampoo and condition as normal.

TIP: An apple cider vinegar rinse after shampoo and conditioner leaves hair sleek and shiny.

ON THE INSIDE

Oils are top of the GLOW food list this week too – a winning combination of oily fish and plant oils with avocado, nuts, seeds and more, chosen to nourish the skin from within, locking moisture into the skin to keep it nourished for longer.

KEY FOODS

- Avocados
- Blueberries
- Edamame beans
- Eggs
- Fermented foods
- Nuts
- Oily fish
- Seaweed
- Seeds
- Spinach, kale and other green leafy vegetables
- Tomatoes
- Turmeric

NOURISHING JUICES

Pineapple Punch *or* Double Green (see page 244)

NOURISHING TEAS

Ginger and Turmeric *and* Matcha Mint Latte (see page 252)

WEEKLY NOURISH PLAN

EVERY DAY

- Nourishing teas
- Nourishing juice
- Turmeric Tonic (page 107)
- 1 tbsp ACV on its own or mixed in warm water
- GLOW Trail Mix

MONDAY

BREAKFAST

Summer Surprise Smoothie (page 156) **OR** GLOW Banana Bread (page 152)

LUNCH/LIGHT MEAL

Courgette and Almond Soup (page 177) **OR** Minted Farro and Three Bean Salad with Goat's Cheese (page 191)

MAIN MEAL

Warming Squash, Red Pepper and Chickpea Curry Bowl (page 218) **OR** other Seasonal Bowl of choice **OR** Sweet Potato, Pea and Courgette Cakes (page 197) with Mango, Pomegranate and Cucumber Salsa (page 171)

TUESDAY

BREAKFAST

Shakshuka (page 163) **OR** Avocado on Toast – one of three ways (page 158)

LUNCH/LIGHT MEAL

Creamy Squash and Red Pepper Soup with a slice of sourdough bread (page 174) **OR** Orange, Walnut and Quinoa Salad (page 186)

MAIN MEAL

Salmon/oily fish – one of three ways (pages 205-8) **OR** Shepherdless Pie (page 202)

WEDNESDAY

BREAKFAST

Overnight Oats with Seasonal Berries (page 146) **OR** Buckwheat Pancakes with Caramelised Banana Bites (page 160)

LUNCH/LIGHT MEAL

Spinach and Broccoli Soup with Flaked Almonds and a slice of sourdough bread (page 181) **OR** Quinoa, Pomegranate and Feta Salad (page 184)

MAIN MEAL

Asian-Style Salmon Bowl (page 211) or other Seasonal Bowl of choice **OR** Shepherdless Pie (page 202)

THURSDAY

BREAKFAST

Maya's Granola (page 145) **OR** Avocado on Toast – one of three ways (page 158)

LUNCH/LIGHT MEAL

Beetroot, Edamame and Orange Salad with a slice of sourdough bread (page 188) **OR** Shakshuka (page 163)

MAIN MEAL

Salmon/oily fish – one of three ways (pages 205-208) **OR** Cannellini Bean Salad with Marinated Alaria (page 192)

FRIDAY

BREAKFAST

GLOW Banana Bread (page 152) **OR** Herby Edamame Omelette (page 143)

LUNCH/LIGHT MEAL

Courgette and Almond Soup (page 177) with a slice of sourdough **OR** GLOW Frittata (page 195) with Mango, Pomegranate and Cucumber Salsa (page 171)

MAIN MEAL

Salmon/oily fish – one of three ways (pages 205-8) **OR** Sweet Potato, Pea and Courgette Cakes (page 197) with Mango, Pomegranate and Cucumber Salsa (page 171)

SATURDAY

BREAKFAST

Shakshuka (page 163) **OR** Summer Surprise Smoothie (page 156)

LUNCH/LIGHT MEAL

GLOW Frittata (page 195) **OR** Avocado on Toast – one of three ways (page 158)

MAIN MEAL

Warming Squash, Red Pepper and Chickpea Curry Bowl (page 218) **OR** other Seasonal Bowl of choice **OR** Salmon – one of three ways (pages 205-8)

SUNDAY

BREAKFAST

Herby Edamame Omelette (page 143) **OR** Shakshuka (page 163)

LUNCH/LIGHT MEAL

Courgette and Almond Soup with a slice of sourdough bread (page 177) **OR** Avocado on Toast – one of three ways (page 158)

MAIN MEAL

Salmon – one of three ways (pages 205-8) **OR** Broccolini Risotto (page 198)

KEY POINTS WEEK 3: NOURISH ACTION

- Morning mantra
- ACV shot
- Nourish oils
- Body brush before showering
- Nourish face mask and massage at least 2–3 times
- Nourish body scrub at least 2–3 times
- Nourish foods, teas, juices
- Turmeric Tonic
- GLOW Trail Mix
- Fermented foods

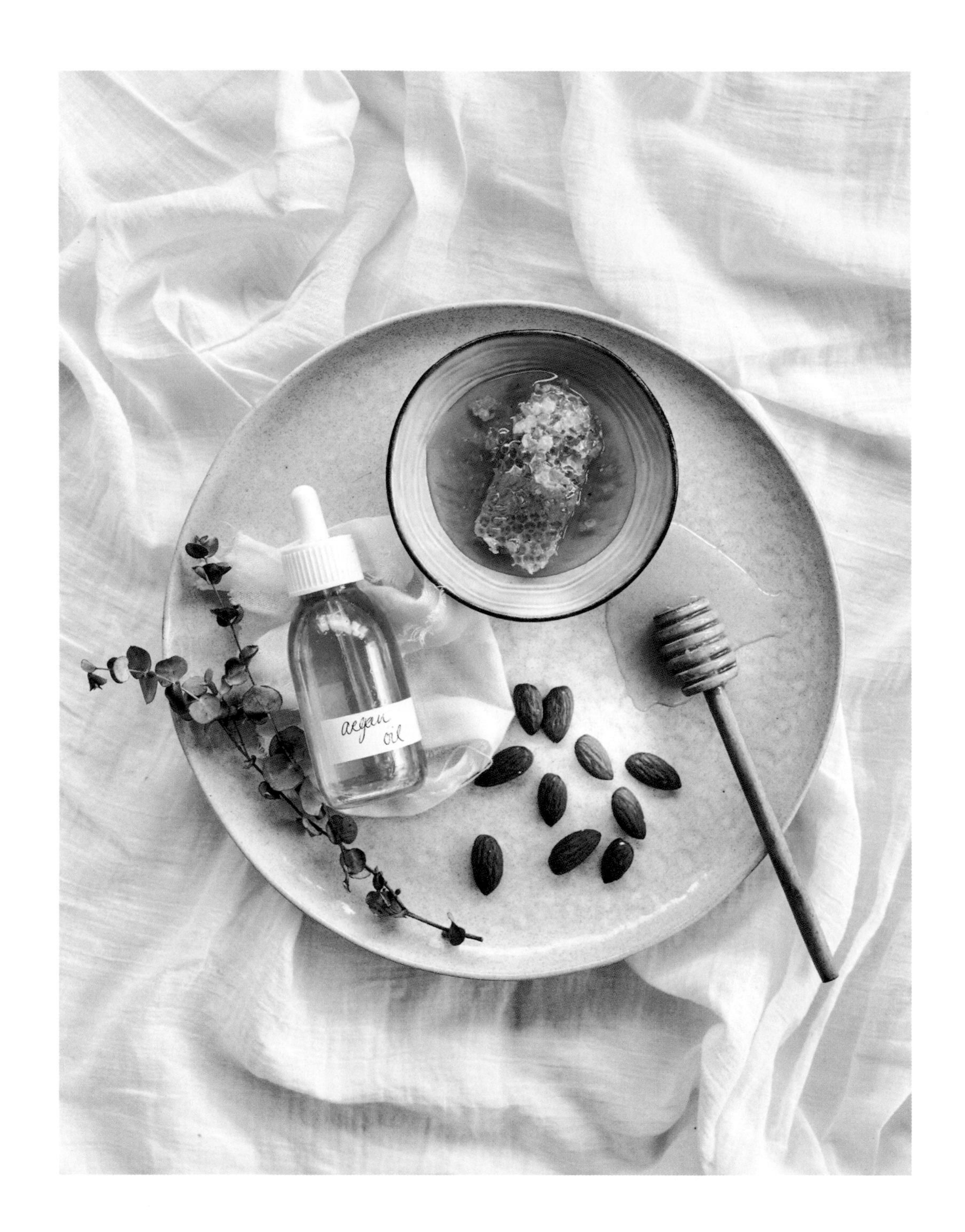
argan oil

WEEK FOUR: GLOW

The key word this week is GLOW. There is no set plan, just a colourful combination of your favourite GLOW foods, oils and skin-nourishing masks and mists. Each of them, without exception, has a role to play in achieving and maintaining that fresh-faced, radiant GLOW.

ON THE OUTSIDE

GLOW OILS: choose your favourite from the previous weeks or try sweet orange oil and rosemary.

THE FACE

Skin Quick Fix: Almond and Honey Facial Scrub

This scrub is mild and gentle so it's a good one to start with.

- 2 tbsp ground almonds
- 2 tsp thick honey
- 4 tbsp natural yoghurt

Mix the almonds, honey and yoghurt. Massage into the face and neck, avoiding the eye area. Leave in place for twenty minutes then rinse off with warm water and a muslin or flannel.

GLOW Face Blend

This simple blend of nourishing oils massaged into the skin will instantly stimulate blood flow and enliven the face. The following recipe can be adjusted for personal preference, how your skin is feeling at a particular time and depending on what oils you have on hand. The key to ensuring optimum benefits lies in using only top-quality oils. No compromise! Although you will pay more, quality oils are worth investing in, as a little goes a long way and the outcome will be better skin.

- 50ml rosehip oil
- 10ml avocado oil
- 2 vitamin E capsules (min. 150mg vitamin E each)
- 2–3 drops of lavender (if skin is feeling a little delicate) and/or rose, argan or prickly pear essential oil (when added nourishment is needed)

First, wash hands and then cleanse and tone the face. Pierce the vitamin E capsules and mix with the essential oils. Adjust according to personal preference and what skin needs at the time.

Take some deep breaths to relax. Pour a few drops of oil into your hand, rub hands together to warm the oil and begin to massage deeply into the skin, primarily with the fingertips – pressing and holding in place for a few seconds before moving over the face.

Don't forget the eyebrows! Press along the brow line, starting from the top of the nose and working out, using a pinch-and-squeeze movement with the tip of the thumb and first finger. Repeat a few times. To complete this area, gently sweep the third (ring) finger of each hand along the eyebrows from the top of the nose and along the socket of the eye to finish with a final press on the inner eye area.

The neck needs attention too – brush up from the bottom of the neck towards the face in sweeping strokes using the full length of your fingers.

Finally, lightly tap your fingertips over your face, starting at the top of the forehead and working down over the eyes to the chin and back up to the forehead. Do this a few more times before finishing.

ON THE INSIDE

KEY FOODS

Choose your favourite recipes from the past three weeks and enjoy every mouthful. No meal plan is required – just mix and match as you please. Be armed with some GLOW Trail Mix when out and about. Snack on the foods included in the plan and enjoy some of the Sweet Things – you deserve it!

Begin every morning this week and from here on in with your morning mantra and Turmeric Tonic. You now know that it works. Make your favourite GLOW teas from the previous weeks or try Green Tea with Mint or Orange and Mint Iced Green Tea. The same applies to GLOW Juices – continue to enjoy your favourites or try Sunshine Skin or Vital Skin.

BETTER SKIN FOR LIFE

The primarily plant-based better-skin plan is packed with oily fish, eggs, vegetables, fruits, nuts, seeds and natural grains. Of course, protein-rich chicken, meat and dairy products can have a role too and should be enjoyed if wanted – but quality is key (free range, grass fed) and twice per week is plenty.

The GLOW guide to better skin has outlined the essence of caring for your skin for these four weeks and for the rest of your life. Remember, GLOW is not about deprivation. Food should be relished and enjoyed. A positive outlook on life really helps too, hence the importance of continuing your daily mantra. A fresh, happy face is an outward sign of a positive mindset too; as we know, the mind exerts huge influence on how we look and vice versa.

This GLOW guide to better skin should be kept on hand to dip into as required. It will benefit your skin and your overall physical and mental well-being for always and especially during stressful periods. Finally, and most important, be kind to yourself. It's the least you deserve.

KEY POINTS

Every Day

- Cleanse, tone, nourish – without exception
- Apply factor 30+ broad-spectrum sunscreen after moisturising and before applying make-up
- Use facial oils suitable for your skin, especially at night
- Set a simple morning mantra/evening gratitude
- Start your day with a Turmeric Tonic
- Aim to have at least one primarily vegetable juice daily
- If you are a meat eater, enjoy top-quality cuts from a trusted source one to two days per week
- Eat fish at least two days each week (especially oily fish)
- Eat some GLOW Trail Mix
- Have some skin-loving fruits – blueberries, strawberries, oranges, pomegranates, etc.
- Eat and drink more fermented foods/drinks – try to make kombucha (page 257)
- Drink plenty of water
- Get enough restful sleep

Every Week

- Cleanse skin with a facial scrub and steam a few times each week if possible
- Use a thorough deep body scrub twice each week
- Use Alexandra Soveral's Honey Cleanse once a week (page 110)
- Apply replenishing facemask – use the recipes in this section or try others using natural ingredients and free from suspect chemicals. If buying a mask, choose a trusted brand and look for natural ingredients – the shorter the ingredient list the less chance of an overload of unwanted toxic extras!
- Dry skin body brush before showering as frequently as possible
- Face massage (Glow Face Blend, page 135) – don't forget the eyes and the neck!

Every 1–2 Months

- Enjoy a cleansing and nourishing facial from a trusted professional to complement your at-home facial massage and mask

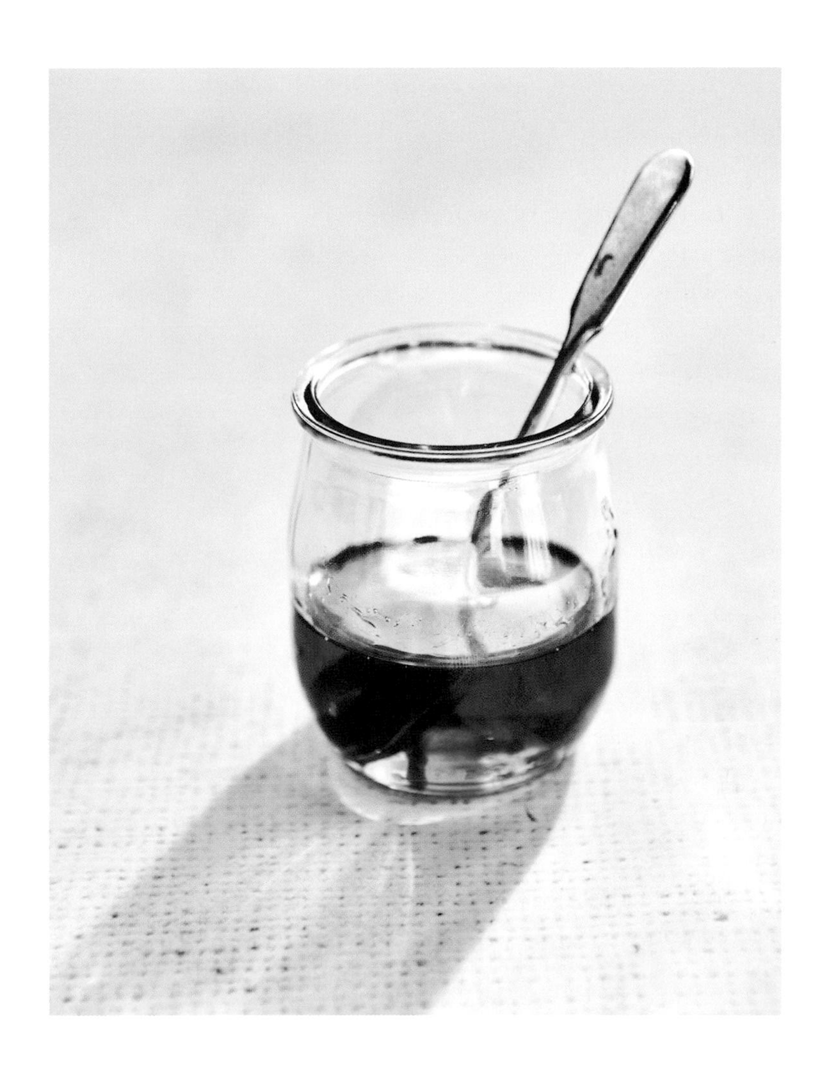

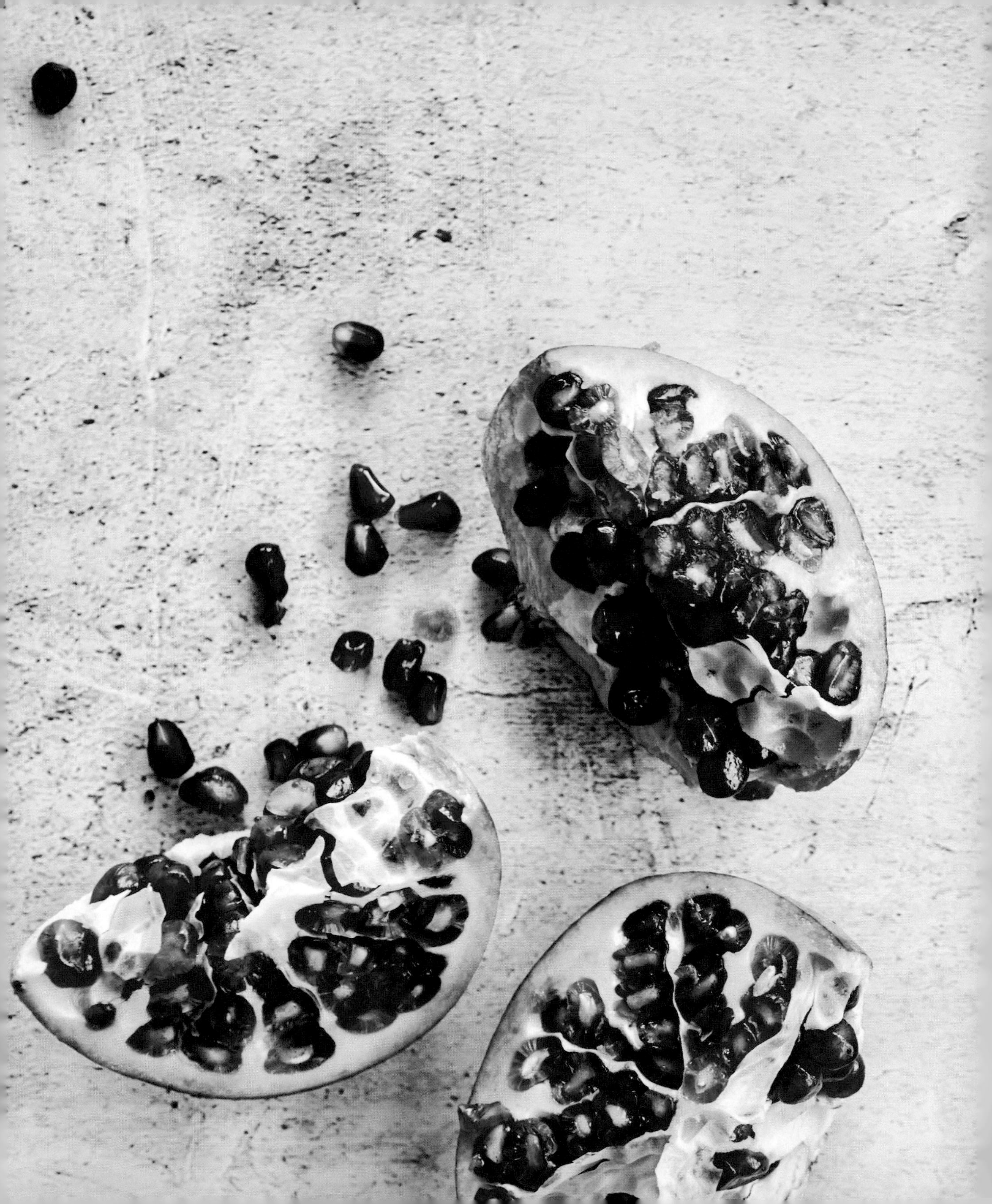

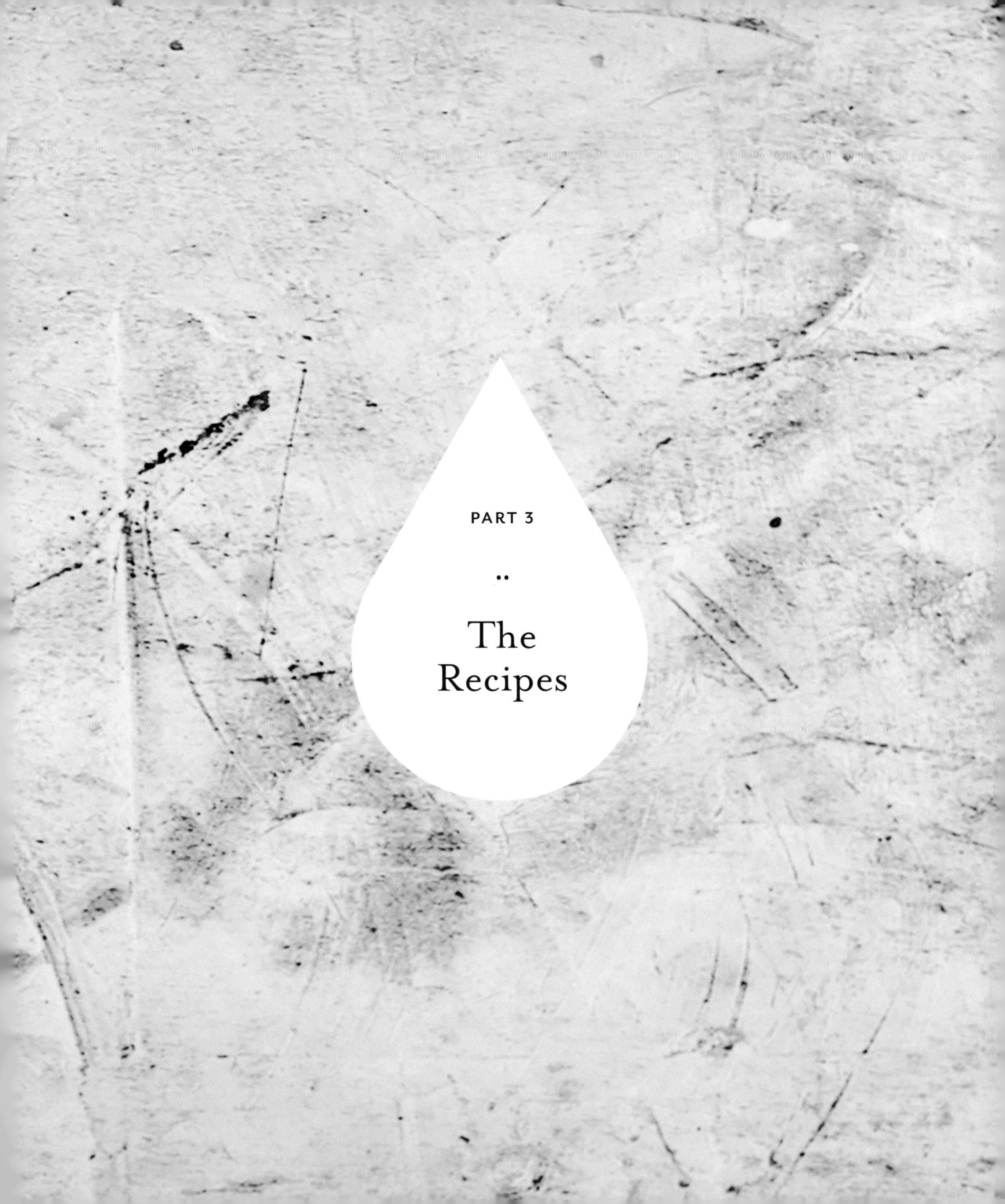

PART 3

The Recipes

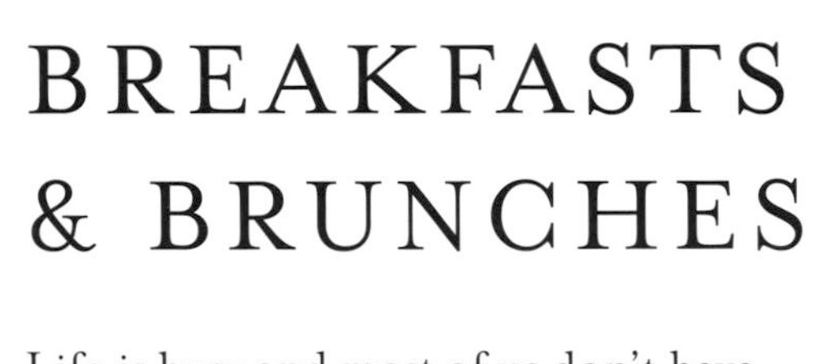

BREAKFASTS & BRUNCHES

Life is busy and most of us don't have time for fuss, especially first thing in the morning, but we do need an energy boost for the day ahead. With this in mind, the following simple recipes will provide your skin with the essential fats and antioxidants needed to nourish and protect it through the day. Think colourful smoothies, overnight oats and granola, and a few ideas that take a little longer for more leisurely weekend mornings.

Herby Edamame Omelette

This super-fast, skin-loving breakfast is delicious. Experiment with herbs, and indeed other legumes, until you find what works best for you.

- 2 eggs
- sea salt and black pepper, to taste
- 1 tbsp finely chopped parsley
- 1–2 spring onions, optional
- 1 tbsp coconut or olive oil
- 1 large handful spinach
- 2 tbsp edamame beans, defrosted and shelled (or other legumes)
- a few cherry tomatoes, to serve

SERVES 1

Crack the eggs into a small bowl with pinch of salt, pepper, the chopped fresh parsley and the spring onions, if using, and whisk. Heat the oil in a large frying pan over a medium heat. Ensure the base of the pan is evenly oiled to prevent the eggs from sticking. Add the eggs, swirling them around the pan to ensure even distribution. When the egg begins to set (after a minute or so) add the spinach and edamame beans to one half of the omelette. Continue cooking for another minute or so before folding the other side of the omelette over the greens to pack them in. Leave for a minute before sliding onto a plate. Serve with cherry tomatoes and a small slice of crusty bread, if wanted.

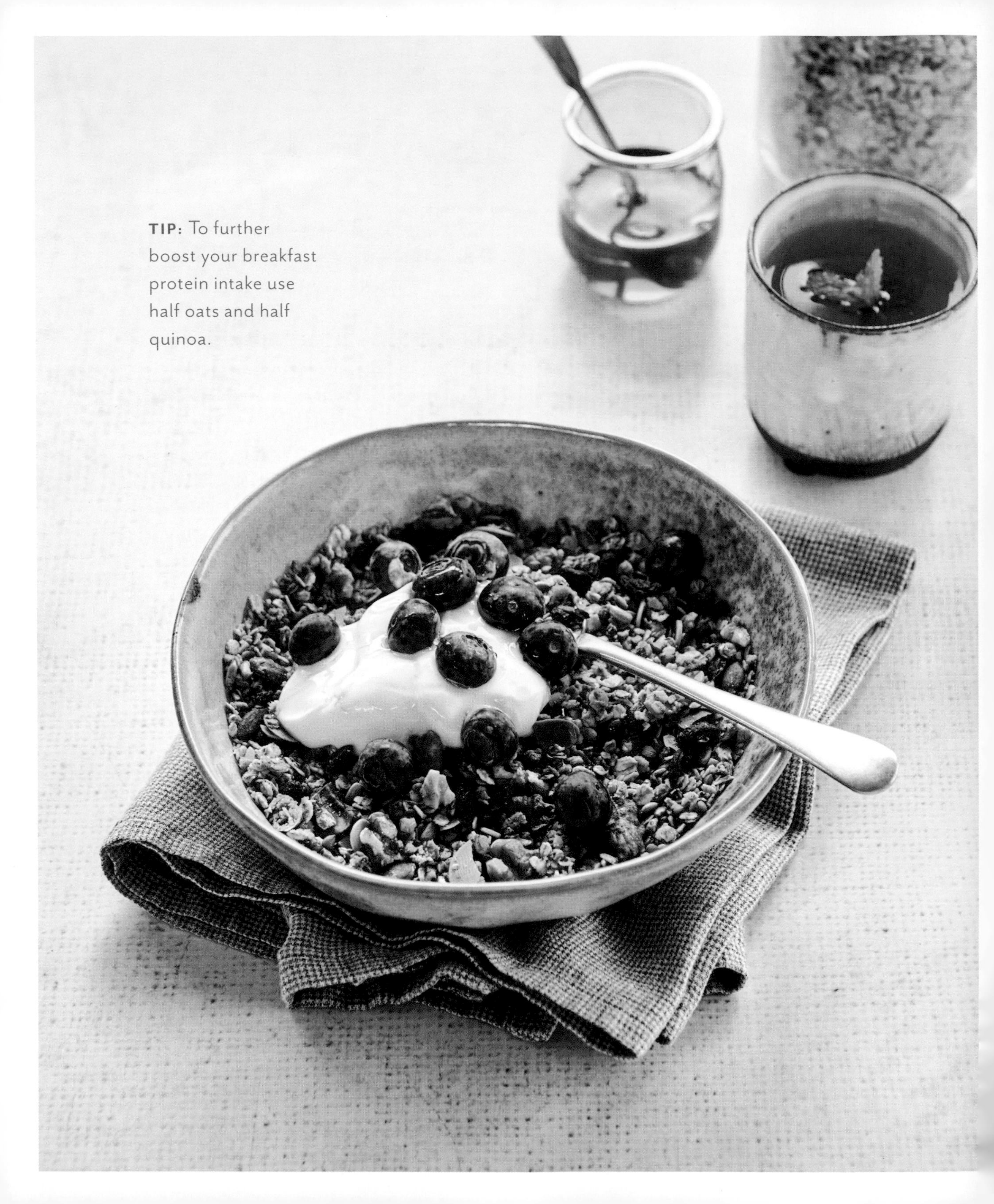

TIP: To further boost your breakfast protein intake use half oats and half quinoa.

Five Ways with Oats

Oats are enjoying a well-deserved revival, with various modern twists making them tastier and even more nutritious than ever before. The type of oats you use can make a difference, with typical rolled oats being slightly larger and more versatile than regular oats.

Maya's Granola

250g buckwheat

250g rolled oats

200g chopped mixed nuts of choice (e.g. almonds, walnuts, hazelnuts, cashews)

100g mixed seeds (e.g. pumpkin, sesame, sunflower, flax, chia)

100g desiccated coconut

70g coconut oil

1 tsp vanilla extract

110ml maple syrup

1–2 tsp cinnamon

6 tbsp add-ins (e.g. goji berries, dried mango, banana chips)

MAKES 1 LARGE JAR

Preheat the oven to 140°C.

Combine all dry ingredients (except add-ins) in a large bowl.

Place the coconut oil, vanilla and maple syrup in a saucepan and heat until the coconut oil has melted. Pour over the dry mix and combine.

Spread out the mixture in a thin layer on two large baking trays and bake for about 70 minutes. Leave to cool before mixing in your add-ins.

Granola can be kept in an airtight jar or container for up to three weeks.

Overnight Oats with Seasonal Berries

The perfect breakfast on the go, overnight oats take just a few minutes to prepare before going to bed and you have deliciously creamy oats in the morning.

4–5 tbsp oats

1 tbsp chia seeds

1 tbsp chopped walnuts

pinch ground cinnamon

dash of maple syrup (if desired)

50–60ml unsweetened almond or coconut milk (depending on preference)

4 tbsp unsweetened natural Greek, sheep's or coconut yogurt

1 tbsp sunflower, pumpkin or mixed seeds

handful fresh seasonal berries of choice

Stir the oats, chia seeds, chopped walnuts, cinnamon, maple syrup (if using) and milk together. Leave overnight in a covered jar or bowl in the fridge. Consistency should be creamy and thick(ish) in the morning. Add more milk if needed. Top with berries and seeds before enjoying the perfect start to your day.

TIP: Don't bin fresh fruit on the verge of going off. Dice larger fruits like bananas, pineapples and mangos and freeze them. Berries can be frozen whole. Use as needed for smoothies and juices or as a sweet and refreshing fruity sorbet (see page 236).

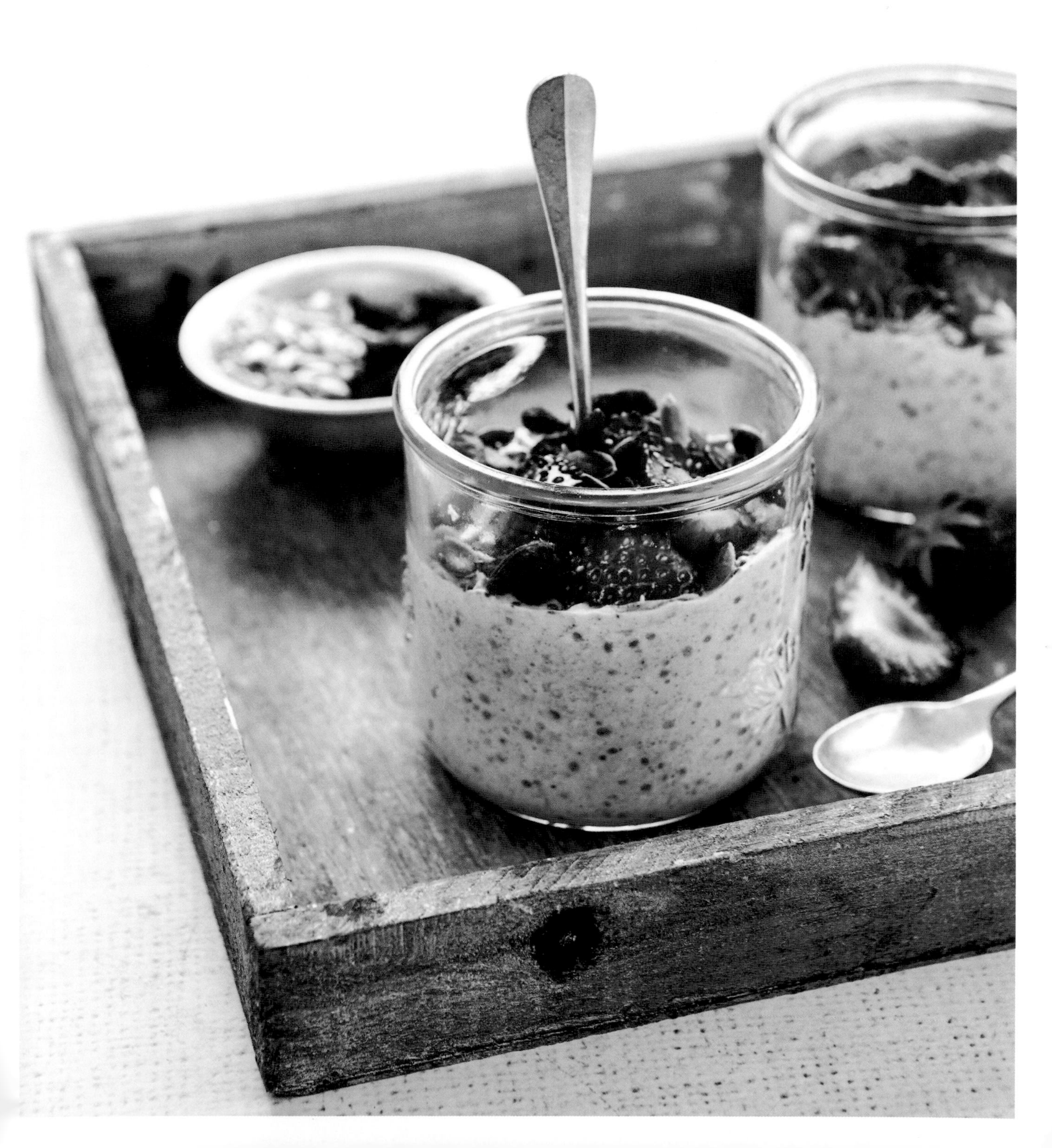

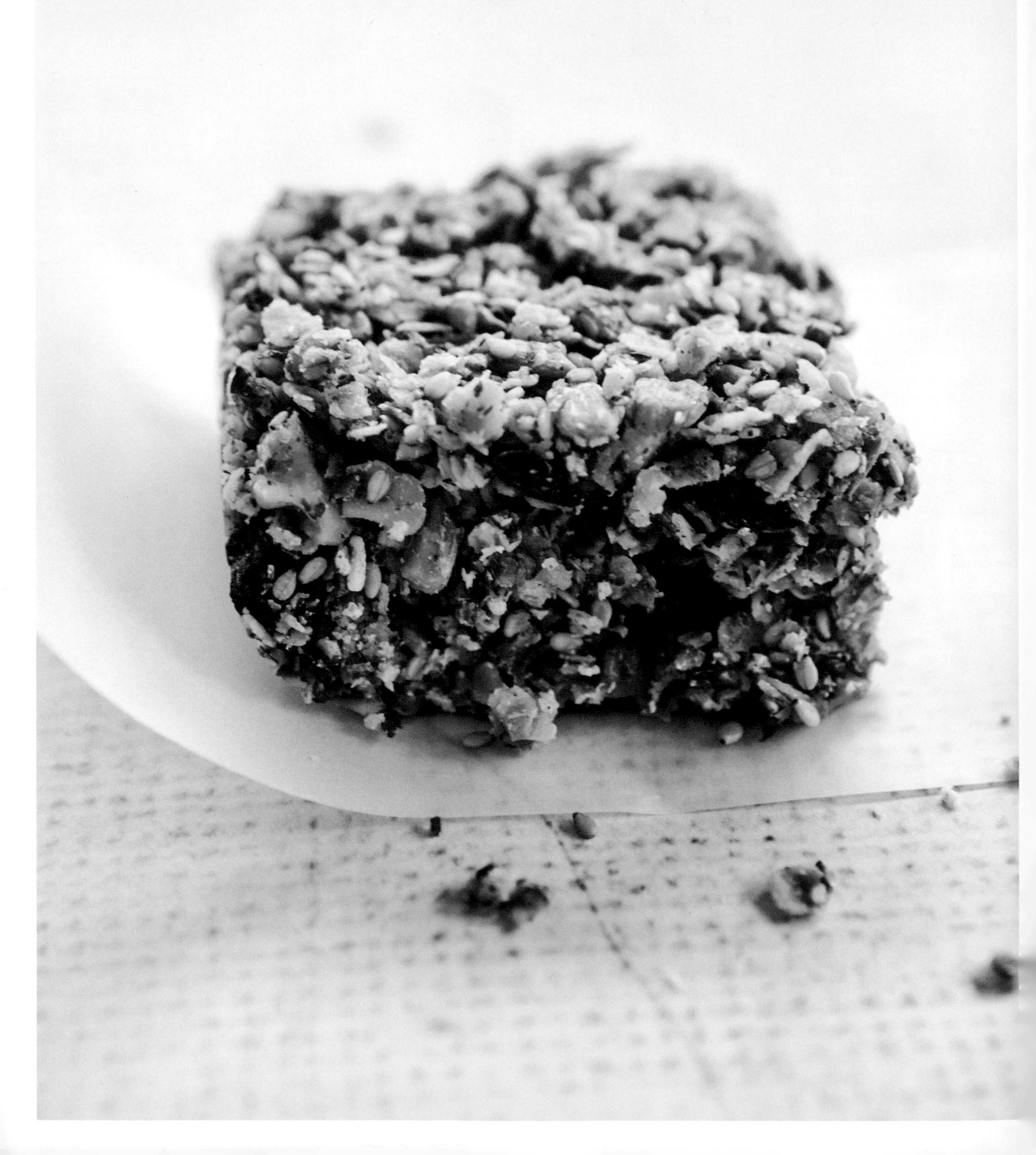

Oaty Breakfast Bars

These super-nutritious oat bars can be customised to taste by simply swapping the nuts or seeds given here for your preferred options. If coconut isn't to your taste then swap it for extra nuts or seeds, but for the right consistency, try to keep the overall quantities as per the recipe.

250g rolled oats

150ml coconut or sunflower oil

50g ground flax/linseeds or milled chia seeds

30g desiccated coconut

40g cashews and/or walnuts, chopped

40g sunflower seeds

40g sesame seeds

20g goji berries

pinch of sea salt

150ml maple syrup or honey

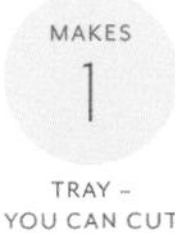

TRAY – YOU CAN CUT THE BARS TO YOUR DESIRED SIZE

Preheat oven to 140°C. Line a deep loaf tin with baking paper. Mix the oats and oil in a bowl until well coated. Add all the remaining ingredients except the maple syrup/honey and stir until everything is well combined. Add the maple syrup/honey and mix. Spread the mixture evenly in the tray, using a potato masher to really squash the mixture in, making it firmer. Bake for about 30 minutes until golden. Leave to cool before cutting. They will keep for up to 4 days in an airtight container.

Oaty Banana Smoothie

2 tbsp rolled oats (ideally pre-soaked in a little milk for 30 mins or overnight to give a creamier taste)

175ml almond milk

1 medium ripe banana

1 tbsp tahini or almond butter

3 ice cubes

generous pinch ground cinnamon

½ tsp vanilla extract

1 level tsp chia seeds, to serve

Combine all ingredients, except chia seeds, in a blender. If it's too thick add a little more almond milk. Top with seeds and enjoy.

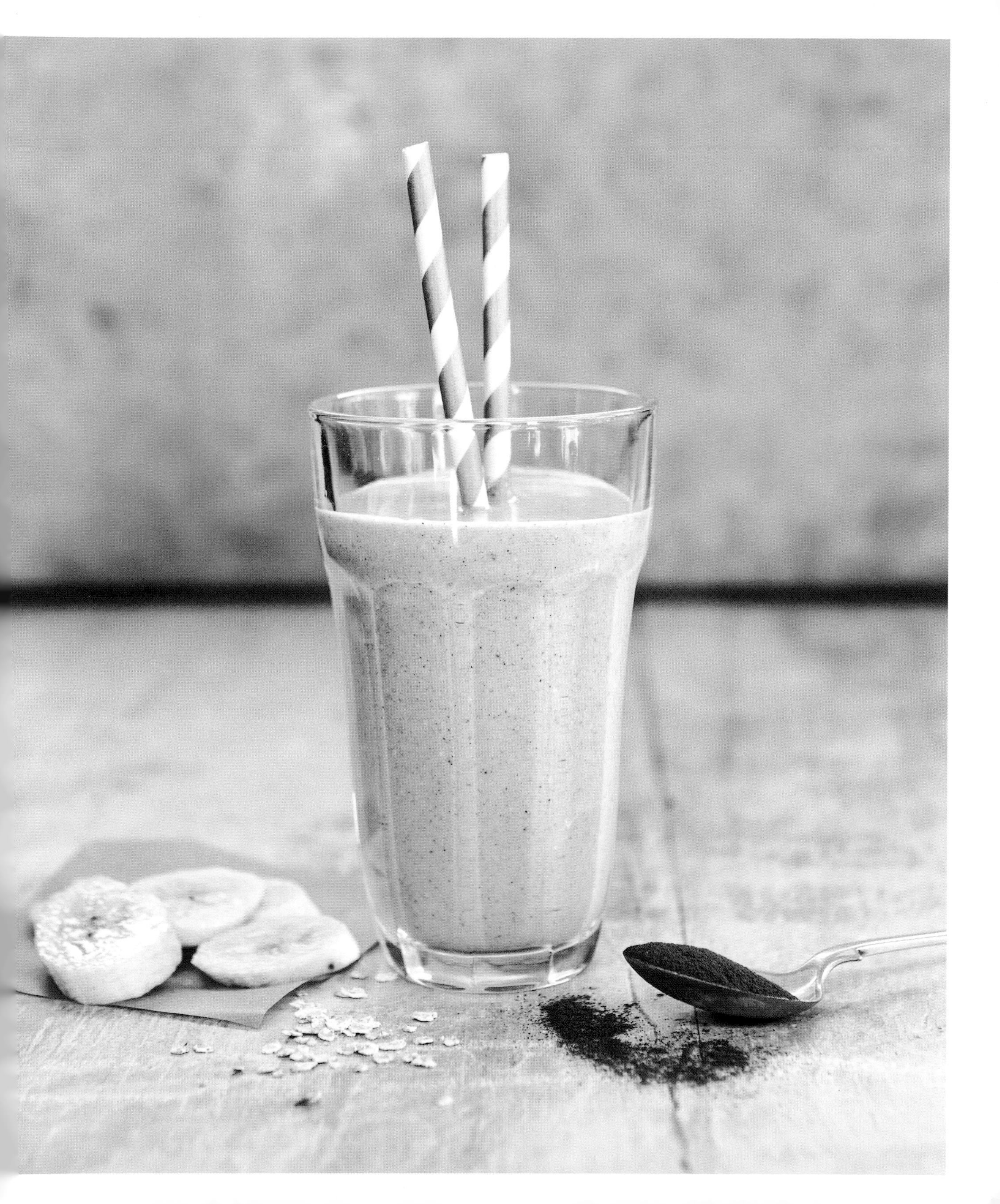

GLOW Banana Bread

This is not a get-up-and-go option – unless it is made in advance, of course. GLOW banana bread is full of skin-loving essential fats, vitamins and more. Most important, it tastes divine! It's delicious toasted and topped with butter or almond butter, and also the perfect snack, giving a boost of goodness when needed.

160g walnuts

200g oats

30g ground almonds

2 tsp baking powder

1 tsp cinnamon

4 ripe bananas

60g coconut oil, melted

180ml maple syrup

100ml almond milk (or milk of choice)

50g dark chocolate, cut into small pieces (optional)

Preheat the oven to 180°C. Line a rectangular loaf tin with baking paper.

Blitz the walnuts and oats in a blender or food processor until they're a floury texture. Add to a bowl with the ground almonds, baking powder and cinnamon. Combine the rest of the ingredients (apart from the chocolate) in a blender. Fold into the dry ingredients and then mix in the dark chocolate (if using).

Pour into the tin and bake for 1 hour and 15 minutes, or until cooked through. Remove from oven and leave to cool.

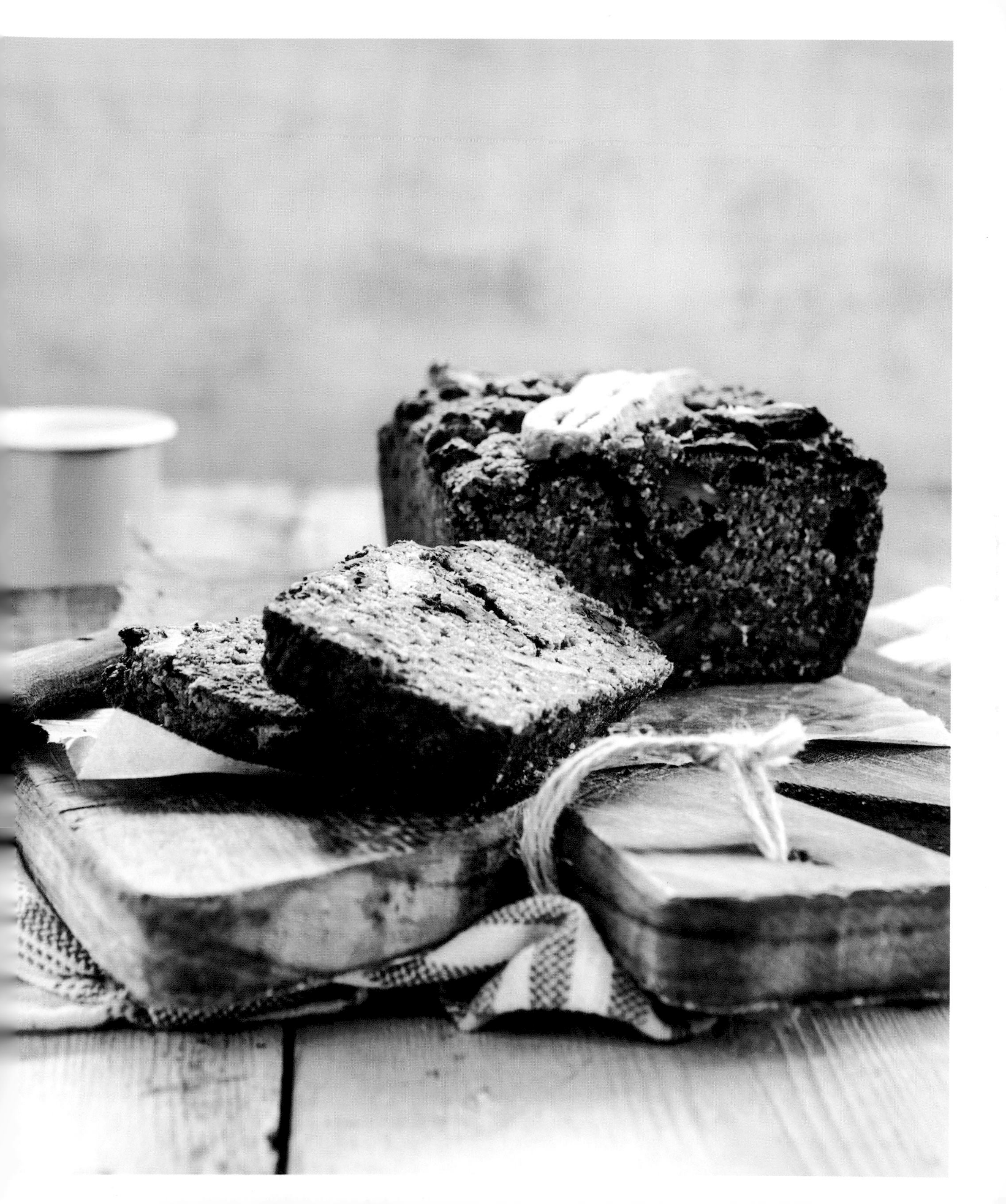

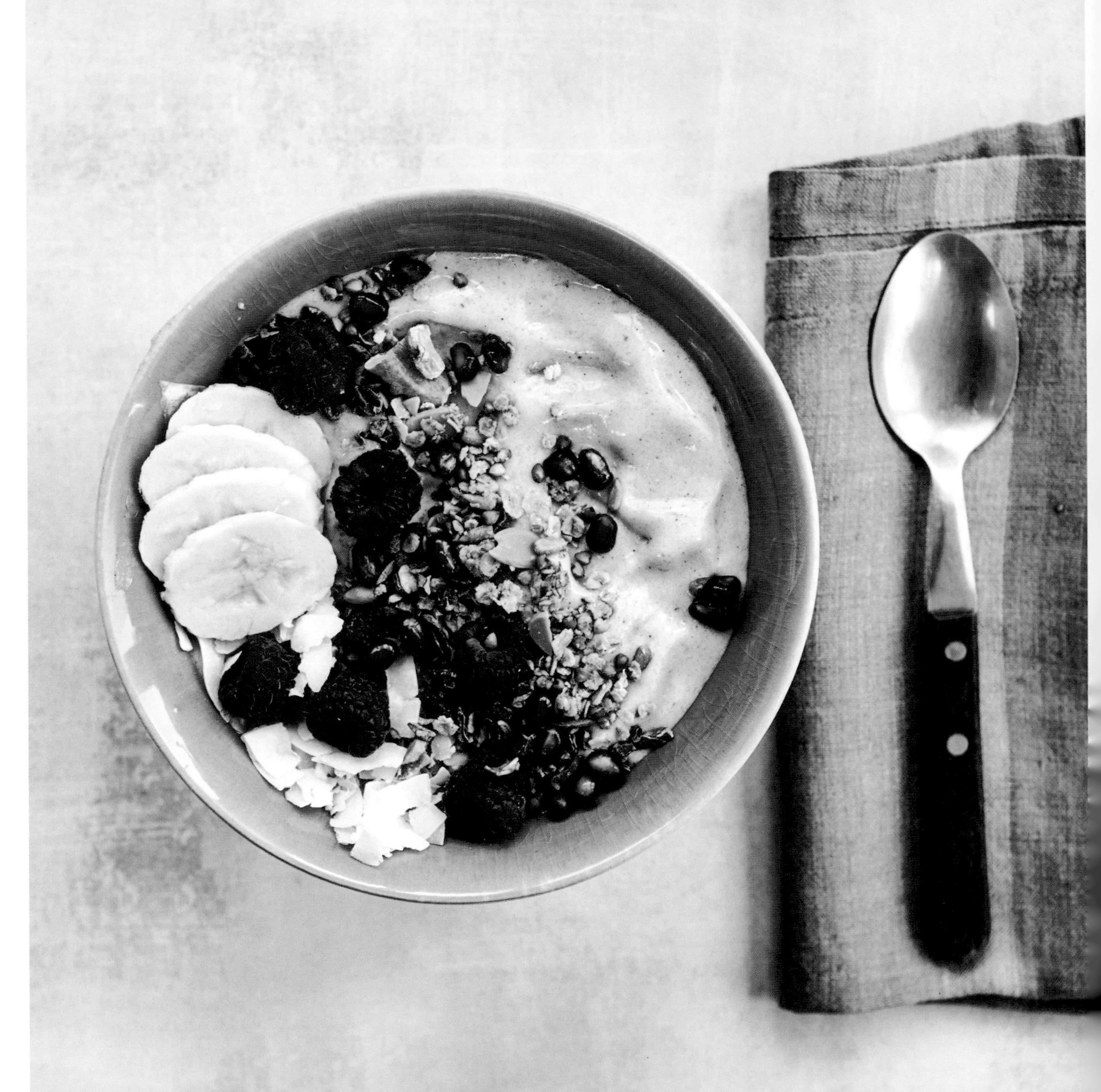

Salted Caramel Smoothie Bowl

2 chopped frozen bananas

1–2 pitted dates, depending on your preferred level of sweetness

1 tbsp nut or seed butter *or* 1 scoop vanilla protein powder

50–75ml almond milk

1 tsp vanilla extract

½ tsp cinnamon

pinch of sea salt

fresh berries, cacao nibs, granola, coconut chips, etc., to serve

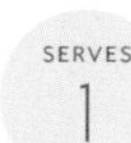

Place all the ingredients, except your toppings, in a blender and blitz. Pour into a bowl, add your preferred toppings and enjoy!

Summer Surprise Smoothie

This invigorating smoothie is made in two parts, swirled deliciously together.

PART 1

100ml coconut milk

½ ripe banana

1 tbsp natural Greek yoghurt

1 heaped tsp milled flax seeds

1 heaped tsp chia seeds

2 ice cubes

PART 2

½ ripe banana

50ml coconut milk

1 large handful mixed frozen berries

Part 1: blend all ingredients and pour into a tall glass

Part 2: blend all ingredients. Pour on top of part 1 and gently swirl both parts together for an inviting, colourful smoothie.

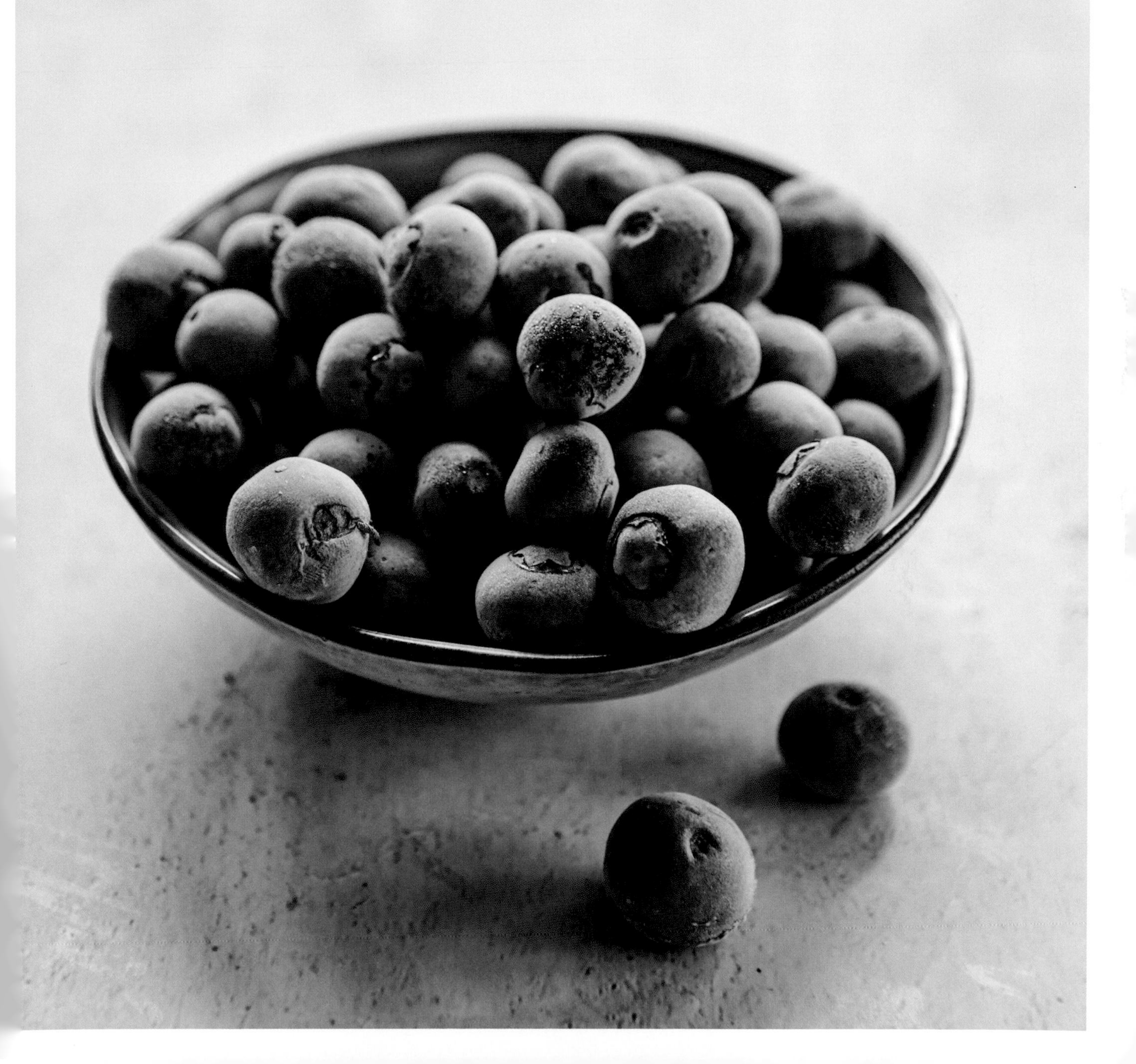

Avocado on Toast – Three Ways

Packed with healthy fats, omega-3 and an antioxidant armoury, avocados sing to your skin. Only buy the best and look for soft, ripe and healthy-looking fruits. They are a great lunch option too, especially when time is tight.

When it comes to bread, sourdough wins every time. Do ensure you are buying genuine sourdough and not some fake alternative. Better still, bake your own. Yes, it takes time and practice (and maybe a few failures!), but it will be worth it all when you eventually get it right. Sourdough is delicious and great for the gut too (see Gut and Skin, page 53) and this means only good things for our skin.

Mash an avocado with a dash of lime juice and black pepper, then pile onto a thick slice of toasted sourdough.

Enjoy on its own or top with any of the three following tasty combinations:

1. Crumbled feta and chopped basil leaves or a dash of basil oil
2. A poached egg and a generous pinch of smoked paprika
3. A handful of defrosted, shelled edamame beans – either mashed into the avocado or served alongside it

TIP: When using avocado, always leave the stone in until it is being eaten as it helps prevent the avocado turning brown.

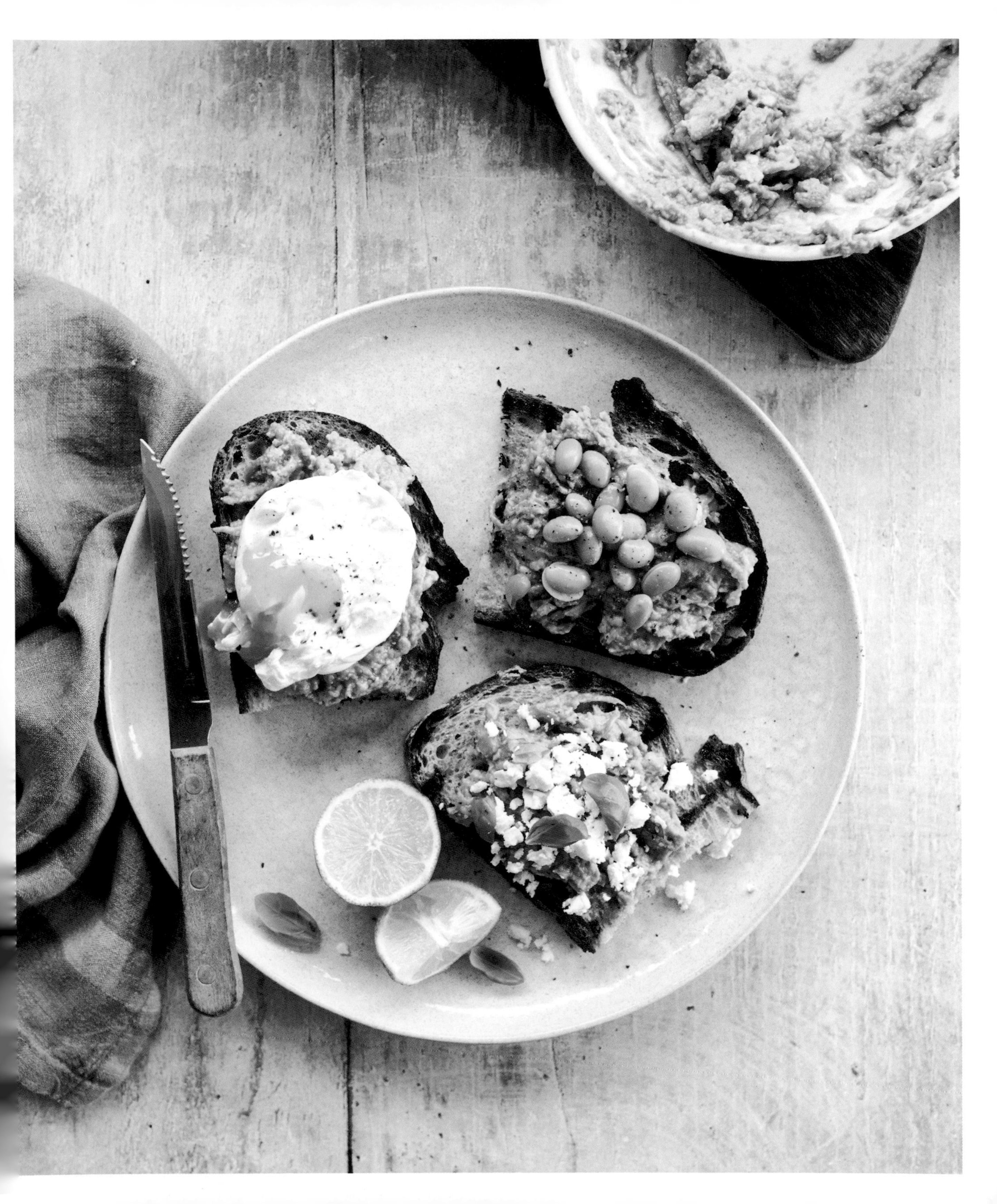

Buckwheat Pancakes with Caramelised Banana Bites

FOR THE PANCAKES

2 eggs

1 tsp baking powder

150g buckwheat flour

150ml almond milk

1 ripe banana

1 tsp vanilla extract (optional)

coconut oil, for frying

FOR THE BANANA BITES

1 large banana, peeled and thinly sliced

1 tsp coconut oil

1 tbsp maple syrup

big pinch cinnamon

TO SERVE

maple syrup

fresh fruit

coconut, sheep's or Greek yoghurt

SERVES 2–3

Whisk the eggs. Stir in the baking powder, flour and almond milk. Mash in the banana and vanilla. Heat a little coconut oil in a frying pan. Add 2 tablespoons of batter for each pancake. Cook over a medium heat until bubbles start to appear, about 1–2 minutes, then flip over and cook for about the same time on the other side. Remove to a warm plate and keep warm while you make the banana bites.

To the same pan, add all ingredients for the banana bites and sauté for 2 minutes, stirring continually.

Top the pancakes with the banana bites, a dash of maple syrup, fruits of your choice and a spoon of yoghurt.

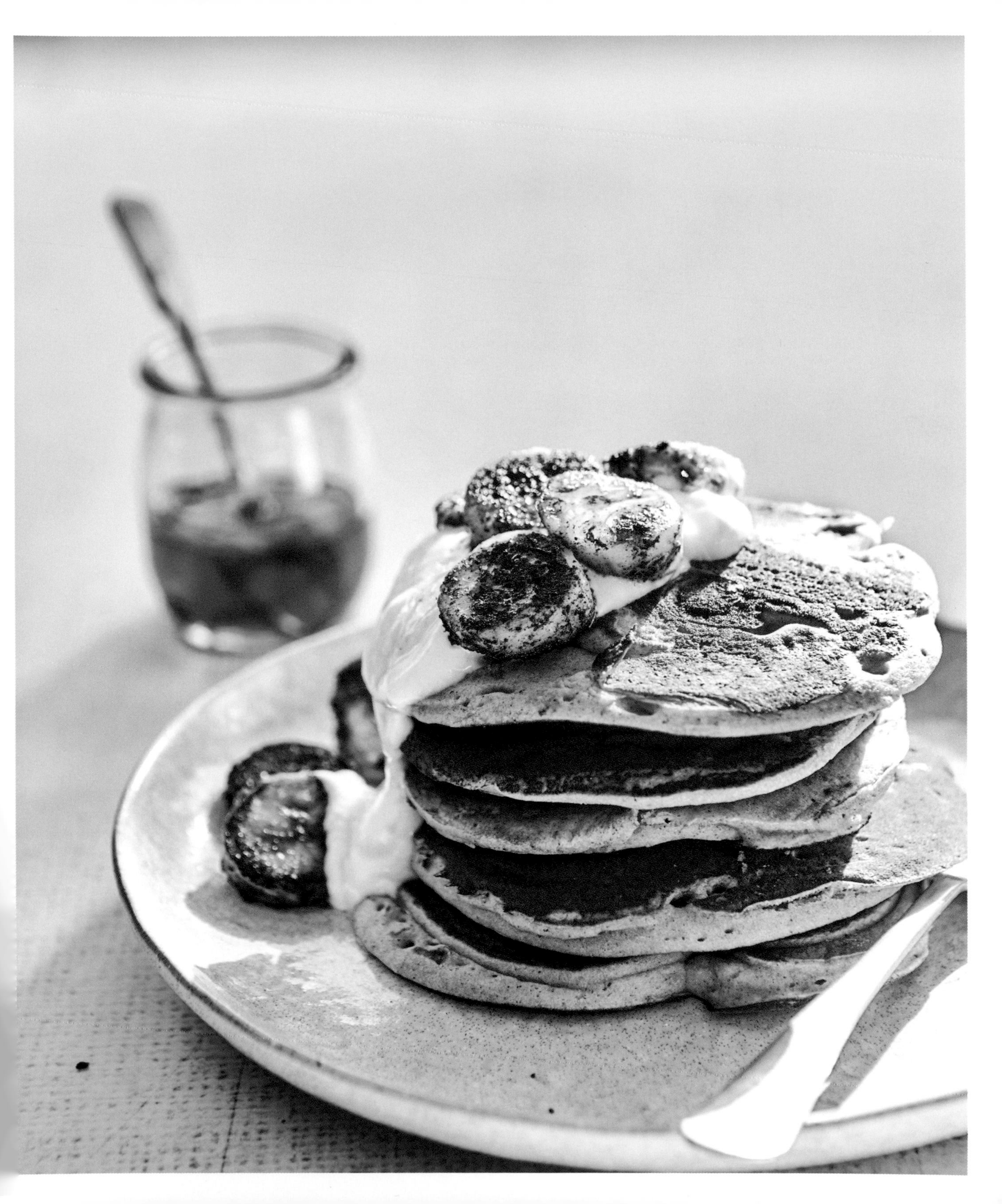

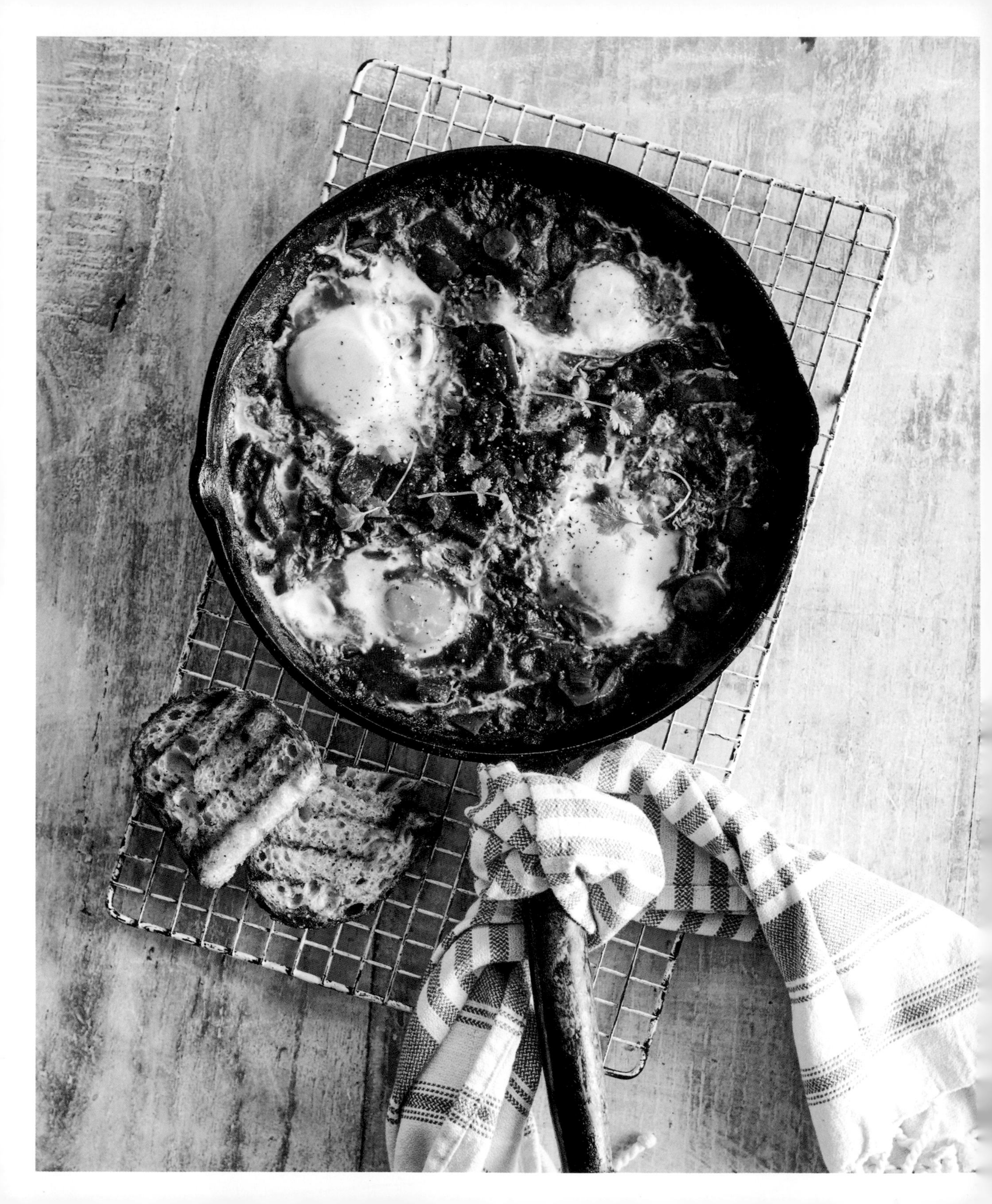

Shakshuka

Shakshuka (or shakshouka) is a staple of North African cuisine. This dish of eggs poached in a sauce of tomatoes, chilli, peppers and onion, often flavoured with cumin and other spices, is traditionally served in a cast iron pan or tagine with crusty bread to mop up the tasty juices.

2 tbsp coconut or olive oil

1 red onion, peeled and diced

1 clove garlic, peeled and finely diced

1 red pepper, deseeded and chopped into chunks

1 carrot, peeled and chopped into little chunks

400g tinned chopped tomatoes

100ml homemade (see page 173) or low-salt vegetable stock

1 tsp smoked paprika

1 tsp ground cumin

good pinch of chilli flakes

large handful of chopped spinach, stems removed

4 eggs

pinch sea salt and black pepper, to taste

handful chopped parsley, to serve

crumbled feta or goat's cheese, optional

First, heat a little coconut or olive oil in a large frying pan. Add the onion, garlic, red pepper and carrot and sauté over a medium heat for about 5 minutes, stirring. Add the chopped tomatoes, stock and spices. Reduce the heat and simmer for 5 minutes.

Add the spinach to the sauce and continue cooking for another few minutes until the spinach is wilted. Make four holes in the mix and crack an egg into each one. Cover the pan and simmer for up to 5 minutes, depending on how well cooked you like the eggs, making sure the whites are cooked through. Add salt and pepper, if desired. Sprinkle with chopped parsley and crumbled feta or goat's cheese (if using). Shakshuka can be eaten from the pan, as is traditional, or divided between two bowls and served with fresh, crusty sourdough bread, pittas or whatever you fancy.

TIP: The tomato sauce can be prepared in advance or made in bulk and frozen to be defrosted as needed.

SERVES 2

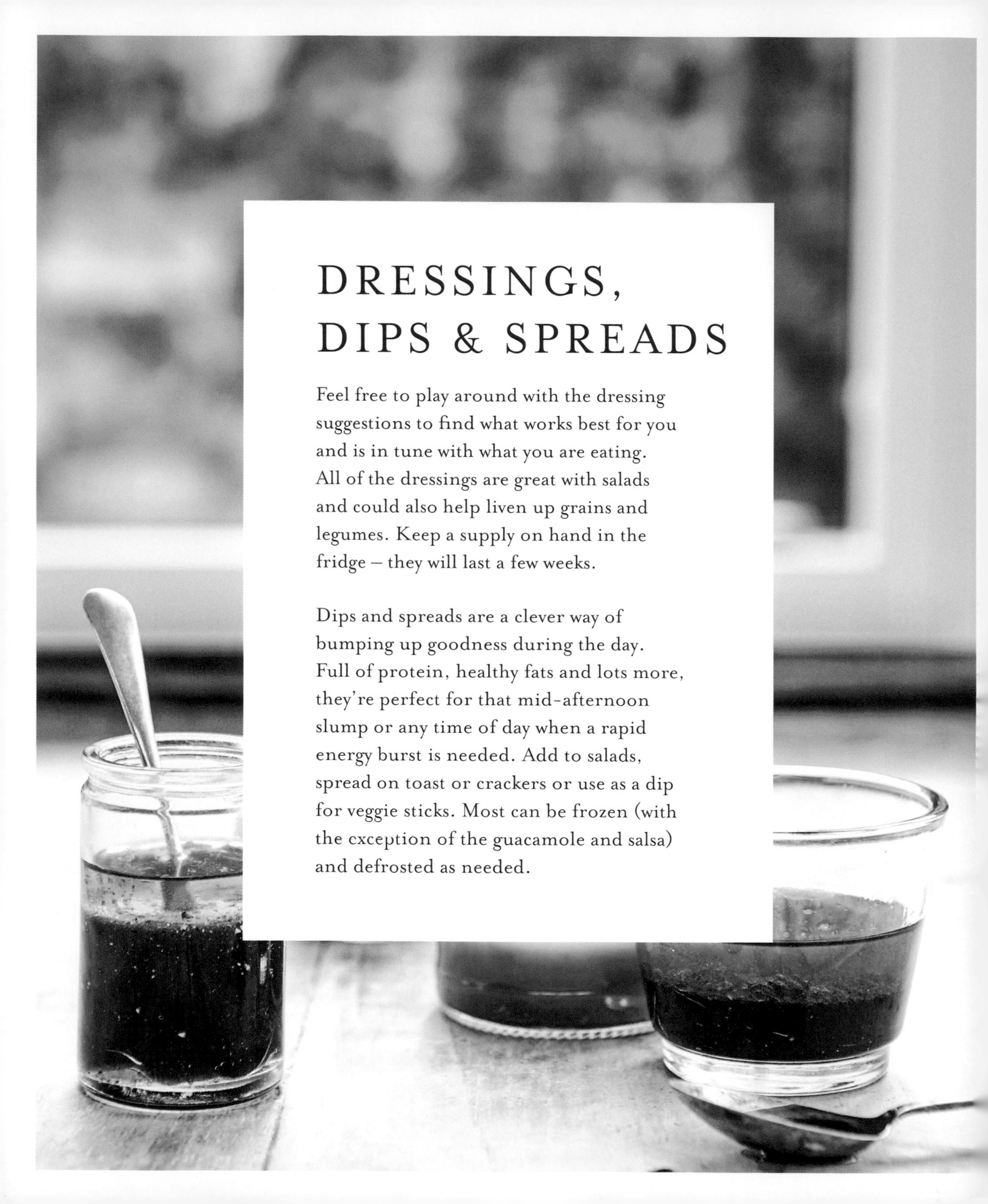

DRESSINGS, DIPS & SPREADS

Feel free to play around with the dressing suggestions to find what works best for you and is in tune with what you are eating. All of the dressings are great with salads and could also help liven up grains and legumes. Keep a supply on hand in the fridge – they will last a few weeks.

Dips and spreads are a clever way of bumping up goodness during the day. Full of protein, healthy fats and lots more, they're perfect for that mid-afternoon slump or any time of day when a rapid energy burst is needed. Add to salads, spread on toast or crackers or use as a dip for veggie sticks. Most can be frozen (with the exception of the guacamole and salsa) and defrosted as needed.

Mustard Dressing

1 tbsp Dijon mustard

3 tbsp extra virgin olive oil

3 tbsp sesame or walnut oil

1 tsp red wine vinegar

2 tsp balsamic vinegar

sea salt and black pepper

Combine mustard, oils and vinegars in a jar, close lid tightly and shake well until combined. Season with salt and pepper to taste, adding a little water if too thick.

MAKES 120 ML

Zesty Apple Cider Vinaigrette

5 tbsp extra virgin olive oil

2 tbsp apple cider vinegar

2 tsp red wine vinegar

1 tbsp fresh squeezed lime juice

1 tbsp honey

1 tsp Dijon mustard

sea salt and black pepper, to taste

Put all the ingredients in a jar, close lid tightly and shake well until combined. Check the seasoning, and add a little water if too thick.

Tahini Dressing

1 heaped tbsp tahini

1 tsp tamari or soy sauce

2 tbsp extra virgin olive oil

1½ tsp honey

sea salt and black pepper

juice of half a lemon

Using a whisk or small blender combine all ingredients, except the lemon juice, until smooth. Add the juice. Whisk again and if too thick just add a little more olive oil. Transfer to a jar with a lid and store in the fridge.

Guacamole

flesh of 2 large avocados

1 large tomato, diced

juice ½ lime

1–2 red chilies (depending on preference), deseeded and finely chopped

handful fresh coriander, finely chopped

1 tbsp extra virgin olive oil

sea salt and black pepper

pinch of paprika

SERVES 4 AS A DIP OR SIDE DISH

Mash the avocado to your desired consistency (leaving it a little lumpy can add more texture). Add the rest of the ingredients, except the paprika, and stir through. Sprinkle with paprika. Enjoy on sourdough toast, crackers, with eggs or any other way you like!

TIP: Guacamole on toast is even more delicious and nutritious topped with pomegranate seeds and roasted sweet peppers. To roast the peppers, preheat the oven to 180°C. Place the peppers on a baking sheet and top with a generous drizzle of olive oil and a sprinkle of fresh rosemary. Roast for 20 minutes.

Walnut Basil Pesto

75g walnuts
3 tbsp almond milk
4 tbsp olive oil
2 tbsp water
2 tbsp nutritional yeast
1 clove garlic
20g basil leaves
juice ½ lime
pinch of sea salt
pinch of pepper

Blend all ingredients until fairly smooth. Can be kept in the fridge for a few days.

Pesto is incredibly versatile – it's a tasty addition to salads and delicious heaped on a slice of toasted sourdough, brown bread or crackers.

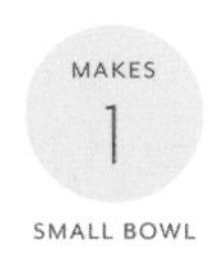

SMALL BOWL

Cashew Cream

200g cashews, soaked in water for at least 6 hours
8 tbsp water
2 tbsp apple cider vinegar
2 tbsp nutritional yeast
2 tbsp tamari or soy sauce
pinch of sea salt

Blend ingredients together until it reaches your desired consistency. Serve on whatever you fancy!

SMALL BOWL

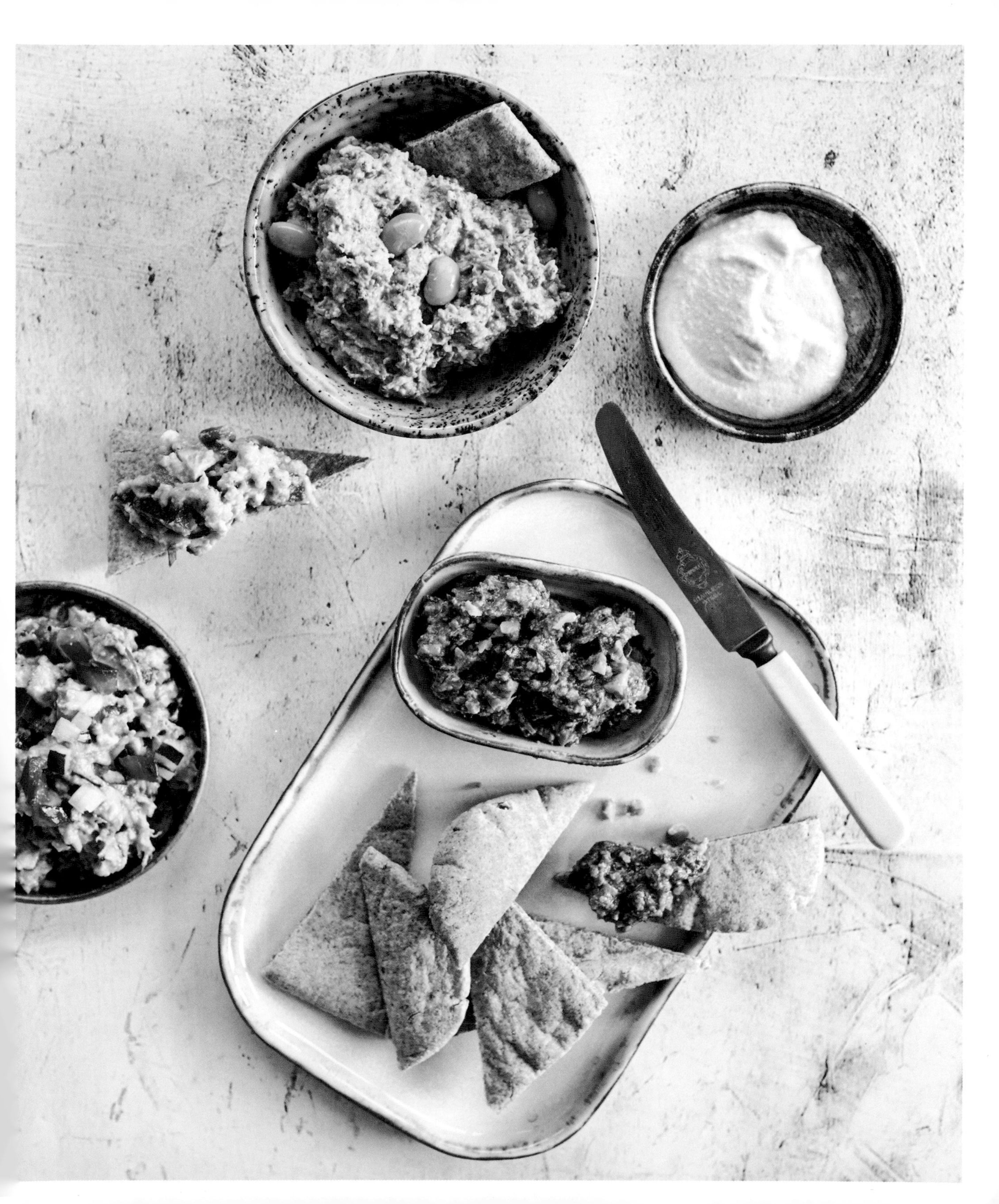

Pea and Edamame Houmous

150g frozen peas, defrosted

150g frozen edamame beans, defrosted and shelled

1½ tbsp tahini

2 tbsp olive oil

1 clove garlic, crushed

2 tsp tamari or soy sauce

juice of ¼ lemon

½ tsp ground cumin

large handful fresh coriander

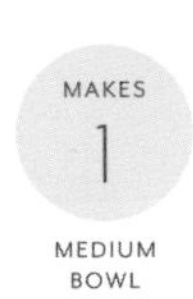

MEDIUM BOWL

Put all the ingredients in a blender/mini food processor and blend into a coarse paste. Spoon into a bowl, cover and leave to chill in the fridge. Serve with salads, on the side, as a dip for vegetable sticks or on bread or crackers.

Mango, Pomegranate and Cucumber Salsa

- 2 mangoes, peeled, stoned and chopped into 1 cm chunks
- ½ cucumber, chopped into 1 cm cubes
- handful fresh mint, chopped
- handful fresh coriander, chopped
- juice ½ lime
- 1 tbsp pomegranate seeds
- ½ tbsp pumpkin seeds

Combine all the ingredients in a bowl. Chill in the refrigerator until needed.

SERVES 2 AS A SIDE DISH

Tzatziki

- 2 tbsp natural Greek or sheep's yoghurt
- ½ cucumber, finely diced
- handful fresh mint, finely chopped
- 1 tbsp apple cider vinegar

Combine yoghurt, cucumber and mint in a bowl. Add apple cider vinegar to taste and for consistency.

TIP: Use ½ tbsp lime juice and ½ tbsp apple cider vinegar for a less assertive sauce, which works well with more delicately flavoured dishes.

SERVES 2 AS A SIDE DISH

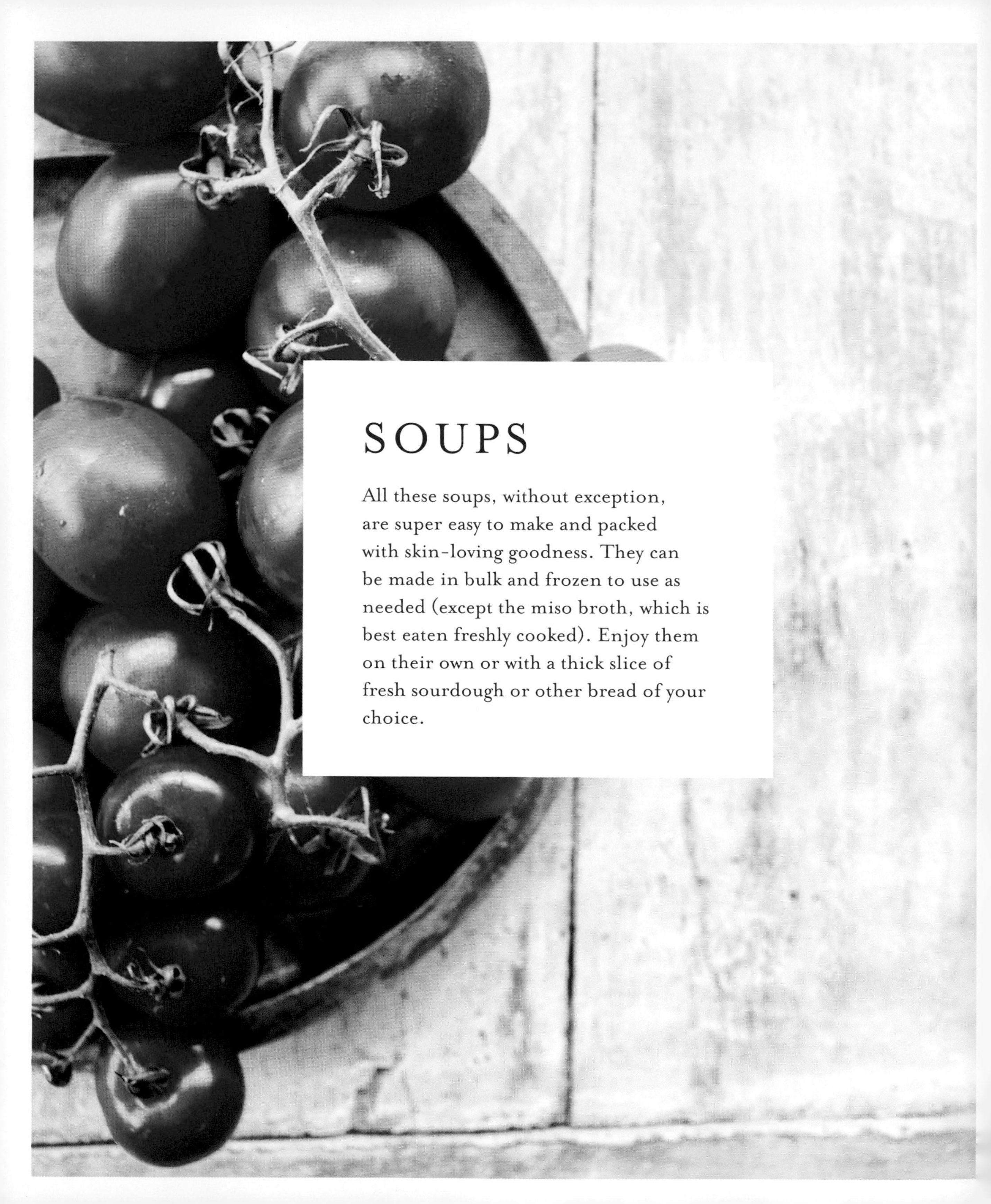

SOUPS

All these soups, without exception, are super easy to make and packed with skin-loving goodness. They can be made in bulk and frozen to use as needed (except the miso broth, which is best eaten freshly cooked). Enjoy them on their own or with a thick slice of fresh sourdough or other bread of your choice.

Quick Homemade Vegetable Stock

Make this simple stock in bulk and freeze in smaller containers to defrost as required for soups and other dishes.

Any leftover cooked or raw vegetables can be used, along with a base of celery (full stalk, including leaves), leeks and carrots.

Chop all vegetables into 2cm pieces and place in a large saucepan. Add one or two bay leaves (depending on how much is being made), some thyme, parsley, lemon peel and other herbs of choice. Cover with cold water (use 1.5l of water for each 1kg of vegetables). Bring to the boil and then cook on medium-high heat for about 30 minutes. Cool, strain and decant into freezer-friendly containers.

Creamy Squash and Red Pepper Soup

1 large squash, peeled, deseeded and cut into chunks

3 large tomatoes, quartered

3 large red peppers, deseeded and quartered

3 tbsp olive oil

few sprigs fresh rosemary

few sprigs fresh thyme

2 red onions, peeled and finely chopped

2 tsp harissa or smoked paprika (depending on taste)

4 stalks celery, chopped (use all of stalk)

1l homemade (see page 173) or low-salt vegetable stock

1 orange, juice and zest

sea salt and black pepper, to taste

natural yoghurt, to serve

Preheat oven to 180°C.

Place squash, tomatoes and peppers on a roasting tray. Toss with 1 tbsp of olive oil and a few sprigs of rosemary and thyme. Place in oven for 20–25 mins or until cooked and starting to brown.

Add 2 tbsp olive oil to a pan and sauté the chopped red onion over a medium heat. Add the harissa or smoked paprika after a few minutes.

Once the onions have started to caramelise, add the roasted peppers, tomatoes and squash, the celery, the stock and the orange juice and zest and bring to the boil. Reduce the heat and simmer for 5–10 minutes.

Remove from the heat and allow to cool a little before whizzing in a blender. Add more stock or boiling water, if required. Season to taste and serve with a dollop of natural yoghurt on top.

TIP: You can play around with this soup mix to keep it tasty and seasonal and find what works best for you. Squash can be replaced with sweet potato, and extra seasonal vegetables can also be added to up the ante nutritionally.

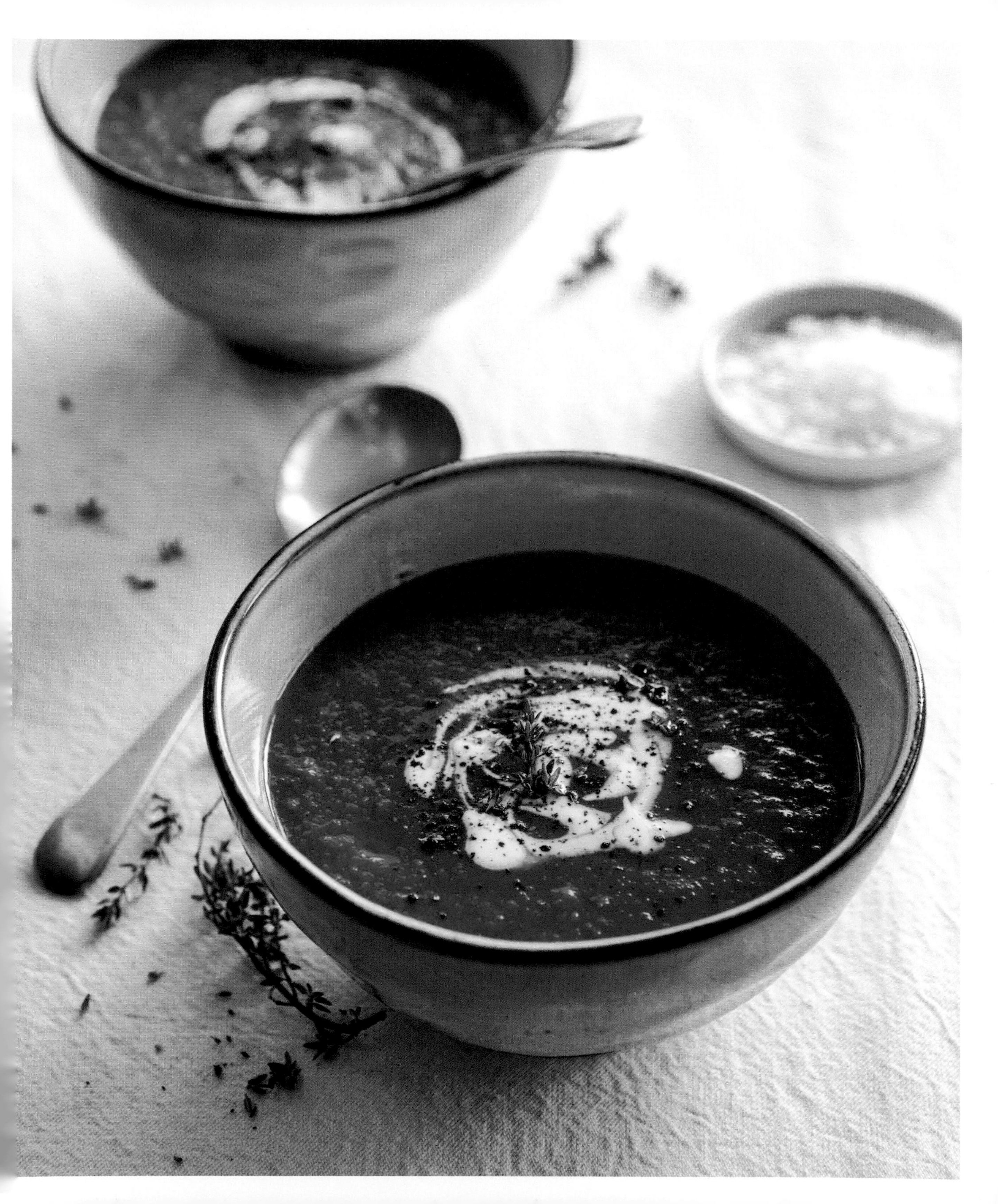

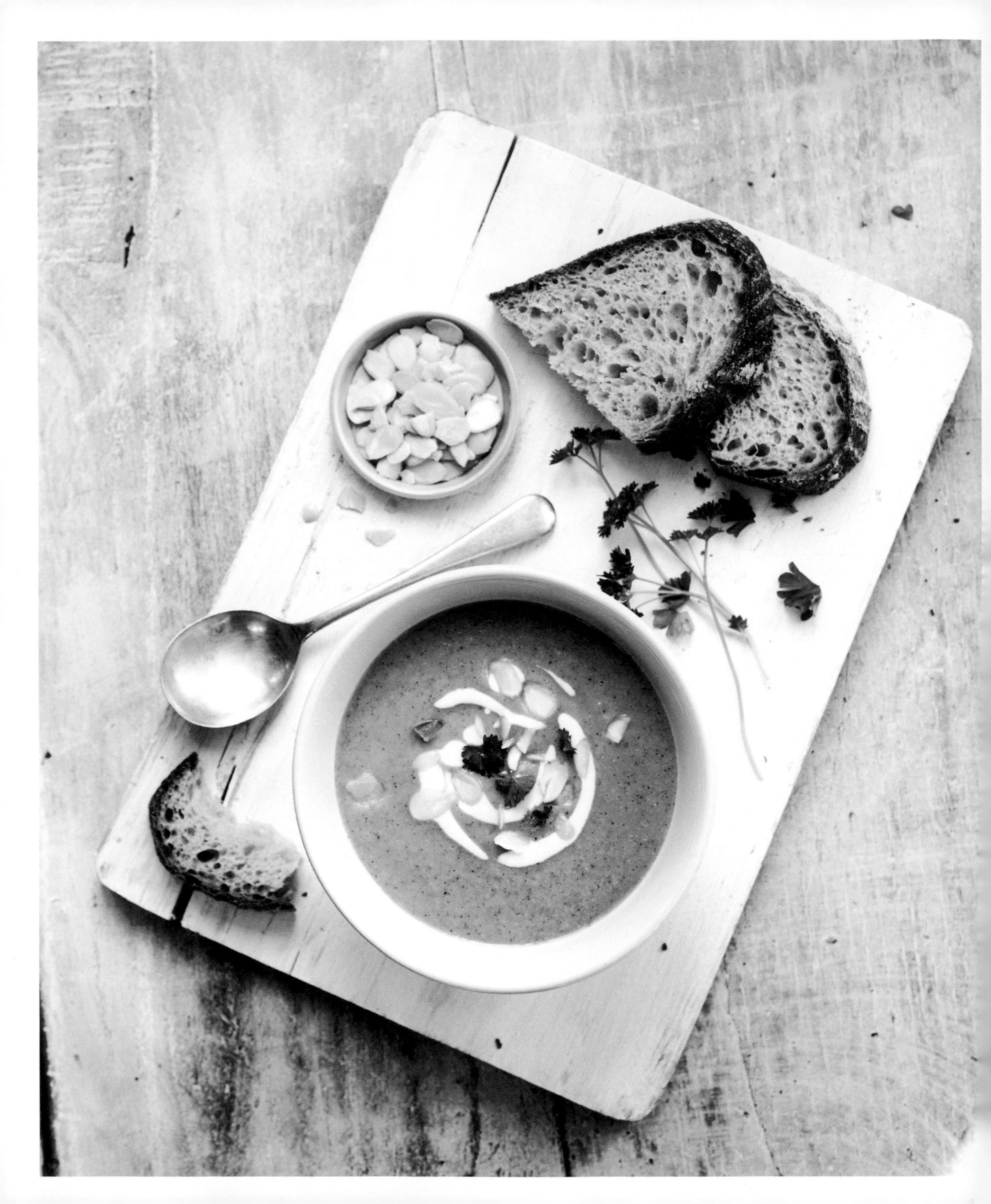

Courgette and Almond Soup

- 2 tbsp olive or rapeseed oil
- 1 large onion, chopped
- 1 large clove garlic, chopped
- 1 large leek, chopped
- 2 medium courgettes, chopped
- 80g flaked almonds
- 600ml homemade (see page 173) or low-salt vegetable stock
- pinch mixed herbs
- sea salt and black pepper, to taste
- natural yoghurt, to serve

SERVES 2–3

Heat the oil in a saucepan over a medium heat. Add the onion, garlic, leek and courgettes and sauté for about 5 minutes or until they start to soften.

Add most of the flaked almonds (reserving a few for decoration), the vegetable stock, a pinch of mixed herbs and some salt and pepper and bring to the boil. Reduce the heat and simmer for about 15 minutes.

Remove from the heat and cool a little before blending until smooth. Reheat over a low heat. Season to taste and top each bowl with a generous dollop of natural yoghurt and the remaining flaked almonds.

Quick Miso Broth with Edamame

Miso is a Japanese seasoning paste produced by fermenting soya beans. It is at the core of traditional Japanese cuisine and is a wonderfully nourishing addition to soups and stews, adding that wonderful umami taste.

The benefits of seaweed speak for themselves (see page 87) but many people struggle with how best to use it in food. Now is the perfect time to experiment! Wakame is ideal for this broth, but use whatever variety you can get. Most need to be soaked prior to use so always check cooking instructions.

2 tbsp olive oil

1 small leek, thinly sliced

1 clove garlic, peeled and finely chopped

2cm fresh root ginger, peeled and finely chopped

5 strips dried wakame (or about 1 small cup (110g) dried nori, thinly sliced, or 5 strands dried sea spaghetti)

140g edamame beans, defrosted and shelled

80g shitake mushrooms, sliced

1 tbsp tamari or soy sauce

1l homemade (see page 173) or low-salt vegetable stock

large handful fresh coriander, chopped

2 tbsp miso paste (superior quality, organic)

2 spring onions, finely chopped, to garnish

SERVES 4

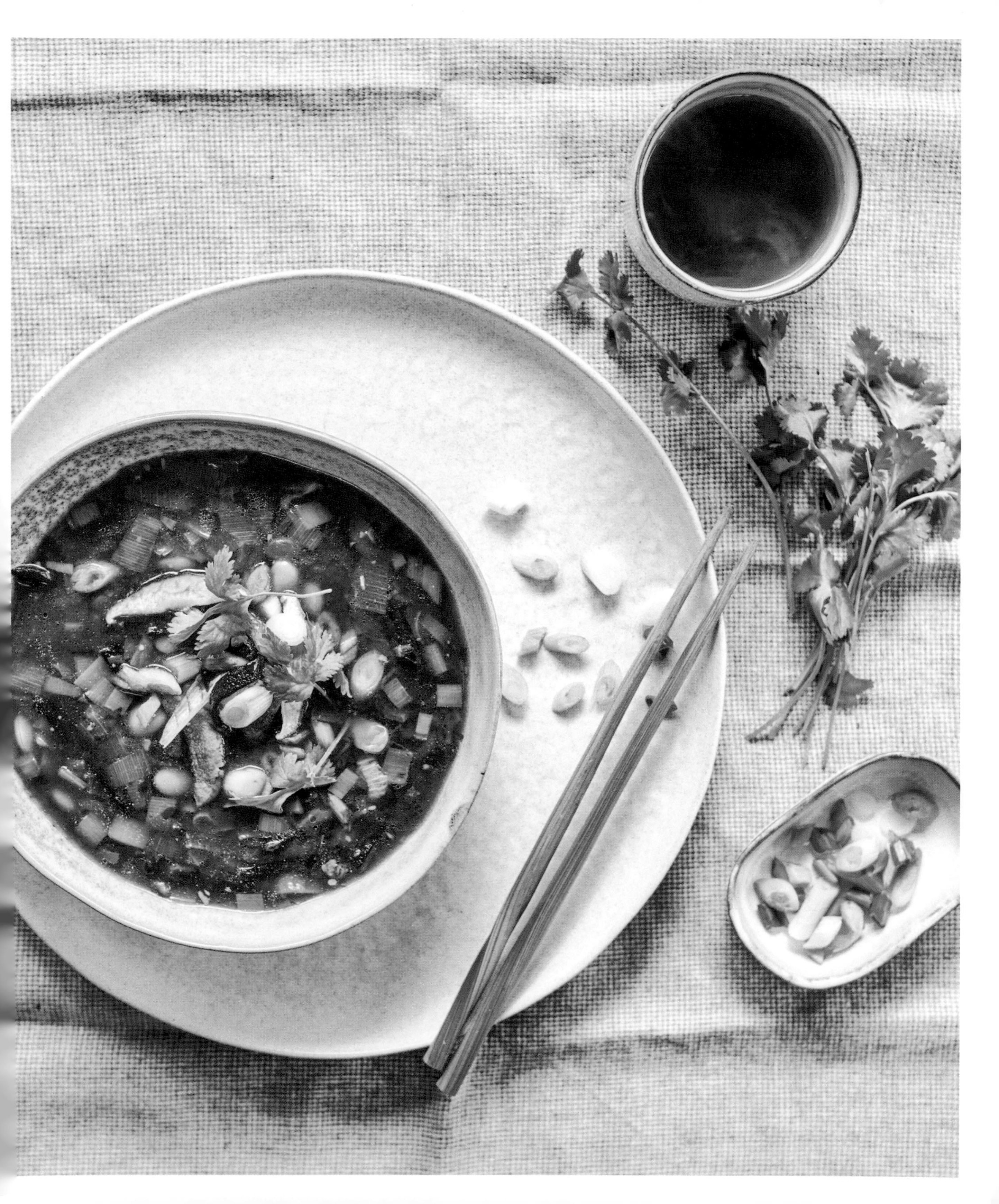

Heat the olive oil in a saucepan and sauté the leek, garlic and ginger. Allow to sweat for about 5 minutes. Add the seaweed, edamame, mushrooms, tamari and stock and ¾ of the coriander. Simmer for about 15 minutes.

Transfer about 300ml of broth from the saucepan into a bowl, Allow to cool a little before stirring in the miso (if the broth is too hot it could kill the active enzymes in the miso). Pour back into the saucepan and mix. Serve in bowls topped with the remaining coriander and the spring onion.

TIP: Varieties of umami-rich miso differ in colour and flavour based on how long they have been fermented. Mellow white miso is a good all-rounder, while yellow miso can have a strong flavour. Robust red miso is most suited to rich braises or marinades.

Spinach and Broccoli Soup with Flaked Almonds

2 tbsp olive or rapeseed oil

1 medium red onion, chopped

2 cloves garlic, crushed

1 large leek, chopped

4 stalks celery, sliced (use all of the stalk)

1 large head broccoli, chopped (use florets and stalk)

1 tbsp lemon juice

large pinch mixed herbs

1 large or 2 small bay leaves

500g spinach leaves

100g flaked almonds

800ml homemade (see page 173) or low-salt vegetable stock

sea salt and black pepper to taste

60g edamame beans, defrosted and shelled (optional)

natural yoghurt, to serve

Heat the oil in a saucepan over a medium heat. Add the red onion, garlic, leek and celery and sauté for about 5 minutes or until the vegetables start to soften. Add the chopped broccoli, lemon juice, mixed herbs and bay leaves and continue cooking for another 7–8 minutes before adding the spinach leaves and flaked almonds. Pour in the vegetable stock and bring to the boil. Reduce heat and simmer for 15–20 minutes.

Remove from the heat and cool a little. Remove the bay leaves and blend in a food processor or blender until smooth. Reheat on a low heat; add the edamame (if using). Season to taste and serve with a generous dollop of natural yoghurt.

TIP: When cooking with broccoli always use the stalk as well as the florets – lots of skin-loving goodness is packed in there.

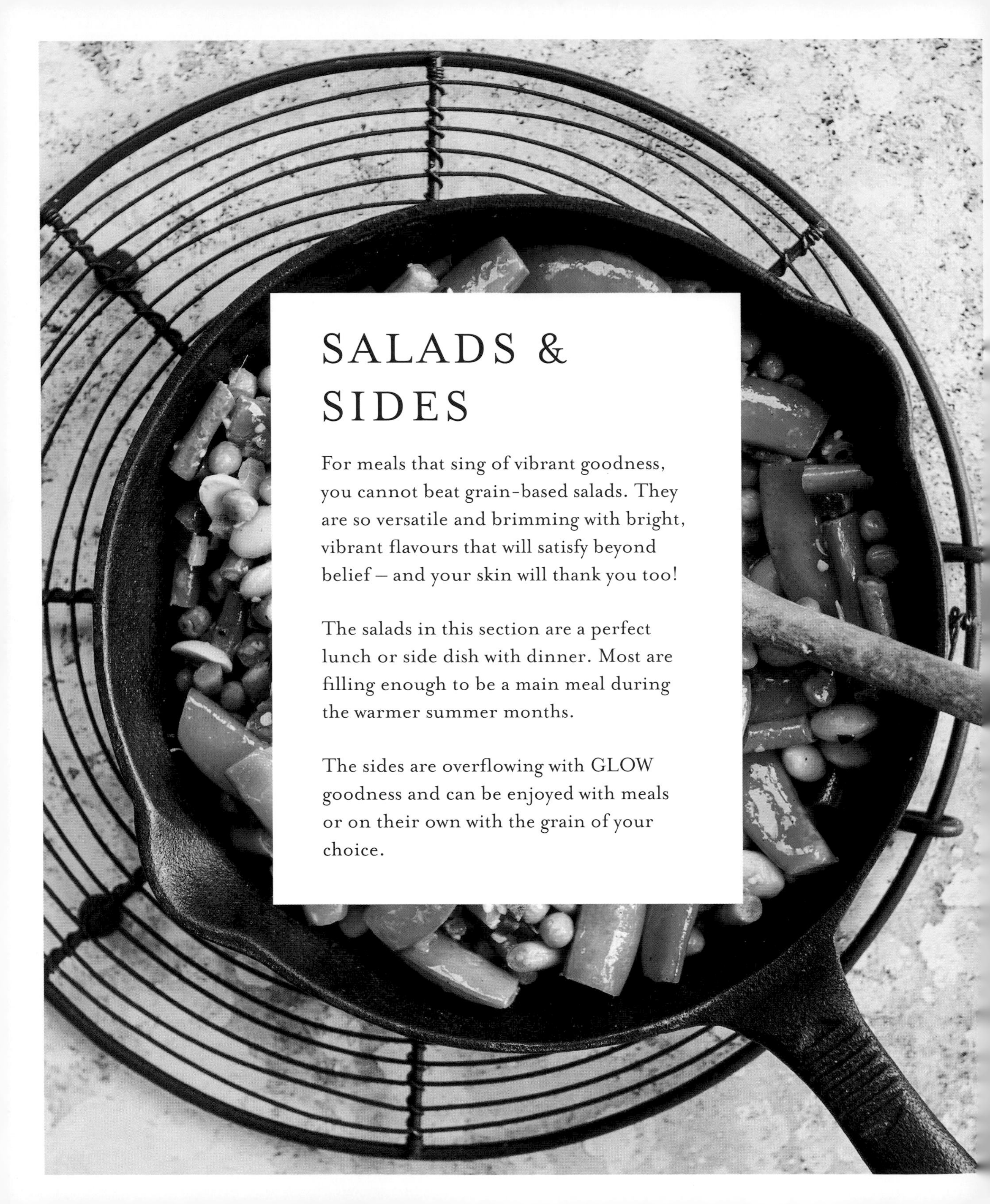

SALADS & SIDES

For meals that sing of vibrant goodness, you cannot beat grain-based salads. They are so versatile and brimming with bright, vibrant flavours that will satisfy beyond belief – and your skin will thank you too!

The salads in this section are a perfect lunch or side dish with dinner. Most are filling enough to be a main meal during the warmer summer months.

The sides are overflowing with GLOW goodness and can be enjoyed with meals or on their own with the grain of your choice.

Spring Medley

Use this recipe as a guide, adding any seasonal vegetables of your choice.

- 2 tbsp olive oil
- 1 red onion, peeled and finely chopped
- 1 clove garlic, peeled and finely chopped
- 100g French beans, rinsed and cut into 3cm pieces
- 100g sugar snap peas, rinsed and tailed
- 100g edamame beans or peas, defrosted and shelled
- 200ml homemade (see page 173) or low-salt vegetable stock
- ½ lemon or lime, juice only
- sea salt and black pepper to taste

SERVES 4 AS A SIDE DISH

Heat 1 tbsp oil in a pan and gentle sauté the onion and garlic for about 5 minutes. Add the other vegetables and stock and bring to the boil. Reduce the heat and simmer for a few minutes until the vegetables are cooked. Drizzle the rest of the oil over, along with the lemon or lime juice. Serve immediately.

Quinoa, Pomegranate and Feta Salad

Goat's cheese could also be used in place of feta.

- 150g uncooked quinoa
- ½ clove garlic, finely chopped
- 350ml vegetable stock or water
- 120g spinach, roughly chopped
- 100g feta cheese, cubed
- 3–4 baby tomatoes or 2 medium tomatoes, chopped
- 1 avocado, peeled and sliced
- 1 small cooked beetroot, cut into chunks
- small handful each fresh mint, coriander and parsley, chopped
- 1 tbsp olive oil
- 1 tbsp balsamic vinegar (or other vinegar of choice)
- large handful pomegranate seeds
- handful chopped walnuts, to serve

SERVES 2

Place quinoa and garlic in a saucepan with vegetable stock or water. Bring to the boil then reduce heat and simmer for 15–20 minutes or until all the water has been absorbed.

Allow the quinoa to cool a little and place in a bowl. Add spinach, cheese, tomatoes, avocado, beetroot and herbs. Drizzle the olive oil and vinegar over the salad and sprinkle pomegranate seeds and chopped walnuts over the top.

TIP: For a taste of the Mediterranean, you can switch the quinoa in any of the recipes for couscous – although the overall protein content will be reduced.

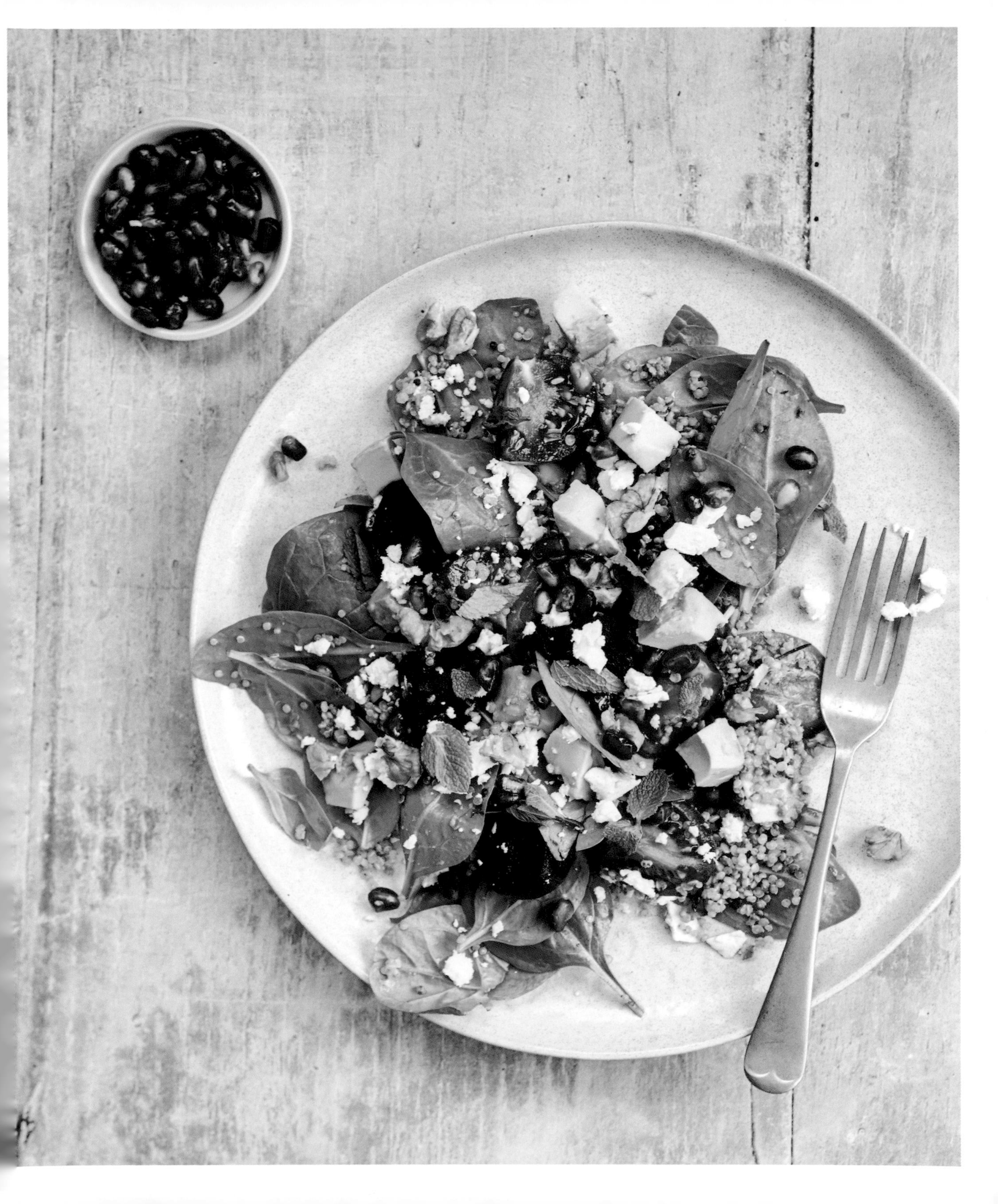

Orange, Walnut and Quinoa Salad

- 170g uncooked quinoa
- 500 ml homemade (see page 173) or low-salt vegetable stock
- 2 oranges, peeled and diced (if pith is thick, remove it first)
- 2 small red onions, peeled and thinly sliced
- 1 stalk celery, finely sliced
- 75g roughly chopped walnuts
- 120g edamame beans, defrosted and shelled
- 2 tbsp pomegranate seeds
- handful fresh coriander, chopped (optional)
- 75g crumbled feta (optional)
- Zesty Apple Cider Vinaigrette (see page 165)
- sea salt and black pepper

AS A SIDE
LIGHT MEAL

Toast the quinoa in a saucepan over a medium heat, stirring often, until the grains begin to pop. Add the vegetable stock and bring to the boil. Reduce heat to a simmer, cover and cook for 10 minutes or until the liquid is absorbed. Leave to cool, then transfer to a salad bowl. Add the remaining ingredients and pour over the Zesty Apple Cider Vinaigrette. Toss to combine, adjusting seasoning to your liking. Serve.

TIP: Pomegranate seeds add a splash of colour and a bucket-load of goodness, so even if they are not included in a salad recipe, add a handful before serving.

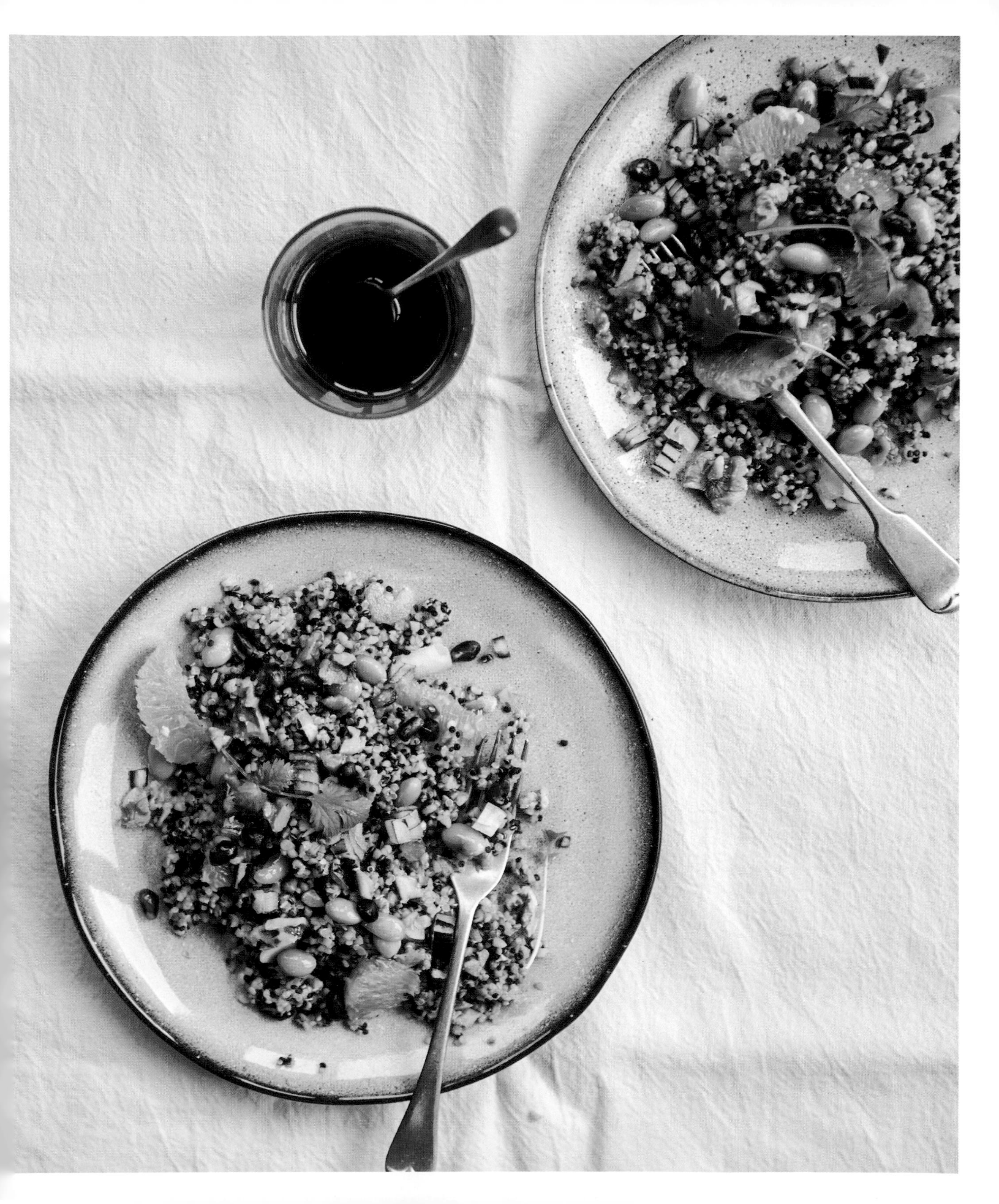

Beetroot, Edamame and Orange Salad

If having as a light meal on its own, feel free to add some extra protein such as a free-range hard-boiled egg, extra edamame or another pulse.

700–800g raw beetroot

2 oranges, peeled

60g pumpkin seeds

60g chopped walnuts

80g baby spinach

120g edamame beans, defrosted and shelled

olive oil

balsamic vinegar

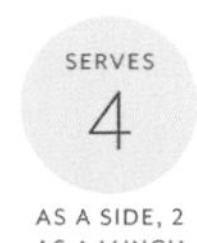

AS A SIDE, 2 AS A LUNCH

Remove all dirt from the beetroot and top and tail it. Scrub the skin but do not peel. Then grate into a salad bowl – you could also try using a mandoline to slice the beetroot paper thin.

Cut the peeled oranges into bite-size segments and mix with the beetroot. Toast the pumpkin seeds in a dry pan for a few minutes until they start to colour. Add to the beetroot along with the chopped walnuts, spinach and edamame beans.

Dress the salad with a mix of 3 parts olive oil to 1 part balsamic vinegar or try the Zesty Apple Cider Vinaigrette (page 165).

Sautéed Spinach with Edamame

2 tbsp olive oil

4 large handfuls spinach

1 clove garlic, finely chopped

large handful edamame beans, defrosted and shelled

sea salt and black pepper, to taste

oyster sauce, to drizzle

SERVES 2 AS A SIDE DISH

Heat the oil in a pan. When hot, add the spinach and garlic and cook over a medium heat for about 2 minutes, until wilted. Add the edamame beans, sea salt and pepper and drizzle a little oyster sauce over. Cook for another minute or so and serve immediately.

TIP: This can also be enjoyed served as a main on a bed of short-grain brown rice.

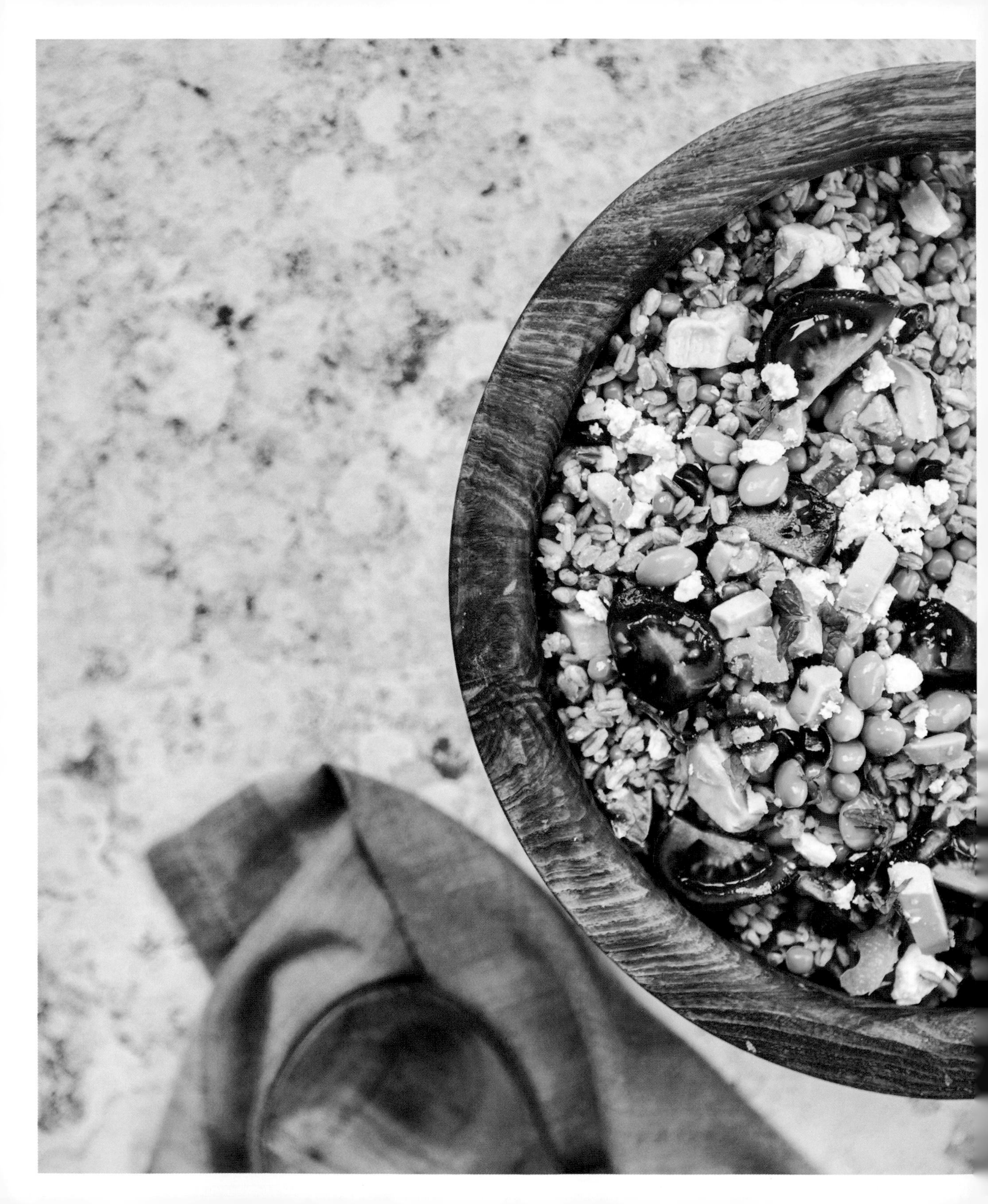

Minted Farro and Three Bean Salad with Goat's Cheese

125g farro

750ml water

large handful fresh mint leaves

150g frozen edamame (or broad) beans, defrosted and shelled

150g frozen petit pois, thawed

200g baby kale or baby spinach leaves

½ lime, juice only

2 tbsp extra virgin olive oil

½ avocado, peeled and sliced

5–6 cherry tomatoes, halved

50g goat's cheese, cubed

2 tbsp pomegranate seeds

handful chopped walnuts

handful fresh coriander, chopped (optional)

sea salt and black pepper

SERVES 3–4

Rinse the farro and place in a medium saucepan with the water, mint leaves and a pinch of salt. Cover and bring to the boil. Reduce heat to low and cook for 20–25 minutes or until the grain is tender. Drain and place in a large bowl, discarding the mint leaves. Meanwhile, put the edamame and peas in small pot of boiling water and cook for 2–3 minutes. Drain and plunge into cold water (to retain colour and maximise nutrient content). Mix with the farro. Add the baby kale or spinach leaves. Drizzle lime juice and olive oil over the salad and toss to combine. Add the avocado, tomatoes and goat's cheese, and sprinkle the pomegranate seeds, chopped walnuts and coriander, if using, on top. For an added flavour hit use the Tahini Dressing on page 166.

TIP: you can substitute buckwheat for the farro – simply cook as for the farro but for a shorter time.

Cannellini Bean Salad with Marinated Alaria

Some people avoid seaweed, as they are not sure what varieties to choose or how best to cook them. This recipe by seaweed expert Prannie Rhatigan of the Irish Seaweed Kitchen is one of my favourites – she is a fount of knowledge on the benefits and uses of this invaluable foodstuff (see page 87 for more).

25g raisins

2 lemons, juice only

100ml olive oil

½ onion, finely chopped

2 garlic cloves, finely chopped

½ red chilli, seeds removed, finely sliced

¼ tsp black onion seeds

450g (or 2 tins) cooked cannellini beans

2 bananas, sliced

½ fresh mango, roughly chopped

Marinated Alaria (see below)

large handful coriander leaves, chopped, plus extra to decorate

SERVES 4

Place the raisins and lemon juice in a small bowl – the raisins will plump up.

Heat the oil in a large frying pan and fry the onion until soft. Add the garlic, chilli and onion seeds and fry for 2–3 minutes. Leave aside and allow to cool.

Rinse the cannellini beans, drain and place in a large bowl. Add the soaked raisins and lemon juice, stirring well. Add the cooled onion and chilli and mix will. Add the bananas, mango, Marinated Alaria and a large handful of coriander. Mix gently. Then decorate with the remaining coriander leaves.

Marinated Alaria

2 x 15cm pieces fresh alaria (or same length of dried) cut into 1–2.5cm pieces

1 tbsp tamari or soya sauce

3 cloves garlic, crushed

2 tsp honey

1 tbsp olive oil

1 tsp grated ginger

dash of toasted sesame oil

Place the alaria in a bowl and cover with tepid water. Soak for about 20 minutes. Combine the rest of the ingredients, except the sesame oil, in a small saucepan and boil for 1 minute. Add the alaria to the saucepan with some of the soaking water and bring back to the boil. Simmer for about 40 minutes or until the tough midrib is tender – add more soaking water if necessary. When cooked, remove from the heat. Add a little toasted sesame oil and more honey if needed.

TIP: Marinated Alaria is a delicious addition to most salads, or you can serve it as a side dish with the grain of your choice.

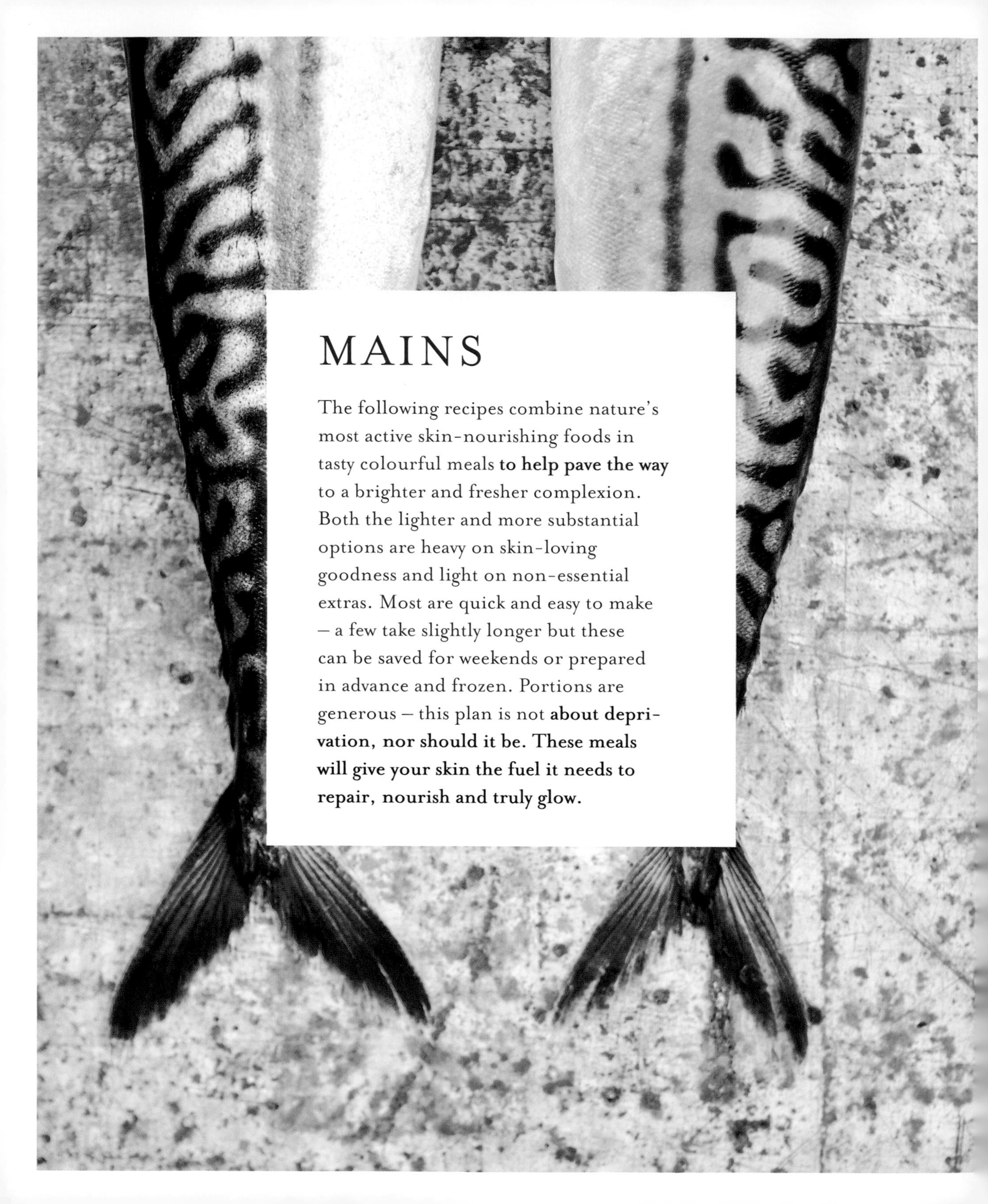

MAINS

The following recipes combine nature's most active skin-nourishing foods in tasty colourful meals **to help pave the way** to a brighter and fresher complexion. Both the lighter and more substantial options are heavy on skin-loving goodness and light on non-essential extras. Most are quick and easy to make – a few take slightly longer but these can be saved for weekends or prepared in advance and frozen. Portions are generous – this plan is not **about deprivation, nor should it be. These meals will give your skin the fuel it needs to repair, nourish and truly glow.**

GLOW Frittata

This is best served hot but any leftovers can be eaten cold.

- 2–3 tbsp olive oil
- 2 leeks, finely chopped
- 1 clove garlic, peeled and crushed
- large handful baby spinach leaves
- 2 medium sweet potatoes, peeled and cut into very thin strips
- 5–6 sprigs of thyme, leaves only
- 10 cherry tomatoes, halved
- 8 eggs
- handful fresh flat-leaf parsley, finely chopped
- 100g Parmesan (or other hard cheese), grated
- 120g frozen peas, thawed
- sea salt and black pepper, to taste

SERVES 4

Preheat oven to 200°C.

Heat 1 tbsp of olive oil in a large pan over a low heat. Add the leeks and garlic and cook for about 5 minutes until softened. Remove from the heat and transfer to a bowl. Rinse the spinach under cold water and drain in a sieve. Add it to the frying pan and cook for 1–2 minutes, stirring continuously, so the leaves steam in the residual water. When the spinach is cooked, but still bright green, transfer it to the sieve and press with the back of a spoon to squeeze any remaining water from the leaves. Add to the leek and crushed garlic and set aside.

Add another 1 tbsp of oil to the pan, followed by the finely sliced sweet potatoes and the leaves from about 4 sprigs of thyme. Cook over a medium to high heat for about 7–8 minutes. Add the tomatoes and cook for another 2–3 minutes until the sweet potato is turning golden. Remove from the heat.

Crack the eggs into a bowl. Add the parsley and whisk together. Add the grated Parmesan and combine.

Put the leek mixture back into the pan with the sweet potatoes and tomatoes. Add the cooked spinach and peas. Pour the egg mixture over this and combine well. Season with salt and black pepper and bake in the oven for about 10–12 minutes or until the top has puffed up and the frittata is fairly firm. If you want a crisper top, finish the frittata under the grill for a few minutes before serving, but be careful not to burn! Serve on its own or with Mango, Pomegranate and Cucumber Salsa (page 171).

Sweet Potato, Pea and Courgette Cakes

1 large or 2 small courgette (about 200g)

1 large sweet potato (about 300g), peeled

150g frozen peas

60g pecorino or Parmesan cheese, grated

3 spring onions, finely chopped

small handful each parsley and chives, chopped

50g breadcrumbs

½ tsp minced garlic

sea salt and black pepper, to taste

2 eggs

3 tbsp olive or light vegetable oil

handful of flour, for coating

1 lime, cut into 4 wedges

200g baby spinach leaves

handful walnuts, chopped

Zesty Apple Cider Vinaigrette (see page 165)

MAKES 12

Preheat the oven to 120°C. Line a baking tray.

Coarsely grate the courgette and sweet potato and place in a colander. Use your hands to squeeze out any excess liquid before transferring to a clean bowl (the more liquid that can be squeezed out the better). Put the peas in a small bowl and cover with boiling water. Leave for about 5 minutes, then drain and mix with the courgette and sweet potato. Add the grated cheese, finely chopped spring onion, parsley, chives, breadcrumbs and minced garlic. Season with salt and pepper and mix. Whisk eggs and add, mixing thoroughly with your hands to ensure everything is well combined.

Heat the oil in a large non-stick frying pan over a medium heat. Divide the mixture into large tablespoon-sized patties. Mould with your hands and place on a well-floured surface to coat on both sides. Place in the pan and cook for about 4 minutes each side or until golden brown and cooked through. Transfer to the lined tray and place in the oven to keep warm. Repeat with the remaining patties. Divide between 4 plates and serve with the lime wedges and a side salad of young spinach leaves topped with chopped walnuts and dressed with Zesty Apple Cider Vinaigrette.

Broccolini Risotto

- 2 tbsp olive oil
- 1 red onion, peeled and finely chopped
- 1 clove garlic, peeled and crushed
- 1 stick celery, finely chopped
- 250g short-grain brown rice
- 1l homemade (see page 173) or low-salt vegetable stock
- 8 stems broccolini
- 1 tbsp fresh parsley, chopped
- 100g edamame beans (or 150g frozen peas), defrosted and shelled
- ½ tsp dried oregano
- 80g pecorino or Parmesan, grated (or choose vegetarian option)
- bunch fresh coriander, chopped, to garnish

SERVES 4

Heat the oil in a pan and sauté the chopped onion and garlic for 1–2 minutes. Add the chopped celery. Continue cooking until it's nicely soft and turning brown. Slowly stir in the rice, followed by the stock. Bring to the boil then reduce the heat and simmer, with the lid on, for about 15 minutes.

Chop the stems of the broccolini, leaving the heads intact. Add the stems and parsley to the rice and continue cooking for another 5 minutes, with the lid on. When the liquid is almost gone, add the broccolini heads and edamame beans (or peas) and simmer for another 3 minutes before mixing in the dried oregano and the grated cheese. Divide between bowls and garnish with chopped coriander.

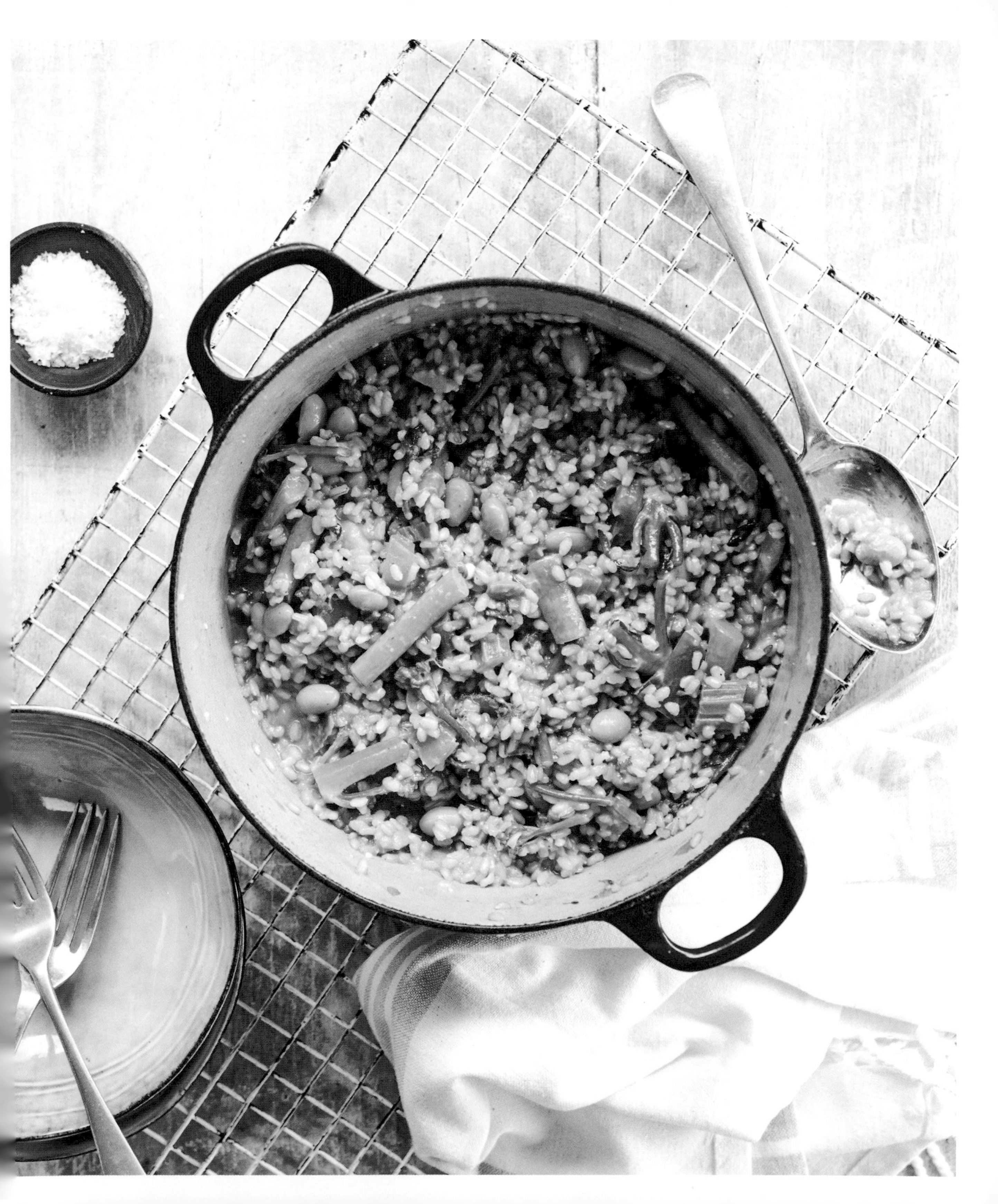

Nachos with a Twist

This delicious twist on nachos is adapted from the brilliant Anna Jones, who would inspire even the least culinarily-inclined to cook with gusto.

- 12 cherry tomatoes, halved
- 1 red pepper, deseeded and cut into thick strips
- olive oil
- sea salt and pepper
- 4 wholemeal wraps
- 1 tsp smoked paprika
- 400g can red kidney beans, drained and washed
- 1 cooked corn on the cob, kernels only
- squeeze fresh lime juice
- 1 ripe avocado, peeled and chopped into cubes
- bunch fresh coriander, chopped
- Cashew Cream (see page 168)

SERVES
3–4
AS LUNCH OR LIGHT DINNER

Preheat the oven to 210°C.

Place the tomatoes and pepper slices on a baking tray, drizzle with some oil and season with salt and pepper. Roast for 20 minutes.

Cut the wholemeal wraps into tortilla-chip shapes. Spread the chips out on a baking tray and make sure they don't overlap. Coat with a little oil and sprinkle with salt, pepper and smoked paprika. Cook in the oven for about 10 minutes, until nicely browned. Transfer to a deep baking dish.

In the meantime, combine the roast peppers and tomatoes with the kidney beans, sweetcorn kernels, a little olive oil, a squeeze of lime juice, sea salt and pepper in a bowl. Mix well. Pour over the chips, with some extra smoked paprika. Put back into the oven for another 10 minutes. Remove and top with avocado, chopped coriander and a few dollops of cashew cream. Serve hot.

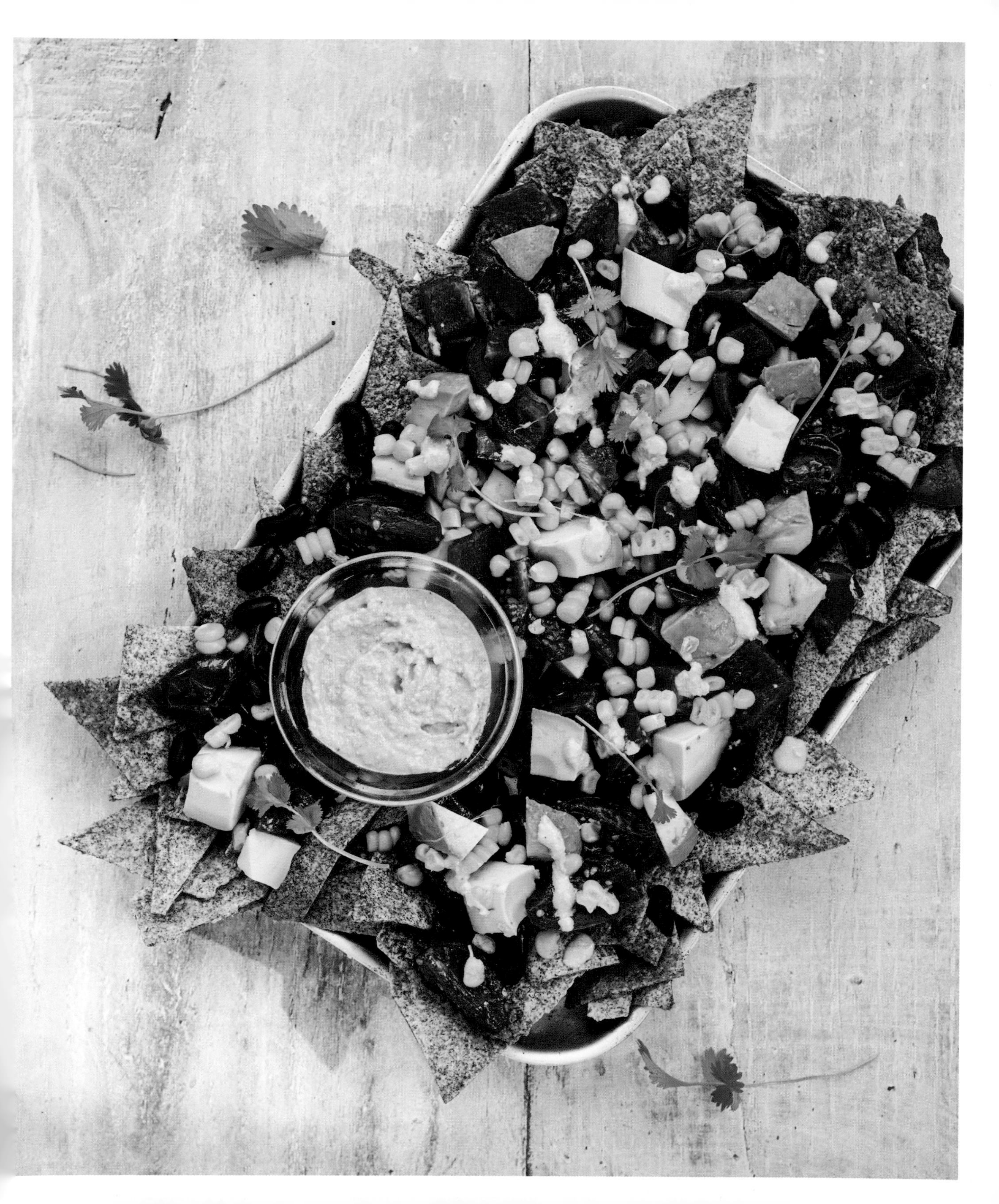

Shepherdless Pie

- 200g uncooked green lentils
- 2 medium sweet potatoes, peeled and roughly chopped
- 2 tbsp olive or rapeseed oil
- 1 red onion, peeled and diced
- 2 cloves garlic, peeled and finely chopped
- 1 large carrot, peeled and diced
- 1 red pepper, deseeded and diced
- 1 courgette, cut into half rounds
- 8 cherry tomatoes, halved
- 400ml homemade (see page 173) or low-salt vegetable stock
- 100ml red wine
- 2 tsp mixed herbs
- 1 bay leaf
- knob of butter (or extra oil)
- sea salt and black pepper

SERVES
3–4

Preheat the oven to 200°C.

Cook the lentils according to the directions on the pack.

Place the sweet potatoes in a pot and cover with boiling water. Bring to the boil, then simmer for 10 minutes or until tender. Drain and leave in the pot, covered with a clean dry cloth to absorb excess moisture.

In a large saucepan, heat the oil and add the red onion, garlic, carrot, red pepper, courgette and cherry tomatoes. Sauté over a medium heat for 10 minutes until softened. Pour in the vegetable stock, red wine, cooked lentils, 1 tsp mixed herbs and the bay leaf. Bring to the boil and reduce to a simmer. Half cover and allow to reduce for 15 minutes. While the lentil mix is reducing, mash the cooked sweet potatoes with a large knob of butter (or a drizzle of olive oil), salt, pepper and 1 tsp of mixed herbs.

Pour the lentil mix into a medium-sized casserole dish and top with the mashed sweet potato. Cook in the oven for 15 minutes. Serve hot.

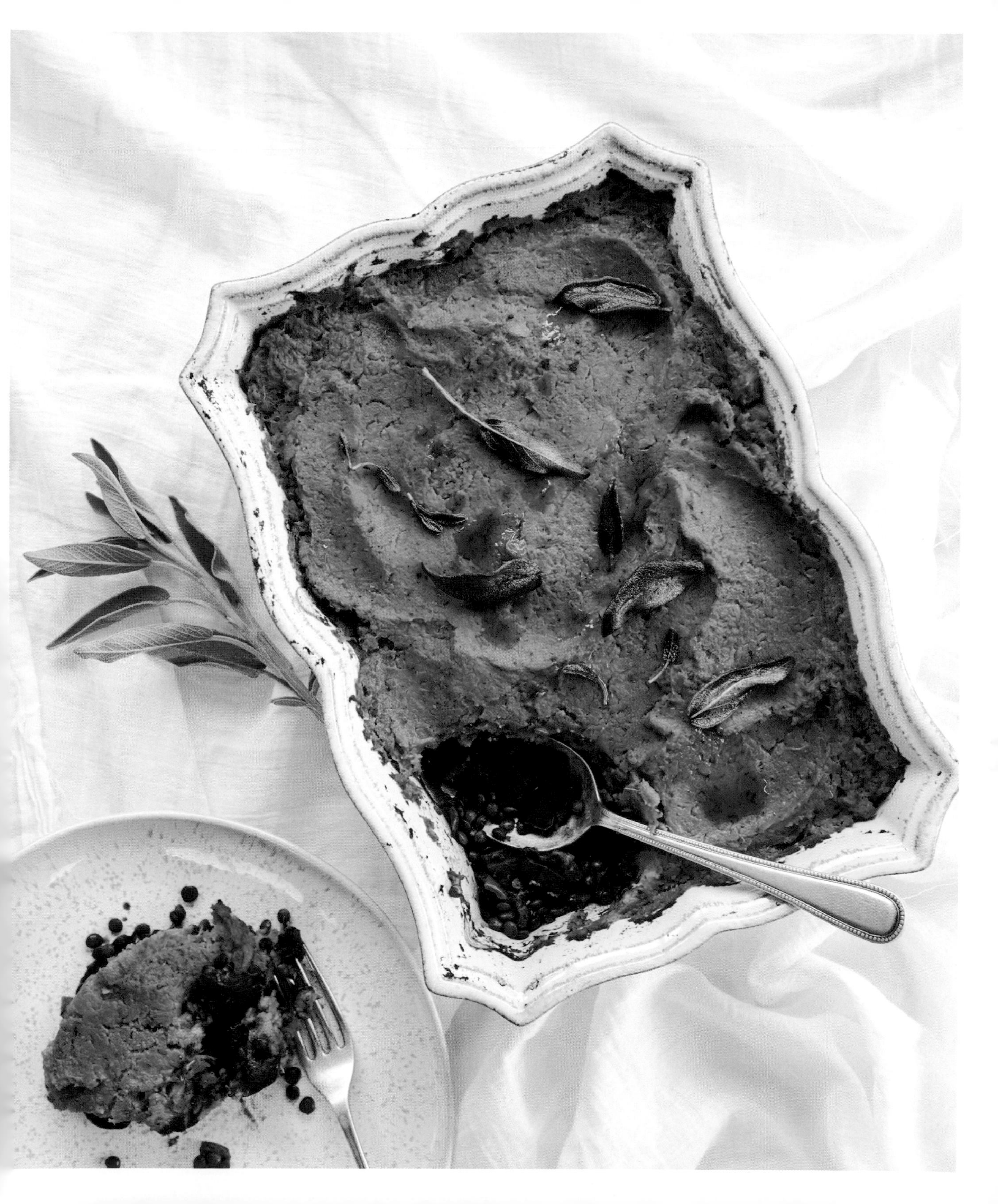

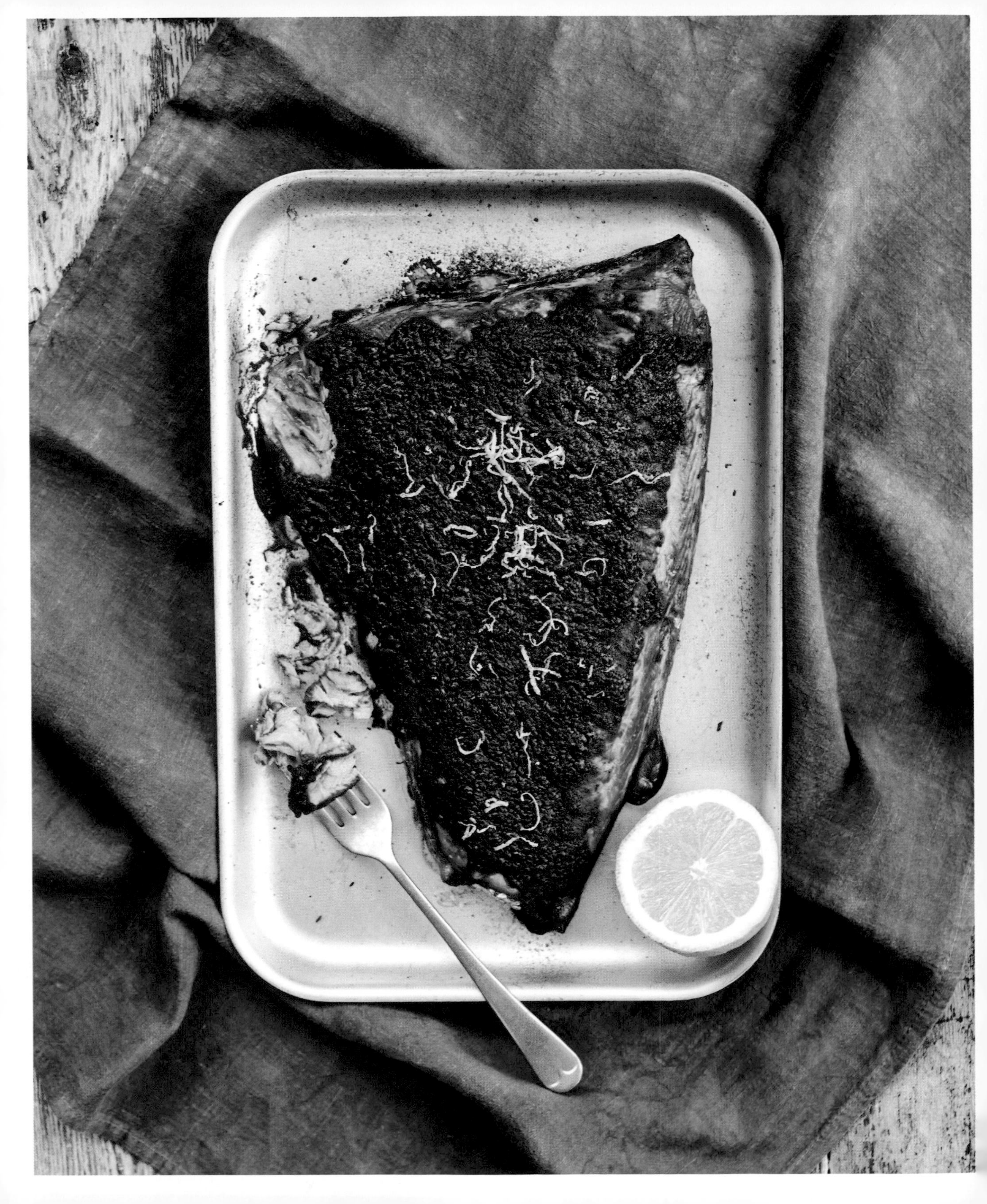

Salmon – Three Ways: Citrus Turmeric Salmon

Inspired by the wonderfully creative Sabrina Ghayour in her cookbook *Sirocco*, this recipe ticks all the boxes for skin vitality. What's more, it is so easy to prepare and can easily take centre stage at dinner parties.

450g (approx.) piece of salmon

1 orange, finely grated zest only

1 tsp black pepper

2 tbsp olive oil

1 tbsp turmeric

pinch sea salt

SERVES 3–4

Place salmon skin-side down on a lined baking tray or oven-proof dish. Combine all other ingredients (except the sea salt) in a small bowl to make a spreadable, smooth paste. Rub the mixture evenly over the salmon flesh. Leave in the refrigerator for at least one hour or overnight.

When ready to cook, preheat the oven to 240°C. Remove the salmon from the refrigerator and season with sea salt. Place in the oven and bake for about 20 minutes. Remove from the oven and serve with couscous, farro, short-grain rice or a salad of your choice.

Flax and Sesame Crusted Salmon with Spinach and Tahini

olive oil

200g baby spinach

60–70g tahini paste

½ lime, juice and zest

4 thick salmon fillets (approx. 180g each)

3 tbsp golden flax seeds

3 tbsp sesame seeds

SERVES 4

Preheat oven to 180°C. Grease a baking tray with a little olive oil.

Heat 2–3 tbsp water in a pot until boiling. Add the spinach and reduce the heat. Stir briefly until the spinach starts to wilt. Remove from heat and cool. Squeeze any excess water from the spinach and leave aside.

In small bowl, mix the tahini paste with the juice of half a lime and a little water if needed. Whisk until well combined. Add the cooked spinach and mix well. Make a large incision in each piece of salmon and fill with the spinach and tahini mix, pushing it in so it stays in place.

Mix the sesame and flax seeds on a plate. Brush the salmon with a little olive oil and roll each piece in the seeds before placing on the greased baking tray. Sprinkle any leftover seeds and the lime zest on top.

Place in the oven and bake for 15–20 minutes. Allow to rest for a few minutes. Serve with a side of your choice (pages 182–93).

TIP: This recipe works well with chicken breasts too – you can make pockets in the breasts by slicing diagonally along each one. Cook for slightly longer – 20–25 minutes.

Moroccan-Style Salmon

150g couscous

pinch turmeric powder

2–3 tbsp rapeseed or vegetable oil

1 clove garlic, peeled and finely chopped

1 medium courgette, cut into bite-sized rounds

1 red pepper, deseeded and cut into small chunks

4 medium cauliflower florets, chopped

10 cherry or sundried tomatoes, halved

1 ear of corn, kernels removed and cooked

1 tsp smoked paprika

1 tsp mixed herbs

sea salt and black pepper

3 salmon fillets (approx. 180g each)

generous handful fresh parsley, chopped

handful pomegranate seeds (optional)

½ lime, juice only

SERVES 3

Cook the couscous according to the directions on the packet, adding a generous pinch of turmeric before adding the water.

Heat half the oil in a saucepan and sauté the garlic over medium heat for one minute. Add the rest of the vegetables and the spices, mixed herbs and salt and pepper. Sauté for about 10 minutes until the vegetables are cooked. Transfer the cooked vegetables to a large bowl.

Heat the remaining oil in the pan. Add the salmon (skin side down) and cook for about 2 minutes before turning over. Reduce the heat and continue to cook until the salmon is just cooked through, about 5 minutes, removing immediately from the heat.

Mix the cooked couscous and vegetables in a large bowl. Add the chopped parsley and pomegranate seeds. Divide between 3 plates and place a salmon fillet on top of each serving of colourful couscous. Squeeze over a dash of lime juice and serve immediately.

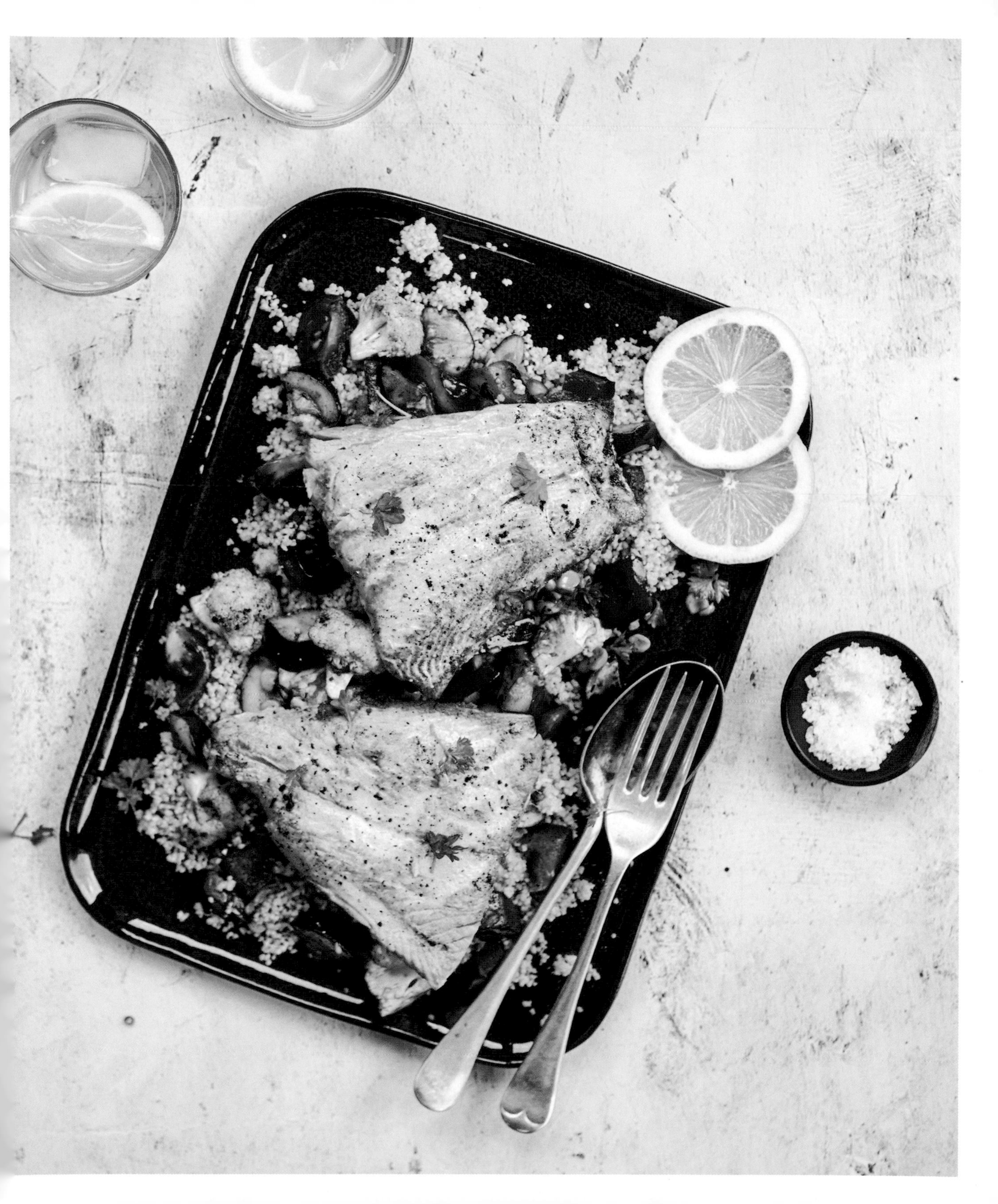

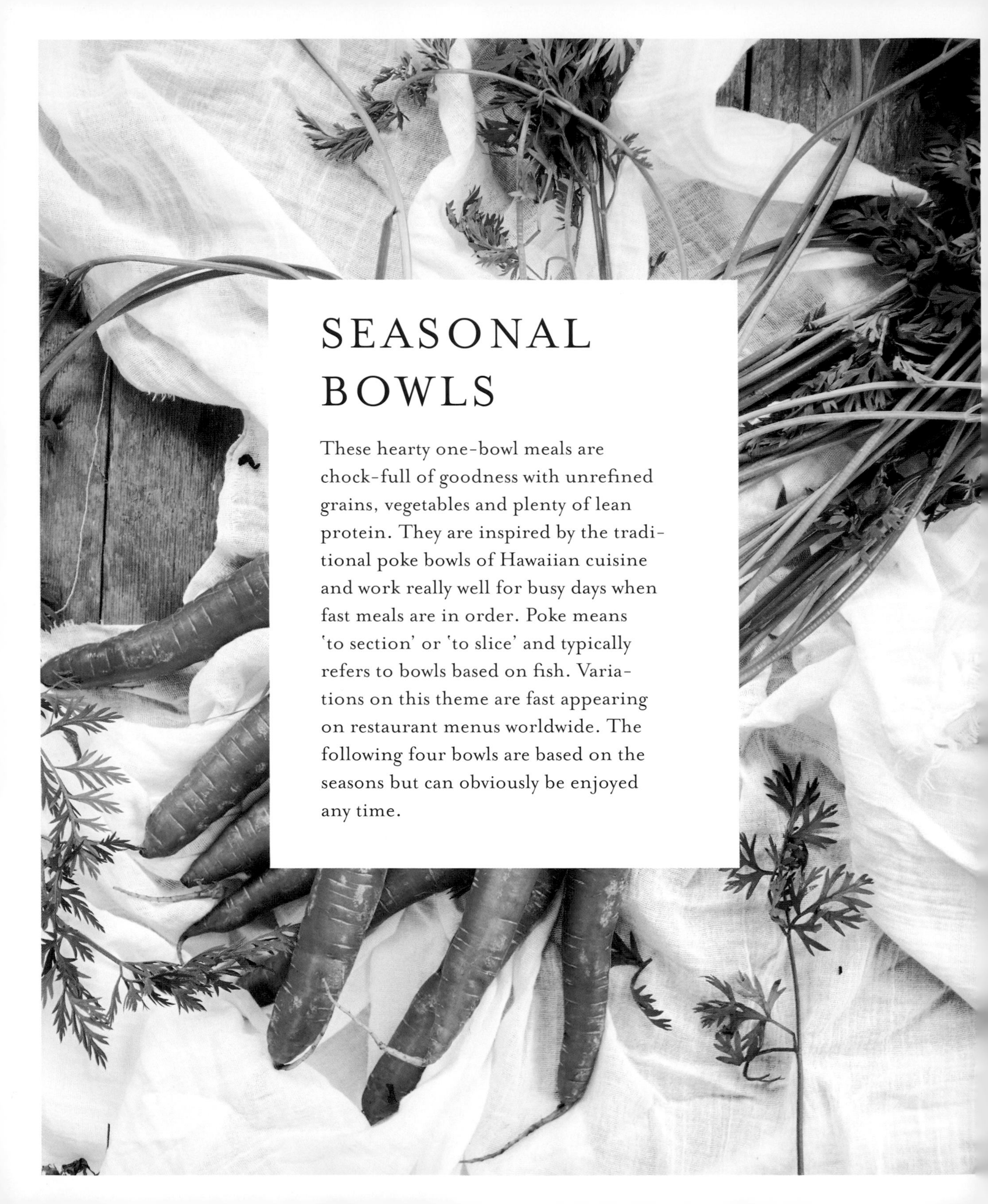

SEASONAL BOWLS

These hearty one-bowl meals are chock-full of goodness with unrefined grains, vegetables and plenty of lean protein. They are inspired by the traditional poke bowls of Hawaiian cuisine and work really well for busy days when fast meals are in order. Poke means 'to section' or 'to slice' and typically refers to bowls based on fish. Variations on this theme are fast appearing on restaurant menus worldwide. The following four bowls are based on the seasons but can obviously be enjoyed any time.

Spring: Asian-Style Salmon Bowl

120g short-grain brown rice

2 tbsp olive oil

2 salmon fillets (150g each)

medium head broccoli, cut into florets

2 handfuls baby spinach

1 ripe avocado, peeled and stoned

50g frozen edamame beans, defrosted and shelled

½ lemon, juice only

TAMARI MISO DRESSING

1 heaped tsp miso paste

2tbsp tamari

1 tbsp sesame seeds, to serve

SERVES 2

Boil the rice for 30–35 minutes until the water is absorbed or as per instructions on the packet. Meanwhile, heat the olive oil in a pan until moderately hot. Add the salmon fillets, skin side down, and cook for 2–3 minutes until lightly browned. Turn them over, reduce the heat to moderate and continue cooking for a further 6–7 minutes until the salmon is just cooked through. Remove from the pan immediately to avoid overcooking.

Boil or lightly steam the broccoli florets for about 5 minutes until al dente. Drain and refresh under cold water. Place a handful of spinach in each of two bowls. Divide the rice, salmon, avocado, edamame beans and broccoli between them.

To make the dressing, dissolve the miso paste in a little warm water, add the tamari and mix.

Drizzle the lemon juice and miso dressing over the salmon. Finish with a scattering of sesame seeds and serve.

TIP: For a veggie twist, simply remove the salmon and add an extra edamame to increase protein.

TIP: For a more intense hit, first rest the salmon in this teriyaki marinade. Add the fish and marinade to a plastic bag and ensure the uncooked fish is well covered with the mix. Leave in the fridge for 1–24 hours.

- 60 ml teriyaki
- 1 tbsp runny honey
- pinch of hot chilli powder/flakes
- 1 tbsp sesame seeds

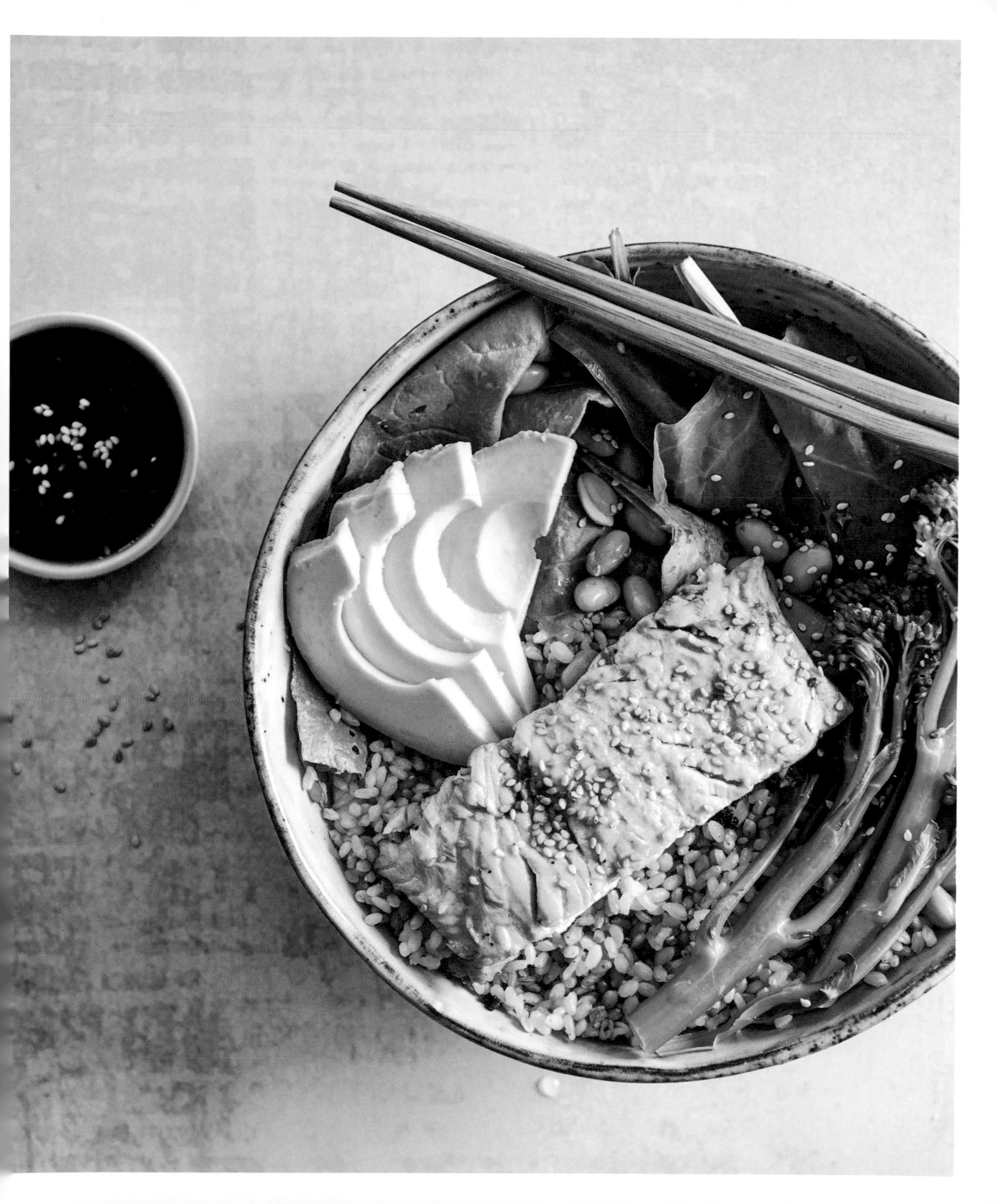

Summer: Cauliflower and Baby Spinach Bowl

- 1 medium head cauliflower, broken into bite-sized florets
- 400g tin chickpeas, drained
- 2 tbsp olive oil
- 1 tbsp dukkah
- sea salt and black pepper
- 1 red pepper, halved and sliced into thin strips
- 100g natural Greek or sheep's yoghurt
- ¼ clove garlic, minced
- 1 tbsp tamari or soy sauce
- ½ lime, juice only
- 1 avocado, peeled, stoned and cut into wedges
- 2 handfuls baby spinach
- 2 tomatoes, cut into wedges, or 4–6 cherry tomatoes, halved
- small handful fresh parsley, finely chopped

SERVES 2–3

OR 4 AS A SIDE SALAD

Preheat the oven to 220°C. Place the cauliflower florets and chickpeas at one end of a large preheated baking tray and drizzle with 1 tbsp of the olive oil. Top with dukkah (or see tip below) and 1 tsp sea salt and toss to combine.

Place the red pepper strips at the other end of the same roasting tray, drizzle with 1 tbsp olive oil and cook alongside the cauliflower.

Roast for 15–20 minutes or until the cauliflower is slightly tender (although still crunchy) and charred. Allow to cool a little.

To make the dressing, place the roasted red pepper strips, yoghurt, garlic, tamari or soy and lime juice in a food processor and blitz. Taste and adjust seasoning as required.

Combine the cauliflower and chickpea mix with the avocado wedges, baby spinach leaves and tomatoes and divide between two bowls. Drizzle some red pepper dressing over each bowl and scatter some chopped parsley over the top.

TIP: Dukkah is an aromatic Egyptian mixture of nuts, seeds and spices. It is now more widely available but if you can't find it, simply mix 2 tsp ground turmeric with 2 tsp ground cumin, 2 tsp ground coriander, 1 tsp ground ginger and ½ tsp chilli flakes.

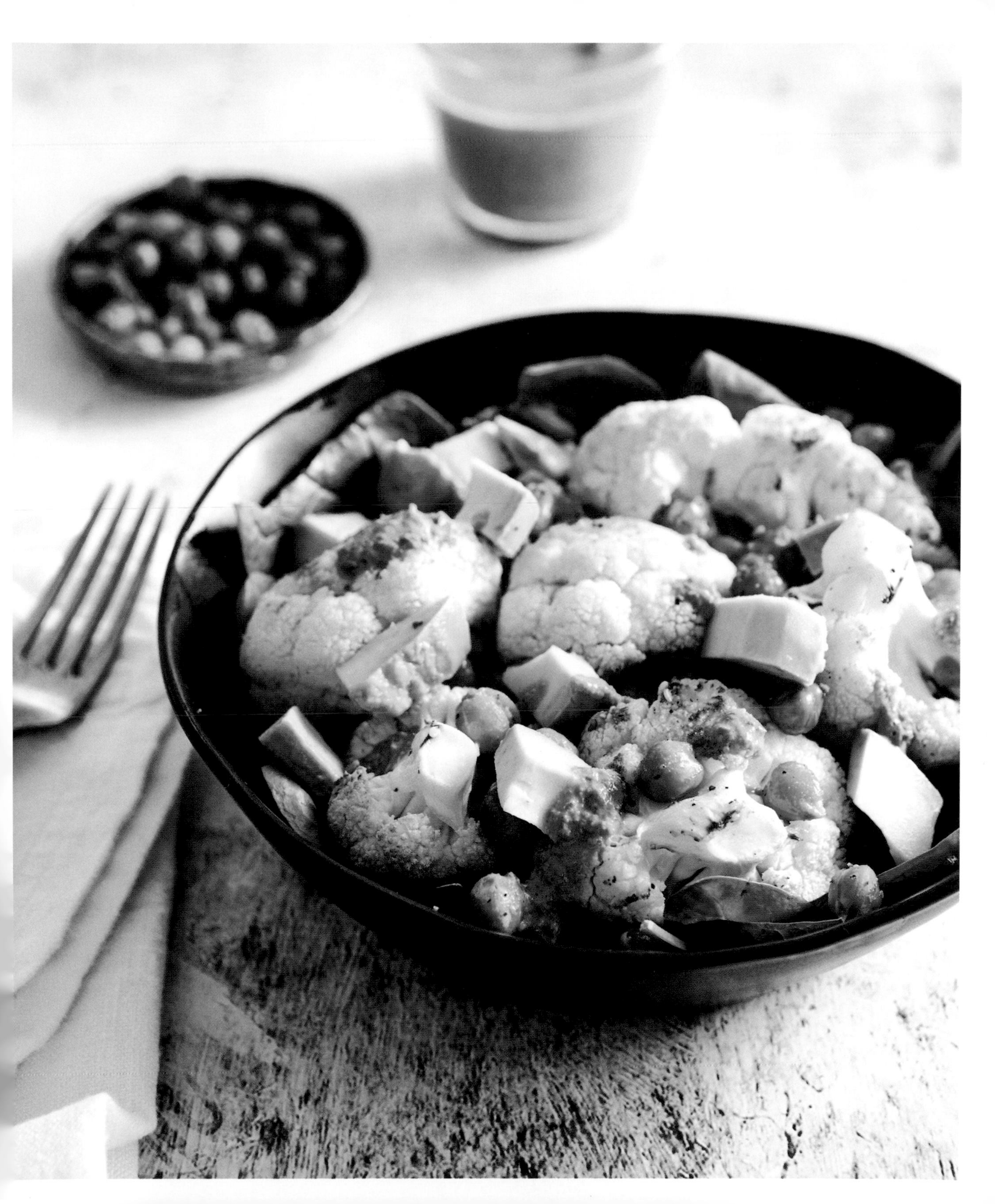

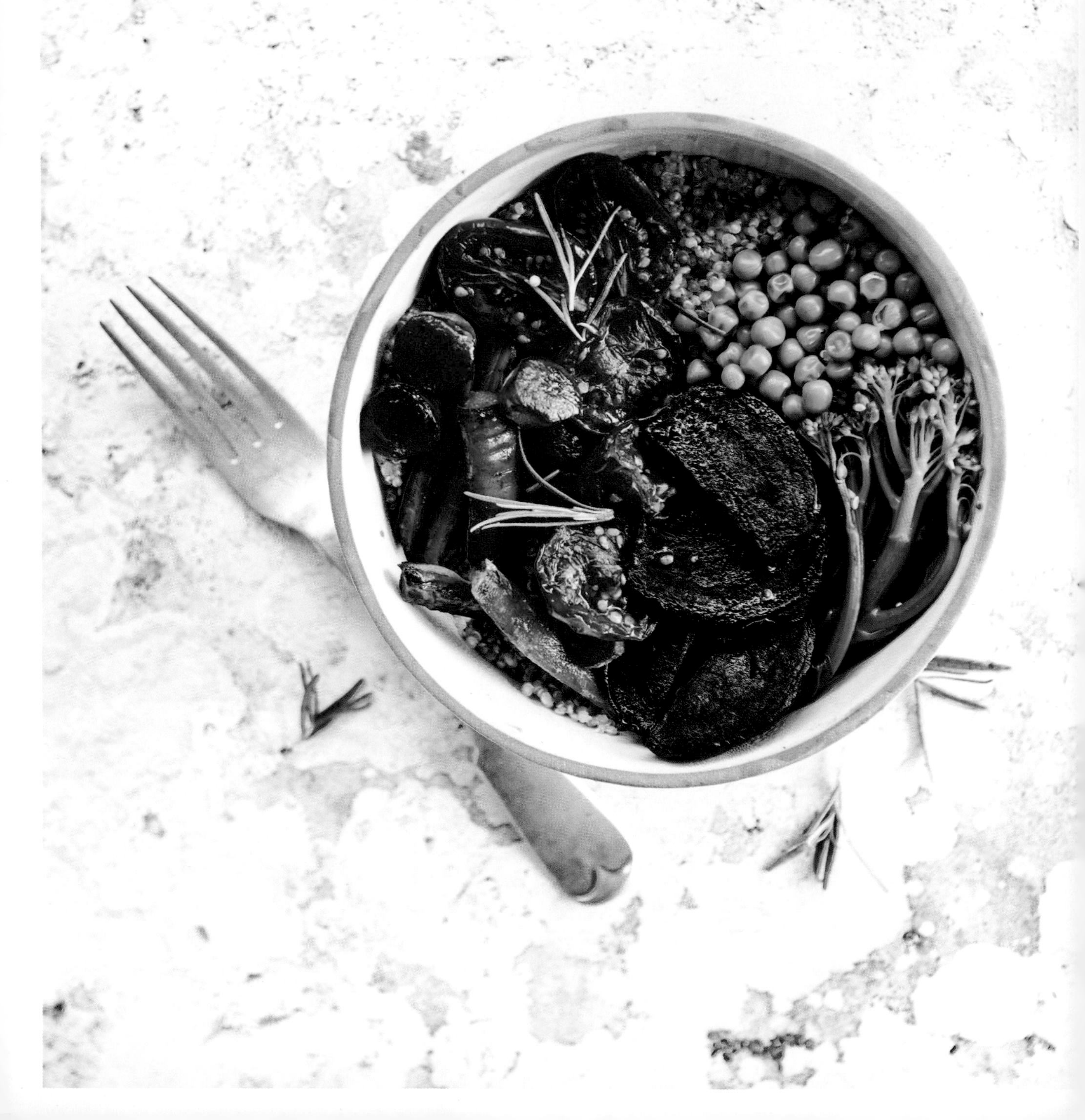

Autumn: Root Veggie Bowl

170g uncooked quinoa

480 ml homemade (see page 173) or low-salt vegetable stock

1 medium raw beetroot (180g–200g), peeled and thinly sliced

6 cherry tomatoes, quartered

1 large carrot, peeled and chopped into rounds

2 tbsp olive oil

few sprigs rosemary

4 stems broccolini

150g frozen peas

2 tbsp Walnut Basil Pesto (page 168)

sea salt and pepper, to taste

SERVES 2

Preheat the oven to 190°C.

Put the quinoa in a saucepan and cover with the stock. Bring to the boil then reduce the heat and simmer for 15–20 minutes, until cooked.

Meanwhile, lay the beetroot, tomatoes and carrots on a warmed baking tray. Drizzle with the olive oil and top with the rosemary. Bake for 20 minutes.

While the vegetables are roasting, cook the broccolini and peas in boiling water for about 5 minutes, until tender.

Divide the quinoa between two bowls and mix 1 tbsp pesto through each. Arrange the carrots, beetroot, peas and broccolini on top. Season with salt and pepper.

Winter: Warming Squash, Red Pepper and Chickpea Curry Bowl

2tbsp olive oil

1 butternut squash, peeled and cut into chunks

1 red pepper, deseeded and cut into small chunks

1 red onion, peeled and diced

2 cloves garlic, peeled and minced

small chunk fresh ginger, peeled and finely chopped

2 tsp smoked paprika

1 tsp ground cumin

1 tsp ground turmeric or small chunk fresh turmeric, minced

1 heaped tbsp curry powder

large pinch cayenne pepper or chilli flakes

400g tinned chickpeas, drained

400g tinned chopped tomatoes

400ml tinned coconut milk

400ml water or vegetable stock

large handful spinach leaves

sea salt and pepper, to taste

200g short grain brown rice

fresh coriander and dash of lime juice, to serve

SERVES
4

Heat the oil in a large saucepan. Add the squash, pepper, onion, garlic, ginger and 1 tsp smoked paprika. Sauté over a medium heat for 8–10 minutes, stirring. Then add the remaining spices, chickpeas, tomatoes, coconut milk and water or vegetable stock.

Bring to the boil, then reduce the heat and simmer for at least 25 minutes (can be left for up to 45 minutes on a very low heat). Stir in the spinach, salt and pepper towards the end of cooking.

Meanwhile cook the rice as per the directions on the packet.

Line each bowl with a bed of cooked rice and spoon over the curry. Sprinkle with chopped coriander and a splash of lime juice.

TIP: The nutty texture of short grain brown rice is a perfect complement to the curry but other grains, such as farro, can be used instead.

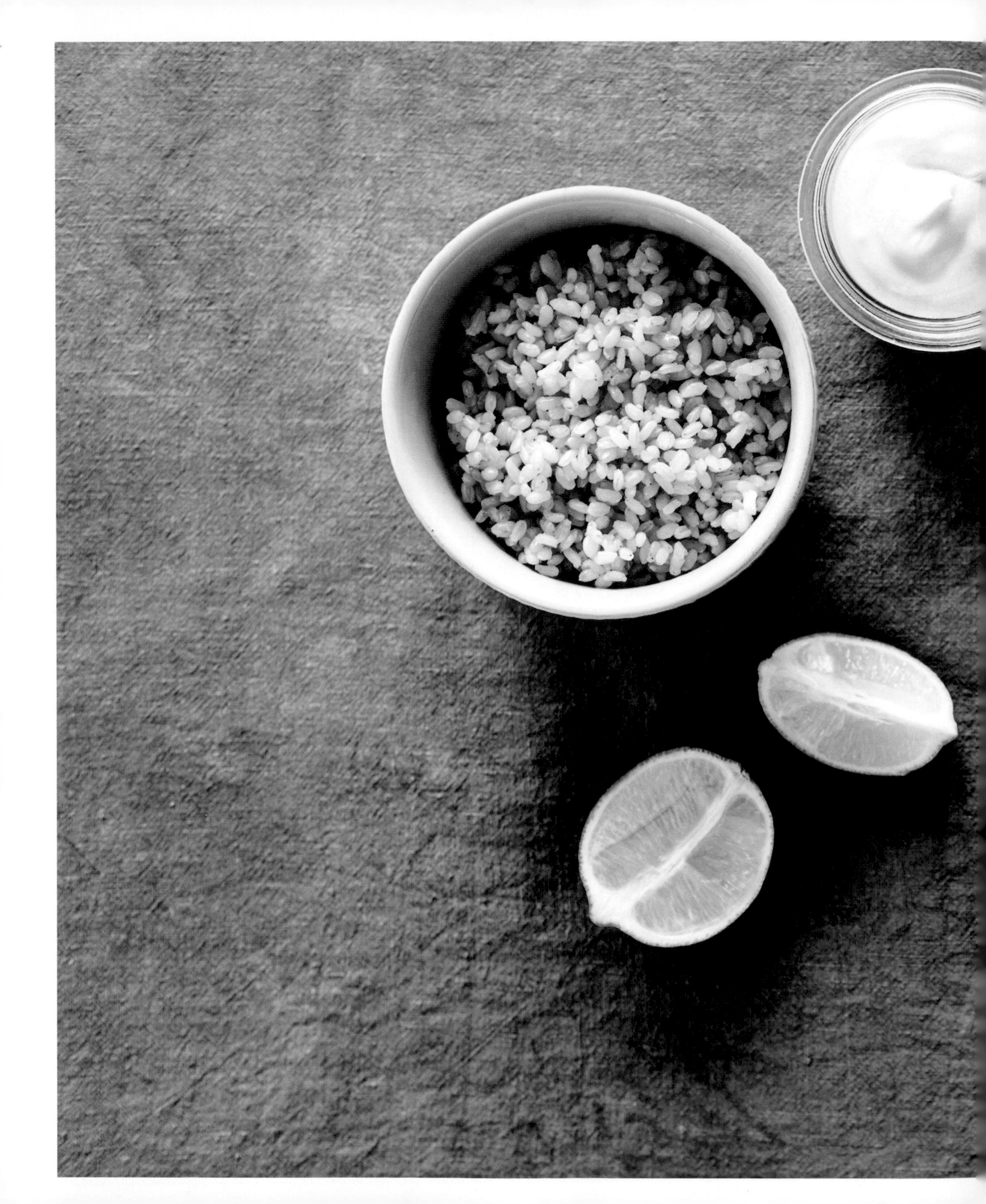

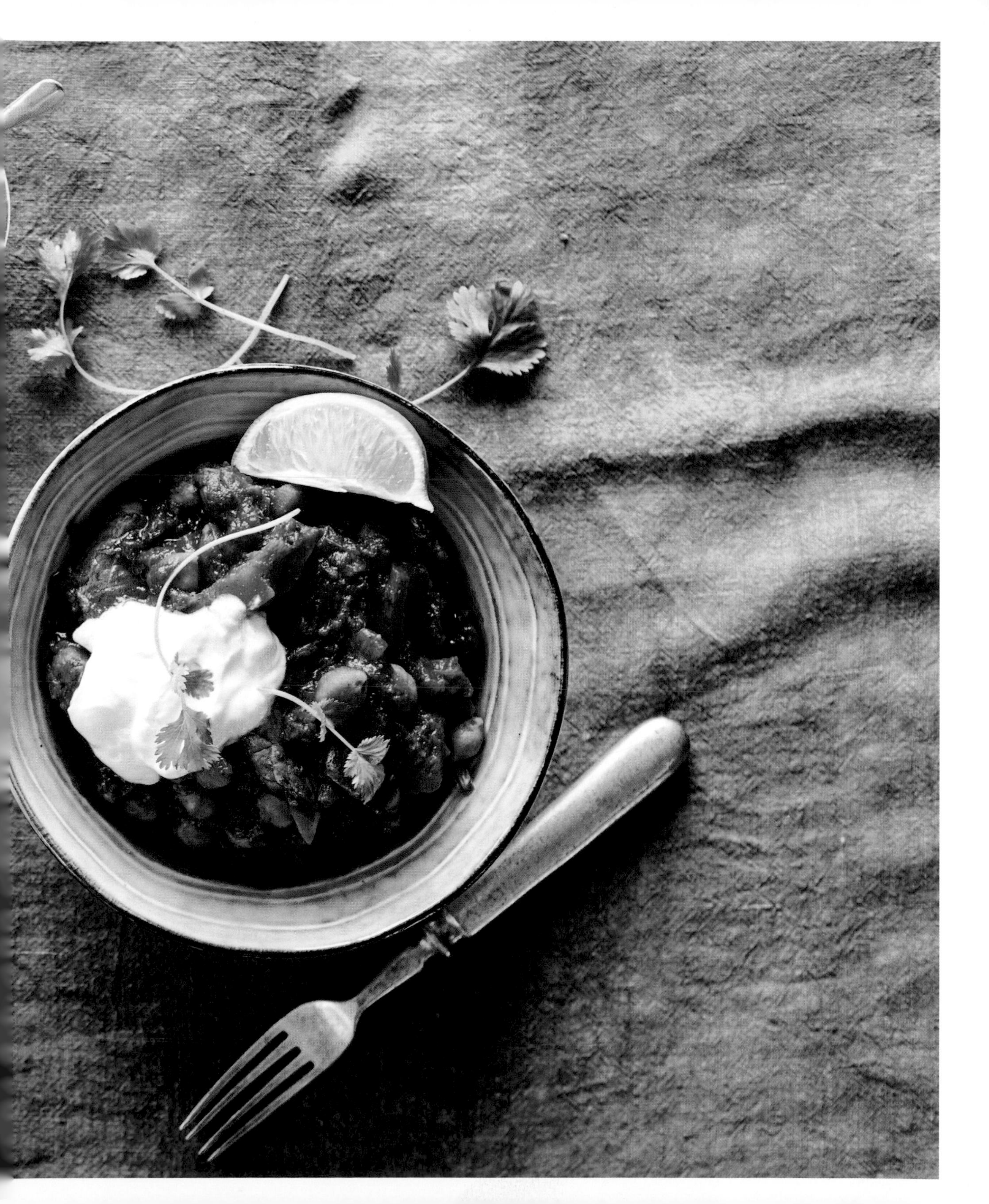

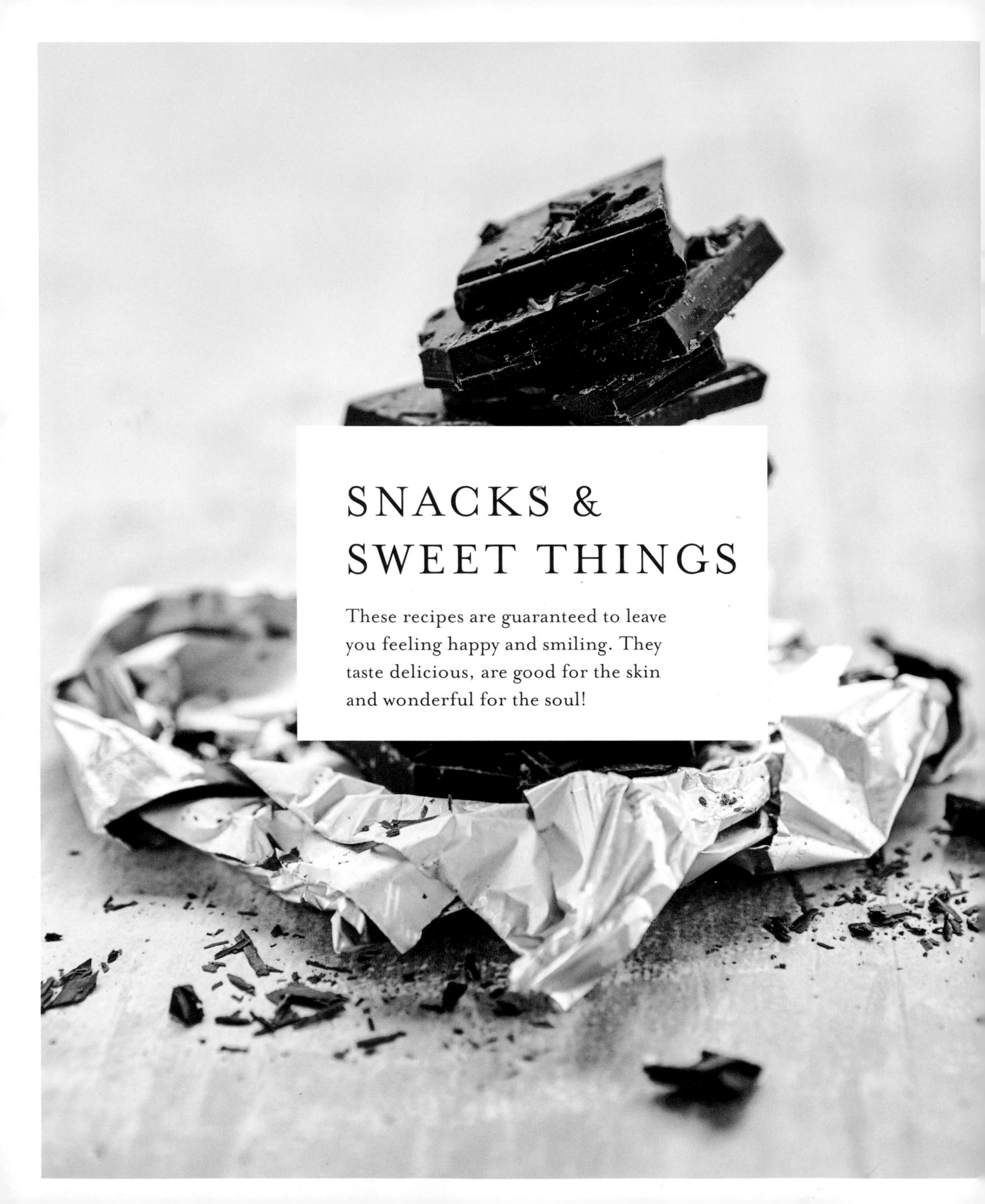

SNACKS & SWEET THINGS

These recipes are guaranteed to leave you feeling happy and smiling. They taste delicious, are good for the skin and wonderful for the soul!

Apple, Pear and Blackberry Crumble

The sheer versatility of crumbles makes them a healthy addition to every meal. Formerly a comforting autumnal dessert, when apples were at their best, crumbles have recently come centre stage in our quest for a healthier lifestyle and better skin. They are a perfect way to use leftover fruits too – simply combine them with granola and a healthy dose of the GLOW Trail Mix for a quick skin-boosting breakfast.

2 large cooking apples (about 200g), peeled and chopped

3 pears, peeled and chopped

handful blackberries

1 large orange, juice and zest

1 tsp ground cinnamon

120ml maple syrup or runny honey

130g oats

75g chopped walnuts

75g pumpkin seeds, roughly chopped

1 tbsp chia seeds

75g flaked almonds

75g shelled pistachios, roughly chopped

generous dollop of natural yoghurt, to serve

SERVES 6–7

Preheat the oven to 180°C.

Put the chopped apple, pears and blackberries in a saucepan. Add the orange zest and juice. Pour a little boiling water over the mix, along with the cinnamon and maple syrup or honey. Bring to the boil and immediately remove from the heat, as we don't want the fruit to cook through.

For the topping, mix together the oats, walnuts, pumpkin and chia seeds, making sure everything is evenly distributed. The mixture needs to be light and crumbly, as it will be heavy and stodgy if it becomes wet.

Place the fruit mixture in a deep baking dish, cover with the crumble and top with the flaked almonds and chopped pistachios. Bake for 30–35 minutes or until the crust is golden brown. Serve warm with some natural yoghurt.

TIP: Other popular crumble variations are

- Pear, blackberry and hazelnut
- Apple, rhubarb and walnut
- Apple, almond and frozen raspberry (about 360g raspberries)

Simply substitute the fruit and nuts in the list for those in the recipe above.

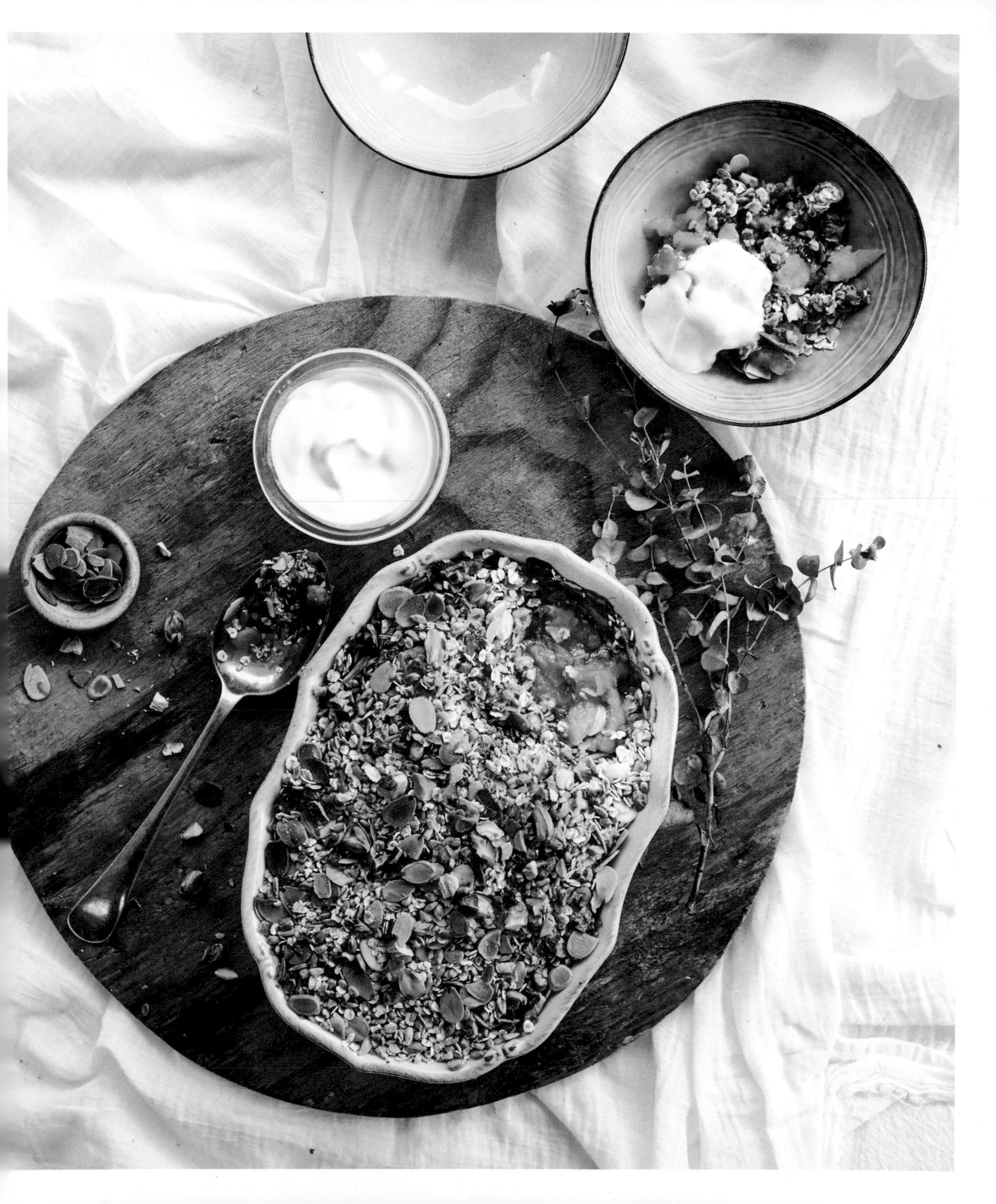

ChocNOlate Chip Cookies

- 100g oats
- 1 tbsp milled flax seeds
- 3 tbsp water
- 130ml maple syrup
- 2 tsp vanilla extract
- 40g coconut oil, softened
- 100g spelt flour
- 1 tsp baking powder
- pinch sea salt
- handful cacao nibs or dark/dairy-free chocolate chips

MAKES 12

Preheat the oven to 180°C. Line a baking tray with non-stick baking paper.

Place the oats in a food processor and blend until they're the consistency of flour. Mix the milled flax seeds and water in a small bowl and leave for 5 minutes to thicken.

In a large bowl, beat together the flax seed mix, maple syrup, vanilla extract and coconut oil. Add the remaining ingredients and mix.

Take small handfuls of the mixture and shape into rounds. Place them on the baking paper, pressing them down slightly.

Cook in the oven for 20 minutes. Leave to cool on a wire rack.

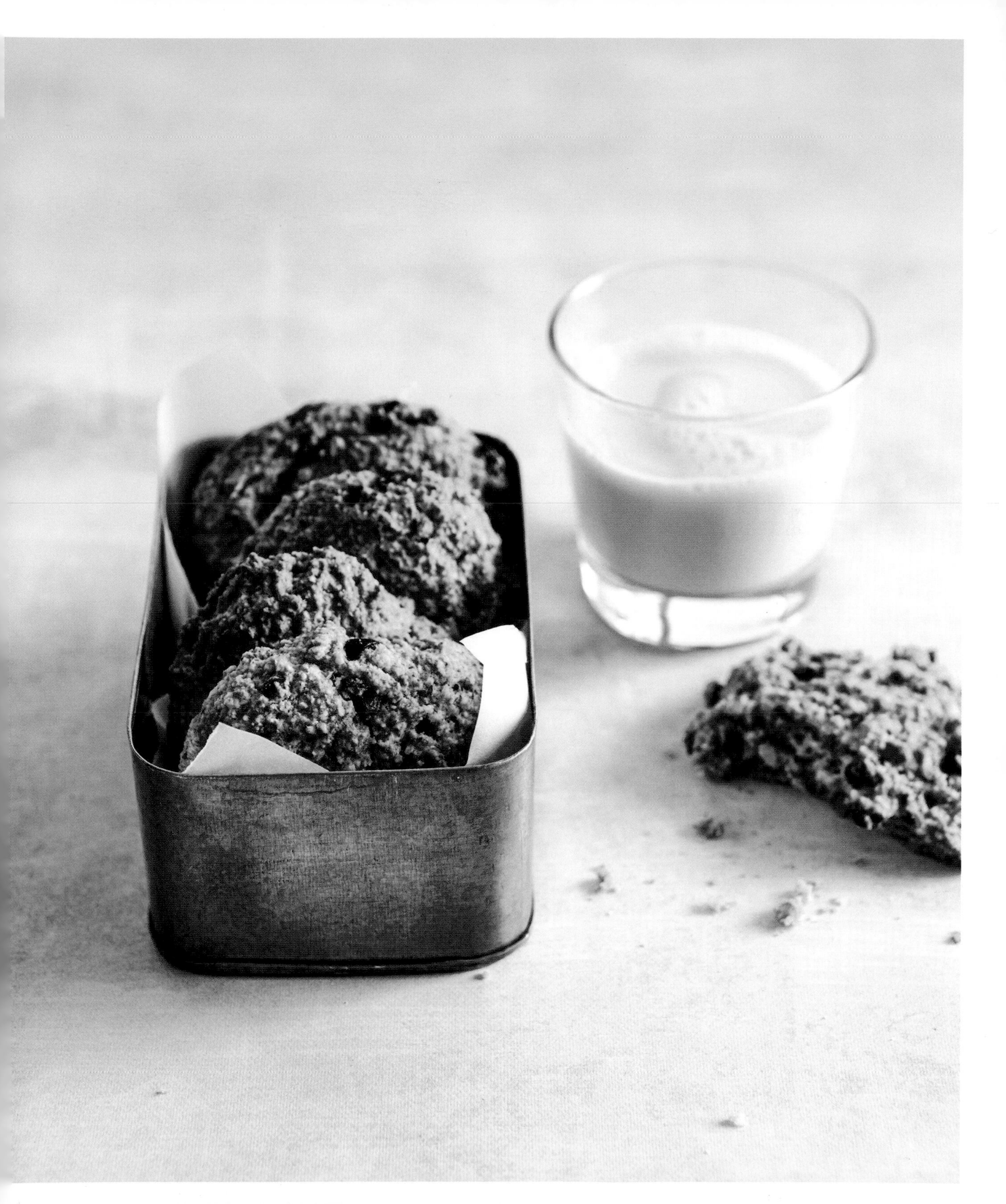

Citrus Delight Cake

2 oranges

1 lemon

butter or coconut oil, for greasing

300g ground almonds

1 tsp baking powder

100g caster sugar

75g desiccated coconut

3 eggs, lightly beaten

150ml maple syrup

2 tbsp pistachios, peeled and chopped

natural yoghurt, to serve

Place the whole oranges and lemon in a saucepan and cover completely with cold water. Bring to the boil and then reduce the heat. Cook for about 1 hour, until tender. Cool a little before transferring to a blender. Blend until smooth, adding a little of the water from the pot for consistency (it shouldn't be solid but it should hold its shape).

Meanwhile, preheat the oven to 180°C. Grease a 24cm round cake tin with a little butter or coconut oil and line with baking paper.

In a bowl, mix the almonds, baking powder, caster sugar and coconut. Pour in ⅓ of the beaten egg and fold into the mixture. Repeat until all the egg is mixed in, and then add the puréed fruit and maple syrup. Combine all ingredients until thoroughly mixed.

Pour the cake batter into the baking tin and bake for about 1 hour, until cooked and springy to the touch. Remove from the oven and leave to cool for about 10 minutes, then gently remove from tin and place on a wire rack. Sprinkle with the chopped pistachios and serve with a dollop of natural Greek yoghurt.

TIP: This can also be made into muffins by dividing the mixture between 14–16 muffin cases. Cooking time will be reduced to about 35 minutes.

Orange and Almond Muffins

200g ground almonds
1 tsp baking powder
100g desiccated coconut
2 oranges, juice and zest
2 eggs, lightly beaten
150g maple syrup
200ml almond milk (or milk of choice)

MAKES 12

Preheat the oven to 180°C.

In a bowl, mix the almonds, baking powder and coconut. Stir in the orange zest and juice, eggs, maple syrup and almond milk. Divide the mix between 12 muffin cases. Bake in the oven for 35 minutes. Remove from oven and allow to cool on a wire rack.

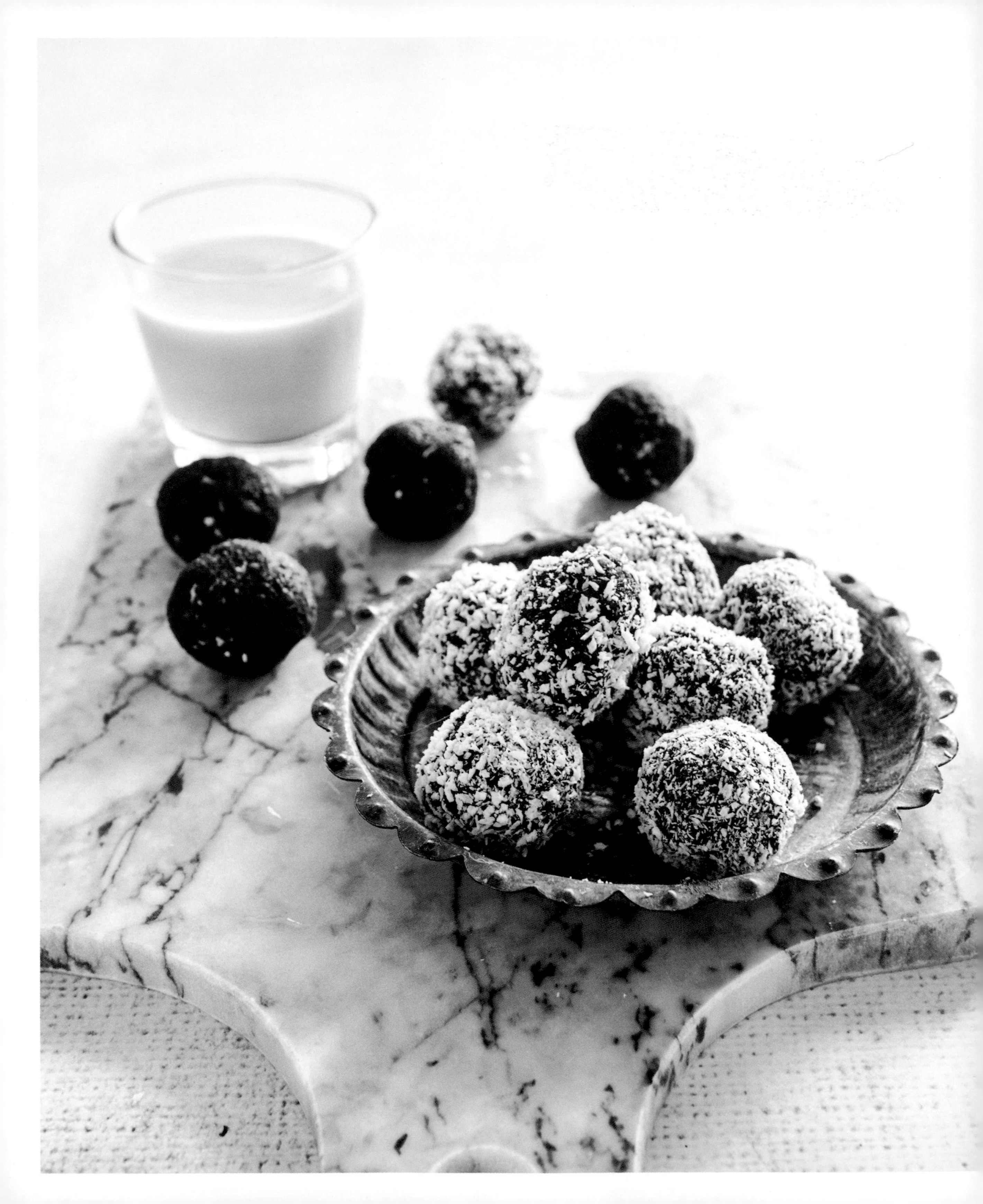

Chocolate Orange Energy Balls

200g dates

150g walnuts

1 heaped tbsp cacao powder

1 orange, zest and 2 tbsp juice

MAKES 12–15

Soak the dates in boiling water for 5 minutes. Drain and add to a food processor along with the rest of the ingredients. Blend until a clumpy mix forms. Roll into balls with your hands. Coat in a little dessicated coconut, if desired. Store in the fridge.

GLOW Trail Mix

This GLOW trail mix is packed with antioxidants, essential fats and protein to keep your skin nurtured and protected through the day. Use liberally on porridge, in yoghurts and smoothies, over salads and in baked goodies. Keep it in the car, in your bag and on hand after exercise if an energy boost is needed.

large handful each of:

linseeds

sesame seeds

chia seeds

sunflower seeds

pumpkin seeds

goji berries

chopped walnuts

chopped roasted almonds

coconut flakes/desiccated coconut

cacao nibs

Use this mix as your starting point, adding and subtracting ingredients to find the taste and texture you enjoy. Combine all ingredients and store in an airtight container for up to a month.

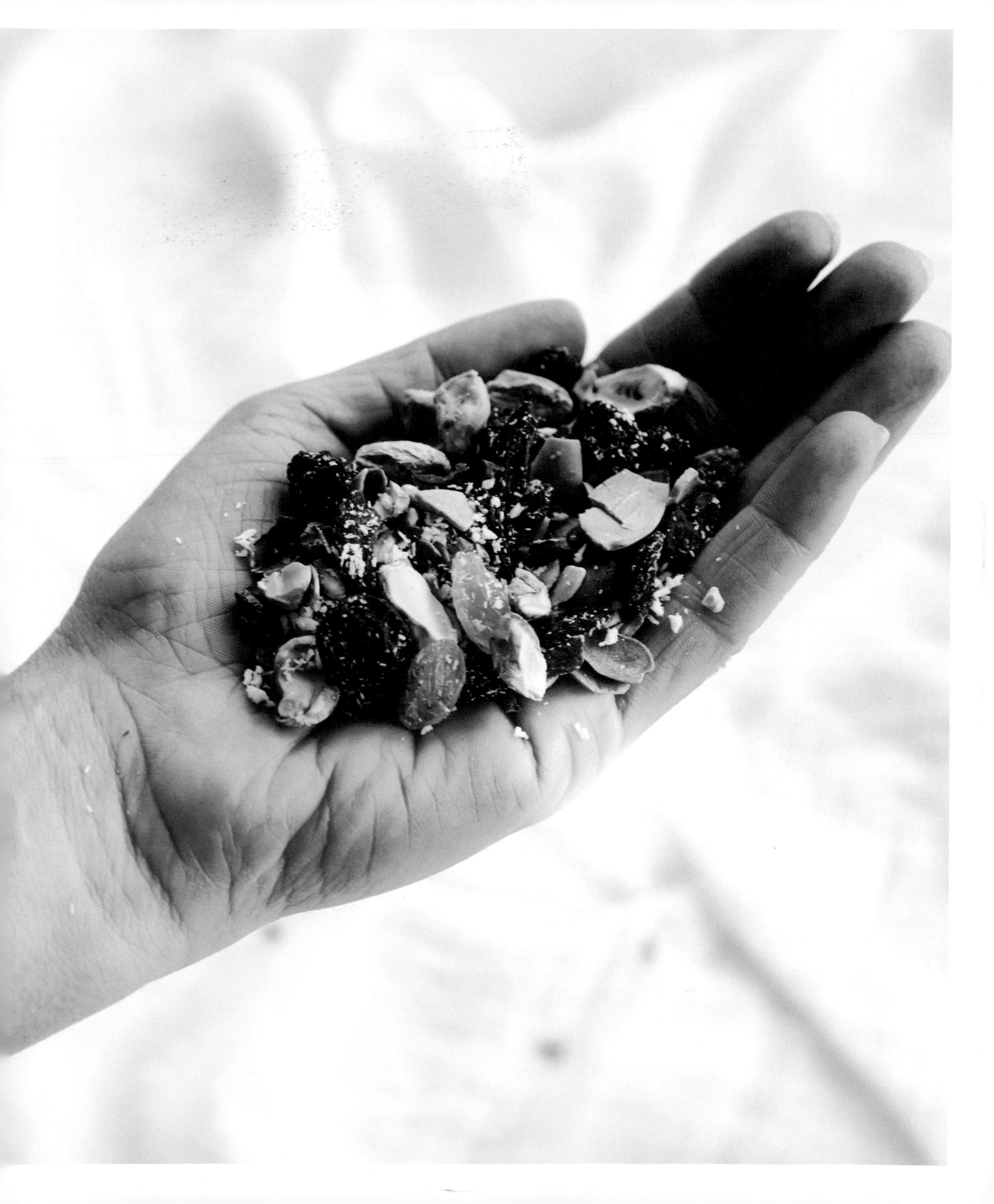

Walnut Brownies

- 160g dark chocolate, mint-flavoured preferably (over 80 per cent cocoa solids)
- 130ml milk of choice
- 140g coconut oil, plus extra for greasing
- 150ml maple syrup
- 1½ tsp vanilla or peppermint extract
- 40g raw cacao powder
- 3 eggs
- 140g plain spelt flour
- 1 tsp baking powder
- 60g chopped walnuts

MAKES 16 SQUARES

Preheat oven to 190°C. Grease a brownie tin (30cm x 30cm or thereabouts) and line with baking paper.

Put chocolate, milk, oil, maple syrup and extract in a pot over a medium heat. Stir gently until everything is melted and combined. Remove from the heat for a few minutes before whisking in the cacao powder and eggs. Fold in the flour and baking powder and, finally, add the chopped walnuts. Pour the mixture into the baking tin and cook for 25 minutes. Remove from the tin and leave to cool before cutting into squares.

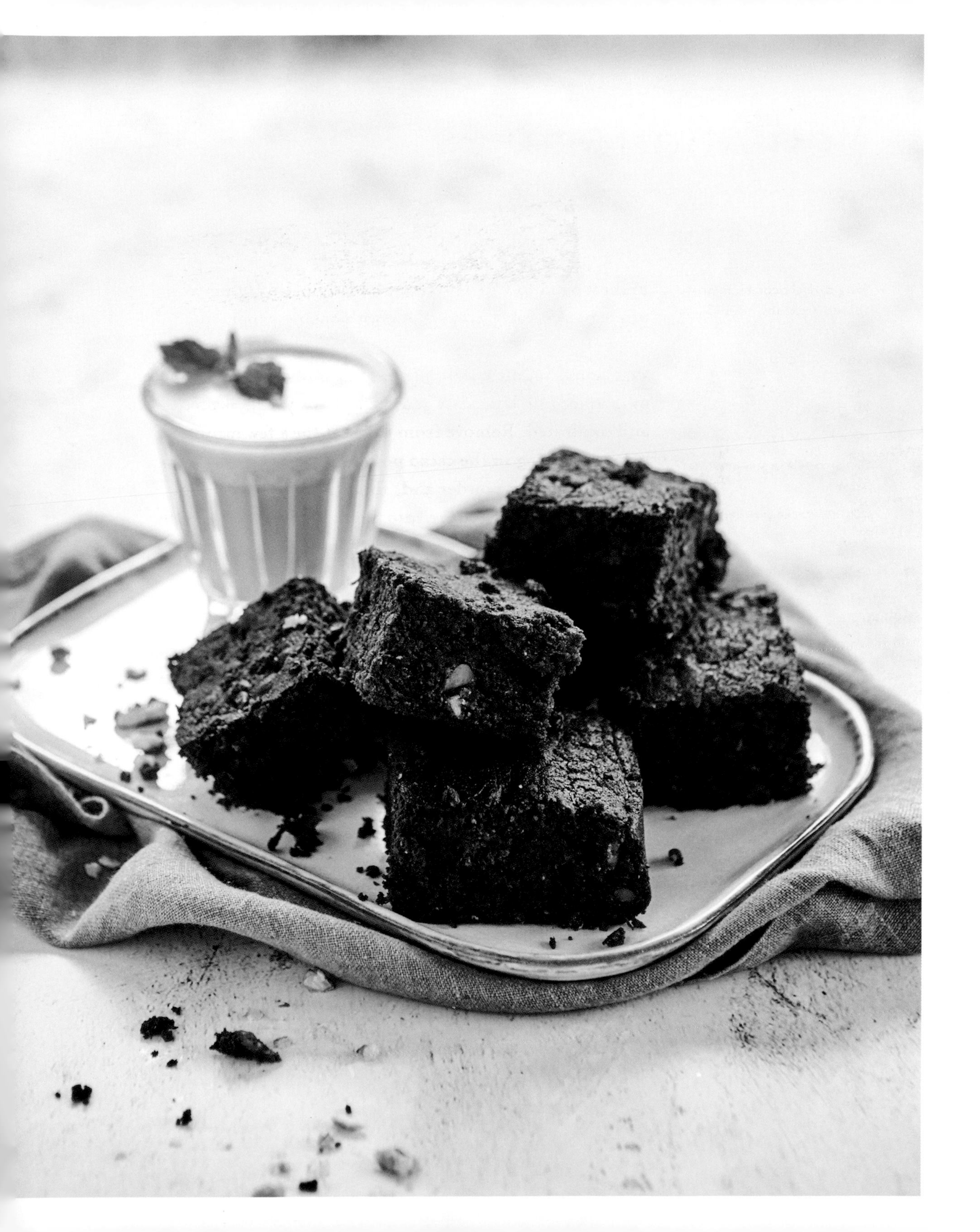

Berry Sorbet

Frozen berries work best for this deliciously fresh and zesty sorbet.

150g frozen strawberries and/or blueberries

2 tbsp Greek or sheep's yoghurt

1 tbsp maple syrup

½ lime, juice only

SERVES 2

Blitz all the ingredients in a blender until smooth.

The sorbet can be frozen in ice-cube trays or small storage pots. If using from the freezer, blend again before serving.

TIP: Top with chopped walnuts and a small handful of blueberries before serving.

Mint Choc-Chip 'Ice Cream'

2 frozen chopped bananas

handful mint leaves

dash almond milk (or milk of choice)

handful chopped dark chocolate (minimum 70 per cent cocoa solids)

Blend all ingredients except for the chocolate in a blender or food processor. Spoon into a bowl and stir through the chocolate.

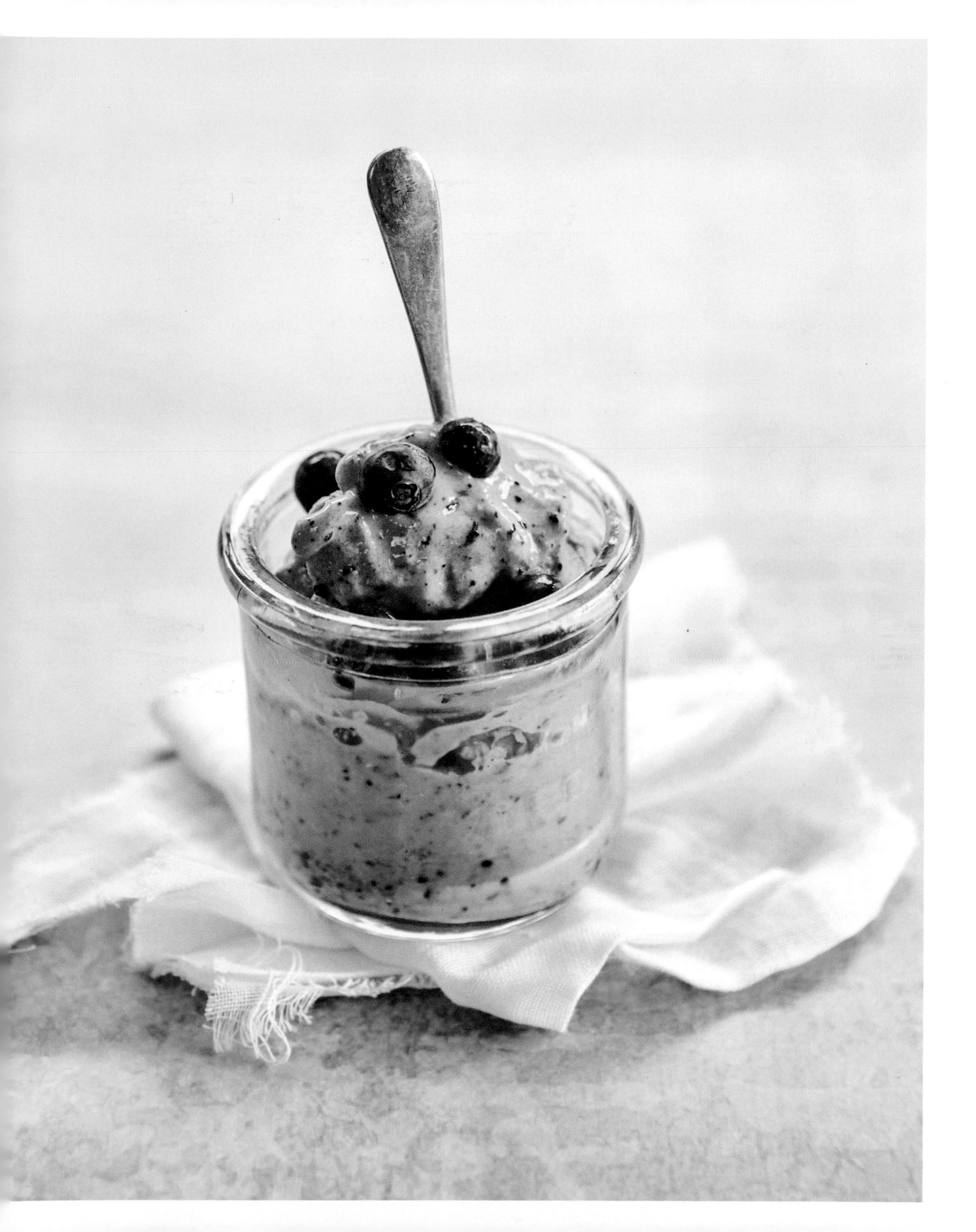

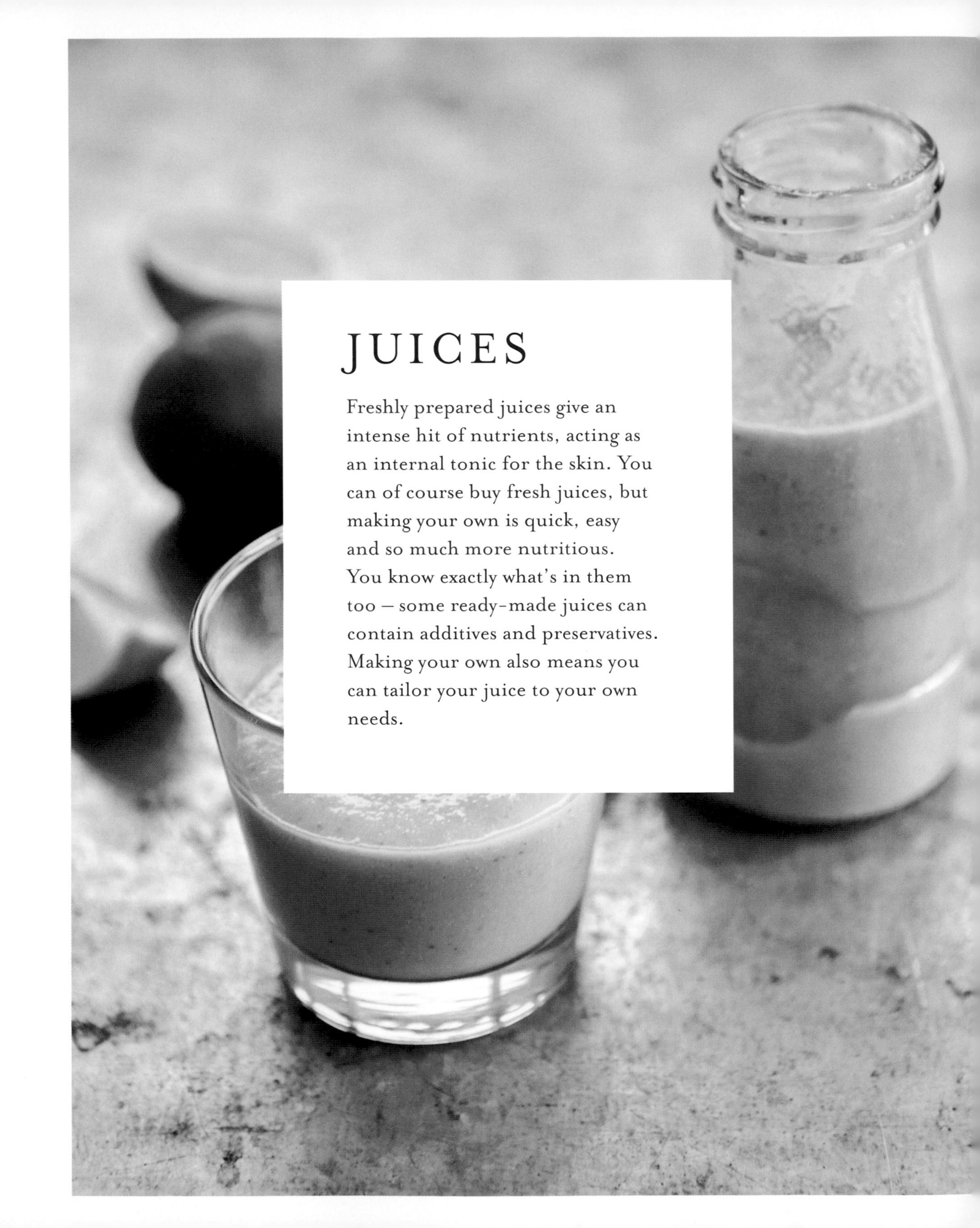

JUICES

Freshly prepared juices give an intense hit of nutrients, acting as an internal tonic for the skin. You can of course buy fresh juices, but making your own is quick, easy and so much more nutritious. You know exactly what's in them too – some ready-made juices can contain additives and preservatives. Making your own also means you can tailor your juice to your own needs.

MORE REASONS TO ENJOY FRESH JUICES

- They are overflowing with antioxidant goodness to protect the body and fight premature ageing.
- They are packed with essential vitamins and minerals.
- They are rich in active enzymes to aid digestion.
- They help cleanse the system and boost vitality.
- They help balance the body internally.
- They are a clever way of getting extra nutrients into children and teenagers.
- They can be relatively low in calories, yet satisfying, so they can help keep hunger pangs at bay, especially if trying to lose weight.
- They can help protect us from illness by providing high levels of easily absorbed nutrients that are specifically needed to strengthen the immune system.
- They are a fast way to maximise our nutritional intake and benefit every cell in the body, while the non-soluble fibre content ensures our gut functions optimally.

TIPS FOR BETTER JUICING

- To maximise nutritional benefits juices should be consumed as soon as possible after blending, as they quickly start to lose enzyme activity and vitality.
- Use raw ingredients or organic if possible. If you can't buy organic fruit and vegetables, give them a good wash in warm water with a mild detergent, then rinse well and dry.
- As a general rule, choose 70 per cent vegetables with 30 per cent fruit, thereby limiting sugar intake.
- Get digestive enzymes flowing by drinking slowly and chewing juices where possible.
- Variety is key. Choose from a wide range of vegetables and fruit and go for different colours.
- If certain fruits and vegetables are not available to you, simply swap for something similar – for example, spinach for kale, orange for kiwi.

TIP: Many routinely used fruits can be kept in the freezer. Bananas, pineapple and berries are perfect – buy frozen fruits when fresh are not in season and use from the freezer as needed.

THE PLAN

While all the juices in this section are packed with skin-friendly nutrients and would be suitable for every stage of the four-week plan, some boast larger quantities of particular nutrients that lend themselves to specific weeks (for example, beetroot and celery for cleansing, avocado and apple cider vinegar for healing).

Drink one large glass of your preferred juice from the options on the following pages every day for the duration of the plan. If time is tight then prepare the ingredients the night before and leave in the fridge so all you need to do is blend it together in the morning. If you don't have some of the ingredients on hand, use what you have and make it as similar as feasible to the recipe.

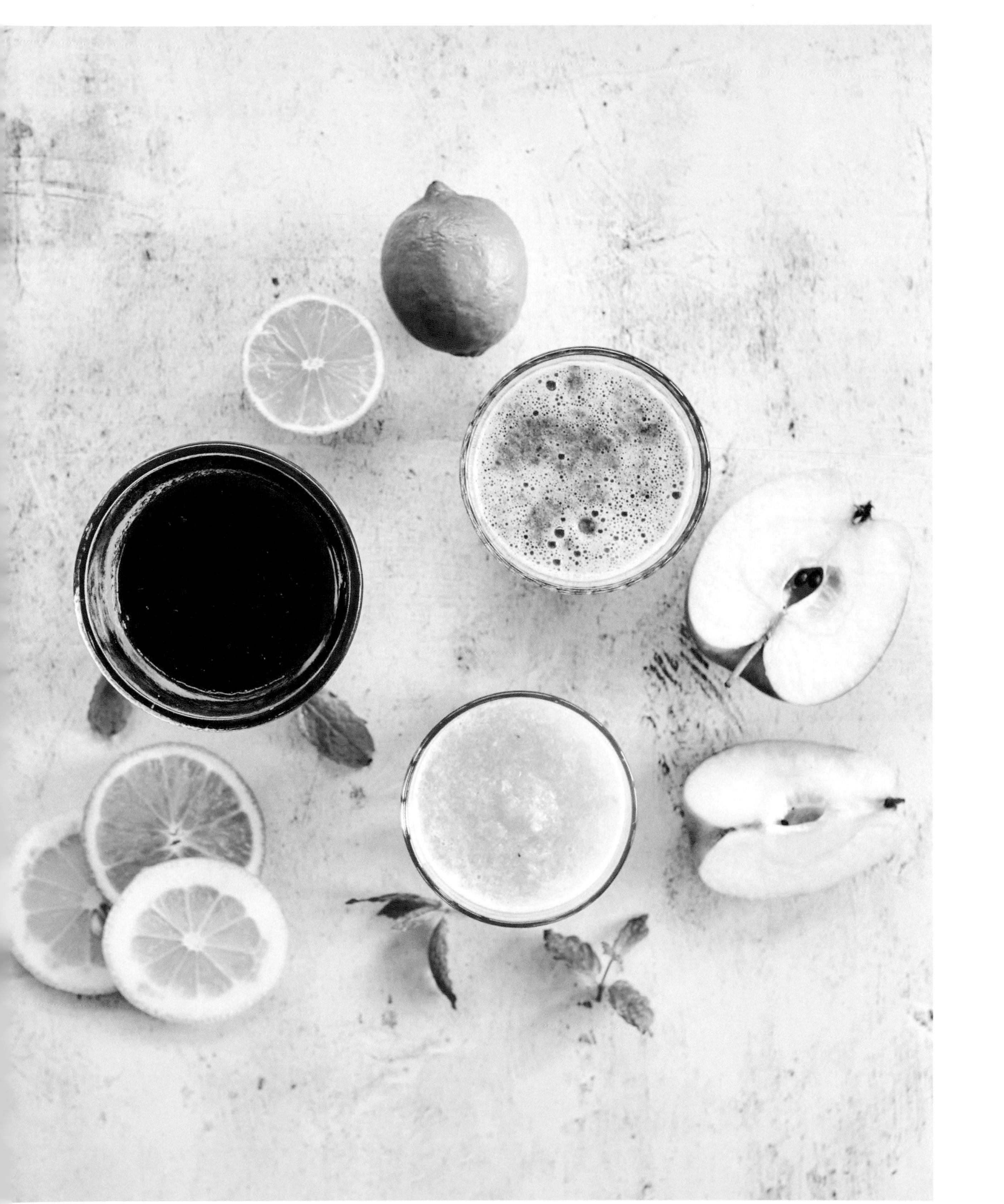

Week 1: Cleanse

FOCUS: Cleanse and restore the liver and skin.

NOTE: The high level of beta-carotene in carrots can give an orange tinge to the skin when taken at very high levels.

EARTHY GOODNESS

The earthy texture and taste of beetroot is softened with citrus fruits and a little ginger for added zing.

2 medium raw beetroot, peeled and roughly chopped

1 carrot, peeled

1 apple

2cm piece root ginger, peeled and roughly chopped

3 stalks celery

½ lime, juice only

250ml coconut water

ZESTY CLEANSER

2 carrots, peeled

½ cucumber

1 orange, peeled

2 stalks celery

handful spinach leaves

handful fresh mint leaves

½ lime, juice only

250ml coconut water

Blend all ingredients thoroughly. If consistency is too thick, add more coconut water or ice. Serve in a tall glass poured over ice cubes.

Week 2: Heal

FOCUS: Top anti-inflammatory and antioxidant ingredients to heal the skin, the gut and the body.

SKIN SOOTHER

½ cucumber

2–3 stalks celery

100g pineapple chunks, skin and core removed, and/or 1 kiwi, peeled

½ ripe avocado, stoned and peeled

handful fresh mint

¼ lime, juice only

1 tsp sunflower lecithin

1 tsp chia seeds

120ml coconut water

2–3 ice cubes

contents of 1 evening primrose oil or borage seed (starflower) oil capsule

INTENSE C

1 pomegranate, seeds only, or small pot pomegranate seeds

1 orange, peeled

2 handfuls blueberries, fresh or frozen

1 tsp chia seeds

1 small banana

1 tsp sunflower lecithin

1 tsp chia seeds

2–3 ice cubes

contents of 1 evening primrose oil or borage seed (starflower) oil capsule (optional)

Blend all ingredients except oil from capsule. Add this at the end. If consistency is a little thick, just add a little coconut water or more ice cubes. Serve in a tall glass.

Week 3: Nourish

FOCUS: Maximise nutrient goodness through green vegetables and other foods overflowing with essential fats and antioxidants.

TIP: Keep pineapple chunks in the freezer, as they add that zesty chill to the juice.

PINEAPPLE PUNCH

100g pineapple chunks, skin and core removed

large handful baby spinach

1 kiwi, peeled

½ avocado, stoned and peeled

½ lime, juice only

1 tsp chia seeds

250ml coconut water

small handful fresh mint leaves

DOUBLE GREEN

handful kale leaves, tough stems removed

handful baby spinach leaves

1 apple, cored and roughly chopped

1 medium cucumber, cut into chunks

1 tsp fresh root ginger, peeled and grated

handful fresh mint leaves

½ lime, juice only

250ml coconut water

Blend all ingredients. If the consistency is a little thick, just add a little more coconut water. Serve in a tall glass poured over ice cubes.

Week 4: Glow

FOCUS: GLOW – vibrant, glowing skin.

SUNSHINE SKIN

2 small oranges, peeled

½ lemon, peeled

1 tsp cinnamon

1 tsp sunflower lecithin

1 tbsp olive or flax seed oil

3–4 ice cubes

VITAL SKIN

2 carrots, peeled

4 stalks celery

2cm piece fresh root ginger, peeled

1 apple

handful blueberries

½ tsp ground turmeric or 1.3cm fresh turmeric (peeled)

1 lime, peeled

1 tsp sunflower lecithin

3–4 ice cubes

Blend all the ingredients. If too thick, add a little coconut water. Serve immediately.

GLOW TEAS

Herbal teas have become kitchen essentials. With such a wide variety on offer there is something for every taste. But making your own is quick, easy and perfect for this four-week plan – all you need are some fresh herbs, select spices, water and a little honey. While the following teas are delicious at any time, certain herbs work particularly well during the various weeks of the plan, so have a pot of freshly brewed tea ready to go when you need a little lift.

The healing Lavender and Rosemary blend (page 248) makes a great hair rinse, as will most other teas in this chapter. So save any leftover teas and simply pour over washed hair while in the shower. For a more concentrated infusion, make a stronger tea, seal in an airtight jar and use on the hair after twenty-four hours.

Week 1: Cleanse

LEMONGRASS, GINGER AND MINT

Ginger, lemongrass and mint are the perfect cleansing combination – packed with anti-inflammatory power to aid digestion and further cleansing.

2 stalks lemongrass, outer leaves and stalk ends removed

1cm piece fresh root ginger, peeled and roughly chopped

handful fresh mint leaves

Bruise the lemongrass a little in a pestle and mortar or bash it with a rolling pin to soften and help extract juices. Cut the stalks in half. Put them into a teapot along with the ginger and mint leaves. Fill with boiling water and leave to steep for up to 5 minutes. Drink and refresh with more boiling water as needed during the day.

NETTLE AND GINGER

Stinging nettles are widely available in lanes and hedgerows in many parts of the world. Nettle tea, as well as having analgesic and anti-inflammatory properties, can help relieve symptoms of acne and skin irritation.

bunch of nettles

1cm piece fresh root ginger, peeled and roughly chopped

honey, to taste

Rinse the nettle leaves (as little stem as possible) and put them in a large saucepan with the chopped ginger and 750ml water. Bring to the boil and simmer for a couple of minutes. Strain into a cup and add honey to taste.

TIP: For more intense cleansing benefits, place a large handful of nettle leaves in a glass jar with 500ml boiling water. Cover with a lid and leave to infuse overnight at room temperature. Strain and drink chilled or warm.

Week 2: Heal

LAVENDER AND ROSEMARY

This aromatic brew helps to heal and enliven the skin. Lavender is a recognised skin healer and rosemary is also great for nourishing hair and scalp. Use any leftover infusion as a hair rinse.

2 sprigs lavender

3 sprigs fresh rosemary

½ lemon, sliced

Put all the ingredients in a teapot. Fill with boiling water and leave to steep for up to 5 minutes. Drink and refresh with more boiling water as needed during the day.

FENNEL AND MINT

This nourishing tea is quick, easy and great for relieving stomach upsets and other digestive issues.

handful fresh mint leaves

½ tsp fennel seeds

1cm piece fresh root ginger, peeled and roughly chopped (optional but excellent for digestive issues)

Put all ingredients in a teapot. Fill with boiling water and leave to steep for up to 5 minutes. Drink and refresh with more boiling water as needed during the day.

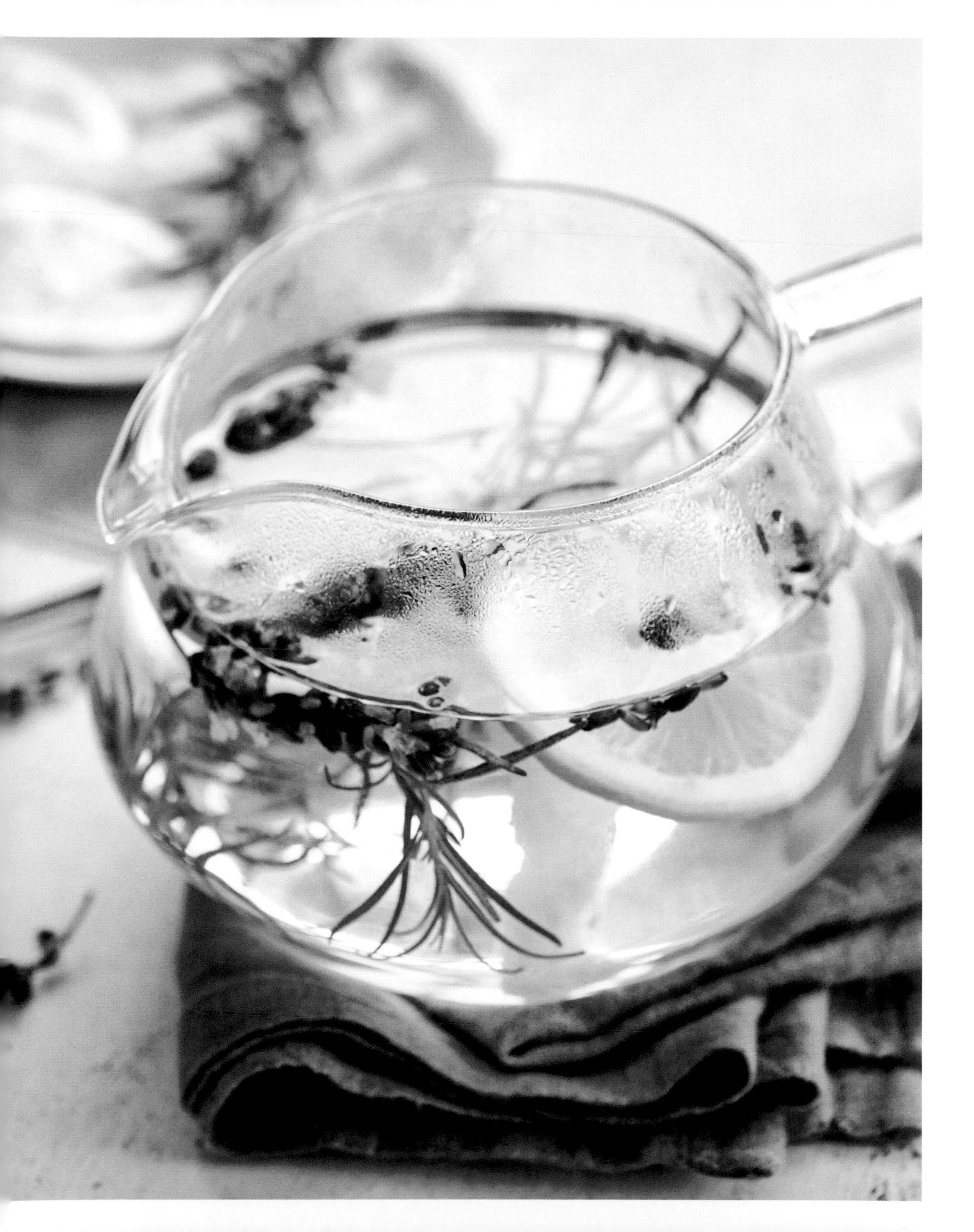

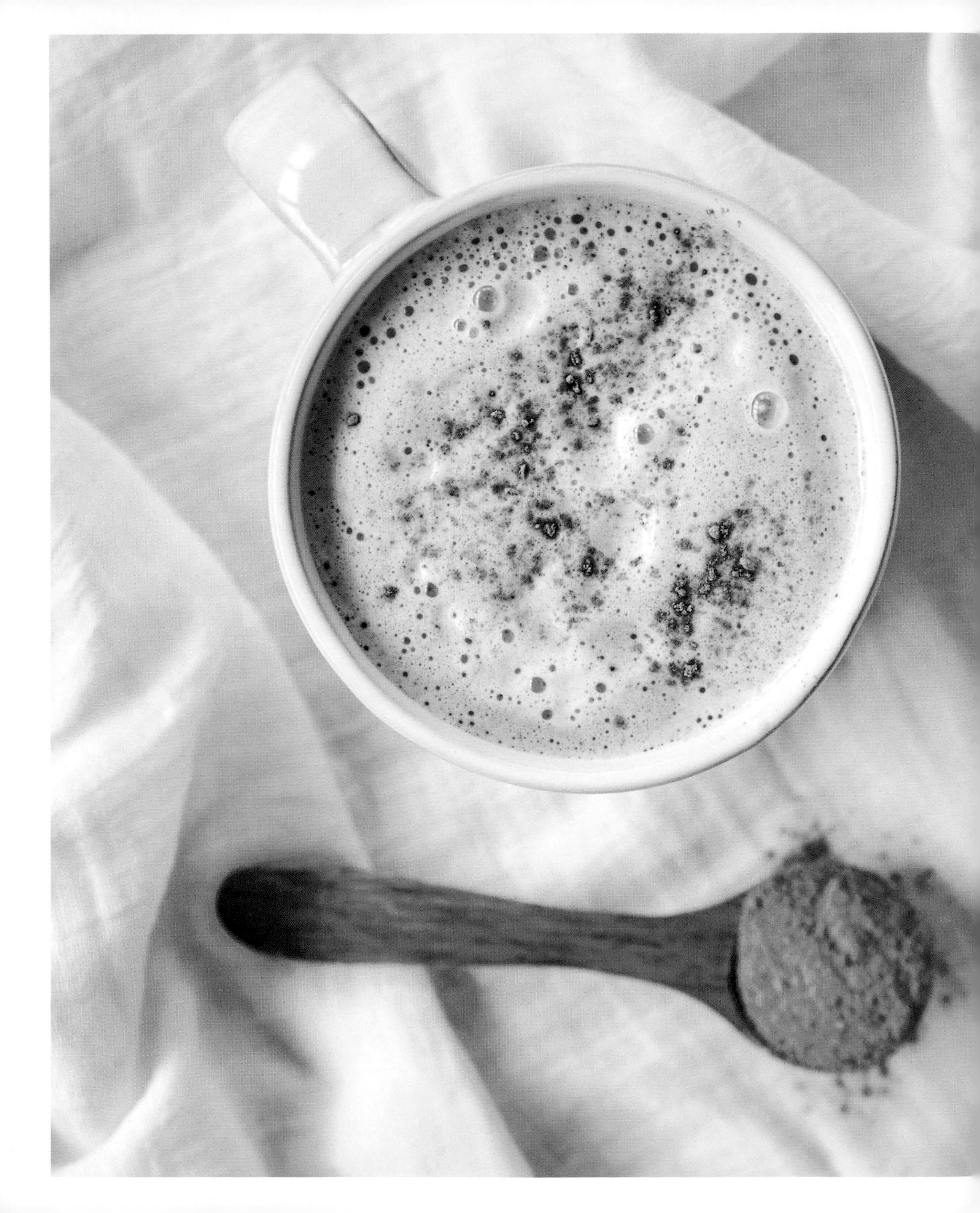

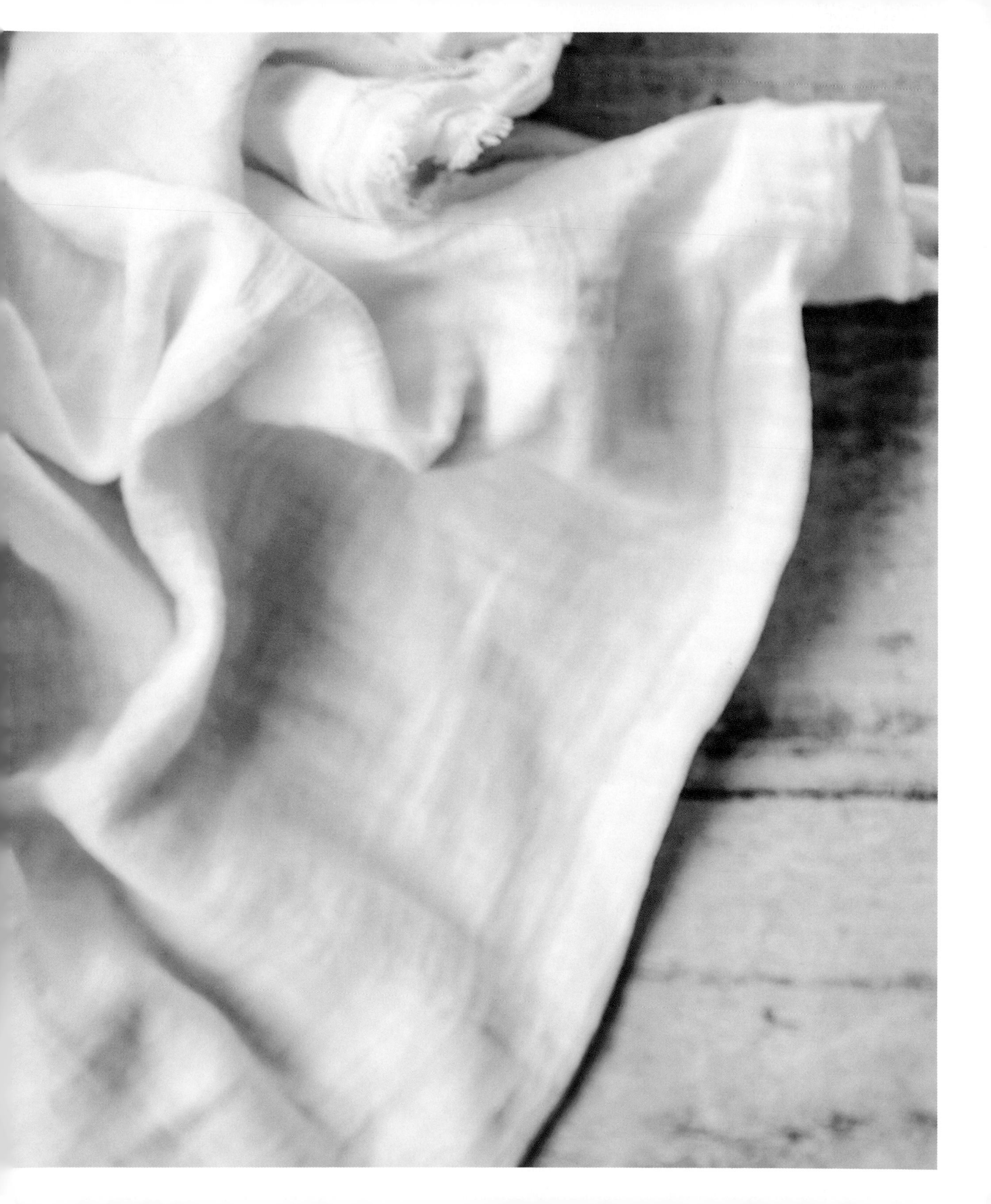

Week 3: Nourish

GINGER AND TURMERIC

1cm piece turmeric, peeled and chopped

1cm piece fresh root ginger, peeled and roughly chopped

honey, to taste

Put the chopped turmeric and ginger in a teapot. Fill with boiling water and leave to steep for up to 5 minutes. Add honey, if needed, to taste. Drink and refresh with boiling water as needed during the day.

MATCHA MINT LATTE

Bright-green matcha powder hails from Japan and is both nourishing and cleansing, being rich in antioxidants and chlorophyll. It is a popular ingredient in facemasks and moisturisers but also great as a tea or latte.

1 mug milk of choice (almond, soya, cashew, coconut or cow's)

handful fresh mint leaves

2 tsp matcha powder

honey, to taste (if desired)

Heat the milk in a saucepan, then transfer to a blender. Add the mint leaves and matcha powder and blend until foamy. Pour into a mug and add honey to taste.

TIP: For an added matcha hit, add a teaspoon of the powder to porridge or smoothies.

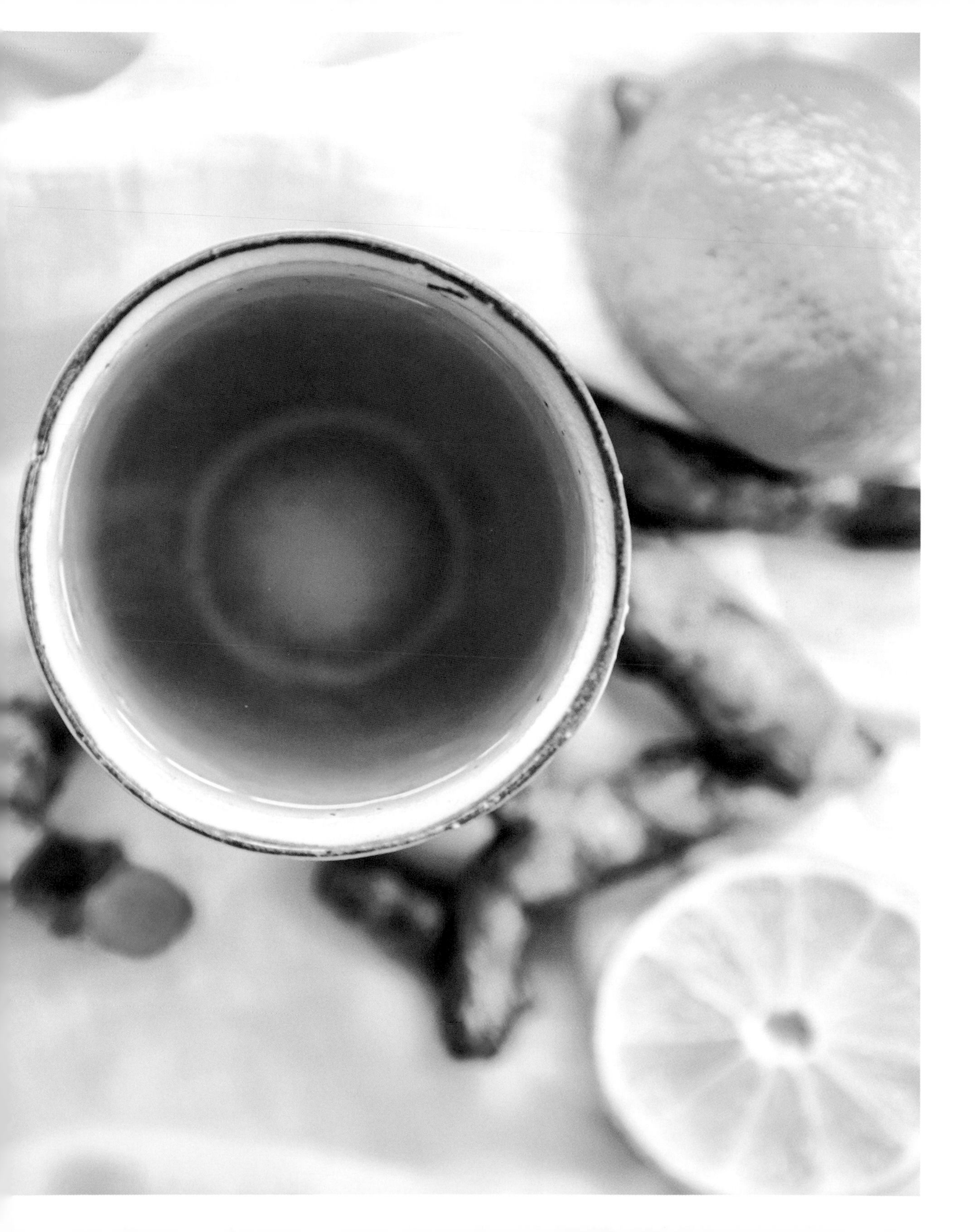

Week 4: Glow

GREEN TEA WITH MINT

Green tea comes from the fresh leaves of *Camellia sinensis* and has long been used in Chinese medicine to help relieve anxiety and depression. Although it naturally contains some caffeine, it can help cleanse and nourish the system when consumed regularly.

4 tsp green tea leaves or 4 teabags

handful fresh mint leaves

1 lemon, sliced

Place tea leaves or bags in a teapot, top with boiling water and let steep for at least 10 minutes (do not squeeze tea bags). Add mint leaves and sliced lemon. Steep for another few minutes before drinking. This can also be enjoyed cold.

ORANGE AND MINT ICED GREEN TEA

This deliciously refreshing combination keeps skin refreshed and glowing through the day.

2 tsp green tea leaves or 2 teabags

handful fresh mint leaves

1 orange, juice only

honey, to taste (optional)

½ lemon, sliced

Heat 750ml water in a saucepan and add tea and mint leaves. Bring to the boil and simmer for at least 5 minutes. Remove from the heat, remove teabags and allow to cool for 10 minutes. Add orange juice and honey to taste. Serve in a tall glass over ice cubes with sliced lemon.

ROSEBUD BREW

2 tbsp dried rosebuds or petals (avoid shop bought, as they are likely to contain pesticides)

a few slices of lemon or a few sprigs of fresh mint (optional)

honey, to taste (optional)

Put ingredients in a teapot. Fill with boiling water and leave to steep for up to 5 minutes. Pour and add honey to taste, if required. Refresh with boiling water as needed during the day.

TIPS:

- Save any leftover tea to make a refreshing facial toner. Simply decant into a clean spray pump bottle and keep at a cool room temperature for one week.
- For a truly Middle Eastern alternative, add 1 tbsp cardamom pods to the tea.

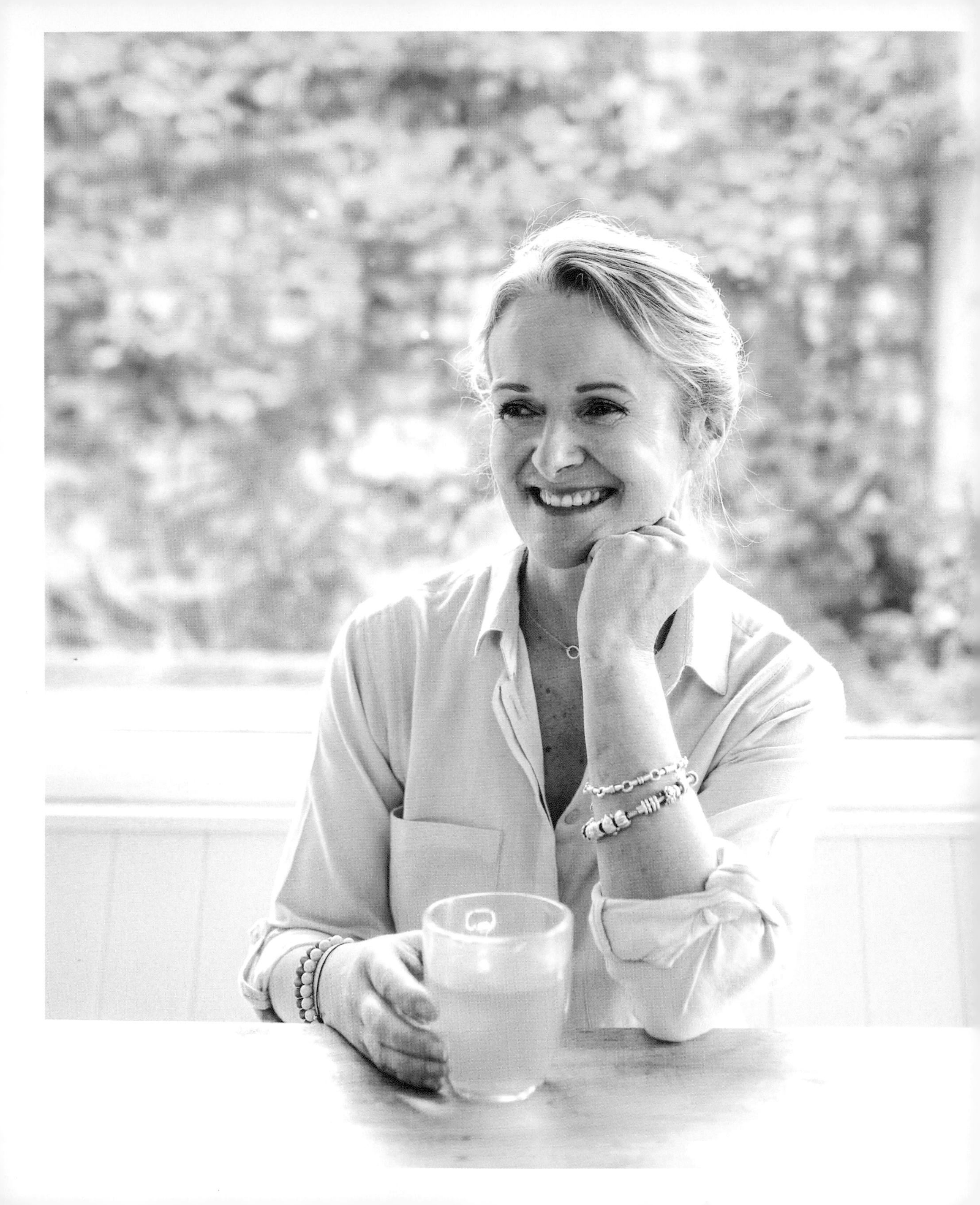

Kombucha

Dearbhla Reynolds is the queen of fermenting and author of *The Cultured Club*. Her easy-to-follow recipes transform simple ingredients into superfoods through the timeless method of fermentation. Here she gives her expert advice on how to perfect your own kombucha.

Kombucha, or 'booch' as it's sometimes called, is a sugar-sweetened fermented green or black tea that is produced by a scoby (aka a symbiotic community of bacteria and yeast). It is a rich source of beneficial probiotic bacteria, supporting gut and overall health.

Although starting out on your kombucha journey sounds a little daunting, once you get your first batch up and running and taste the flavoursome brew, you will soon realise just how easy it is to have your own kombucha on tap to enjoy through the day.

100g raw cane sugar

8 bags of black tea, green tea or a mix (or 2 tbsp loose tea)

250ml starter tea from the last batch of kombucha (or from a bottle of kombucha from a reputable manufacturer)

1 kombucha scoby

2 litres filtered water

Add the sugar to one litre of boiling water to dissolve it. Drop in the teabags and allow them to steep until the water has cooled. Once the tea is cool, remove the teabags (or pour the tea through a sieve to remove loose leaves) and stir in the starter tea.

Pour the mixture into a clean 2-litre jar and top up with another litre of filtered water. Gently slide the scoby into the jar with clean hands. Cover the jar with a few layers of tightly woven cloth, coffee filters or kitchen paper secured with a rubber band. Make sure this cover doesn't let any insects through, as they will be attracted to the sweet brew.

Keep the jar at room temperature, out of direct sunlight, and allow to ferment for at least seven days. It's not unusual for the scoby to float at the top, bottom or even sideways during fermentation. However, a new cream-coloured layer of scoby should start forming on the surface of the kombucha within a few days. You may also see stringy brown bits floating beneath the scoby or sediment collecting at the bottom. These are all normal signs of healthy fermentation.

After about one week, begin tasting the kombucha daily by pouring a little out of the jar and into a cup. When it reaches a balance of sweetness and tartness that is pleasant to you, the kombucha is ready to bottle.

Prepare and cool another pot of strong tea for your next batch of kombucha, as outlined in the first step. With clean hands, gently lift the scoby out of the kombucha and set it on a clean plate. Measure out your starter tea from your freshly brewed batch of kombucha and set it aside for the next batch, which you can begin to make now.

Transfer the fermented kombucha into clean bottles using a small plastic or glass funnel.

SECOND FERMENTATION

Kombucha loves a second ferment. This stage enhances both carbonation and flavour and the options are endless: simply add any juice, herbs or fresh or frozen fruit (diced or blended) and keep the bottles at room temperature, out of direct sunlight, for a further one to three days.

If you would rather drink the fresh brew without a second ferment then store the freshly bottled brew either in the fridge or at room temperature, where it will last for some weeks (as long as the temperature is not too high).

TIP: The flavour of the kombucha will be influenced by the tea used at the initial stage of fermenting. Choose from black, green, white, oolong, pu-erh, lapsang souchong or even a mix of these. They all make especially good kombucha.

NOTE: Do not use metal objects at any stage during the fermentation process. The bacteria do not like it.

Kombucha tastes great on its own, served over ice cubes, but the following recipes are the perfect way to make this skin-loving drink taste even better.

Pineapple Crush

200g (about ½) fresh pineapple, peeled and cut into chunks

50ml coconut water

500ml kombucha

fresh mint leaves, to serve

SERVES 3

Put pineapple chunks and coconut water into a blender. Blend until smooth. Pour into an airtight container with the kombucha. Store in the fridge and drink as desired, topped with fresh mint leaves. Shake before pouring.

Booch Mojito

200ml sparkling water

large handful fresh mint leaves

3–4 ice cubes, plus extra for serving

1 lime

800ml kombucha

SERVES 4

Put the sparkling water, mint leaves, ice cubes and the juice of ½ the lime in a blender. Blend until smooth. Add the kombucha and mix well.

Cut the remaining ½ lime into 4 wedges.

Pour into 4 glasses with more ice and serve each with a lime wedge.

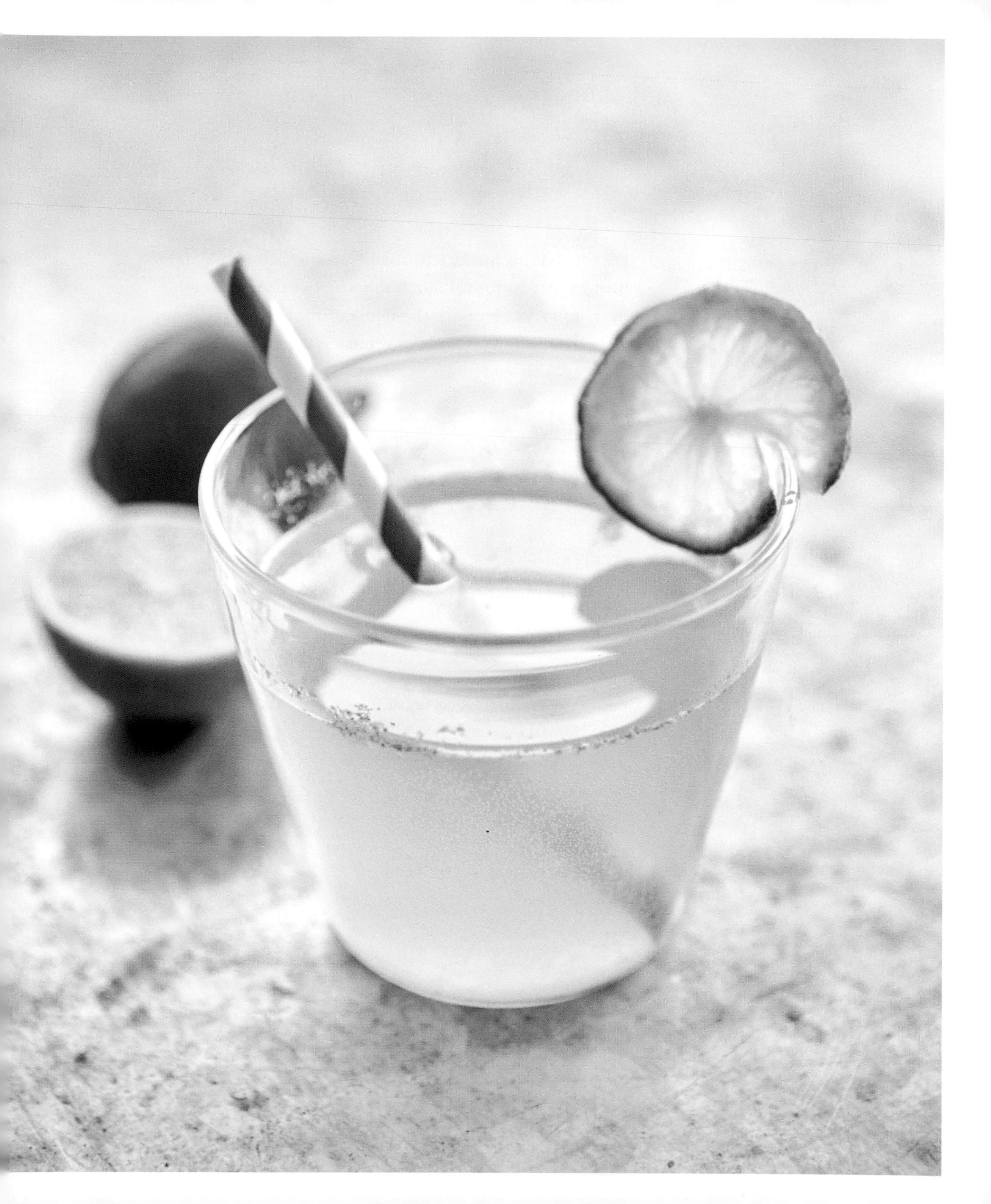

Blackberry Rose

100g blackberries

1 tsp dried rose petals, plus extra for serving

400–450ml kombucha

ice cubes, to serve

SERVES 2

Put the berries and dried rose petals into a blender. Add enough kombucha to blend. Pour the mixture through a sieve. Split between 2 glasses with a couple of ice cubes in each. Top with kombucha and scatter a couple of rose petals over each.

TIP: Raspberries can be used instead of blackberries.

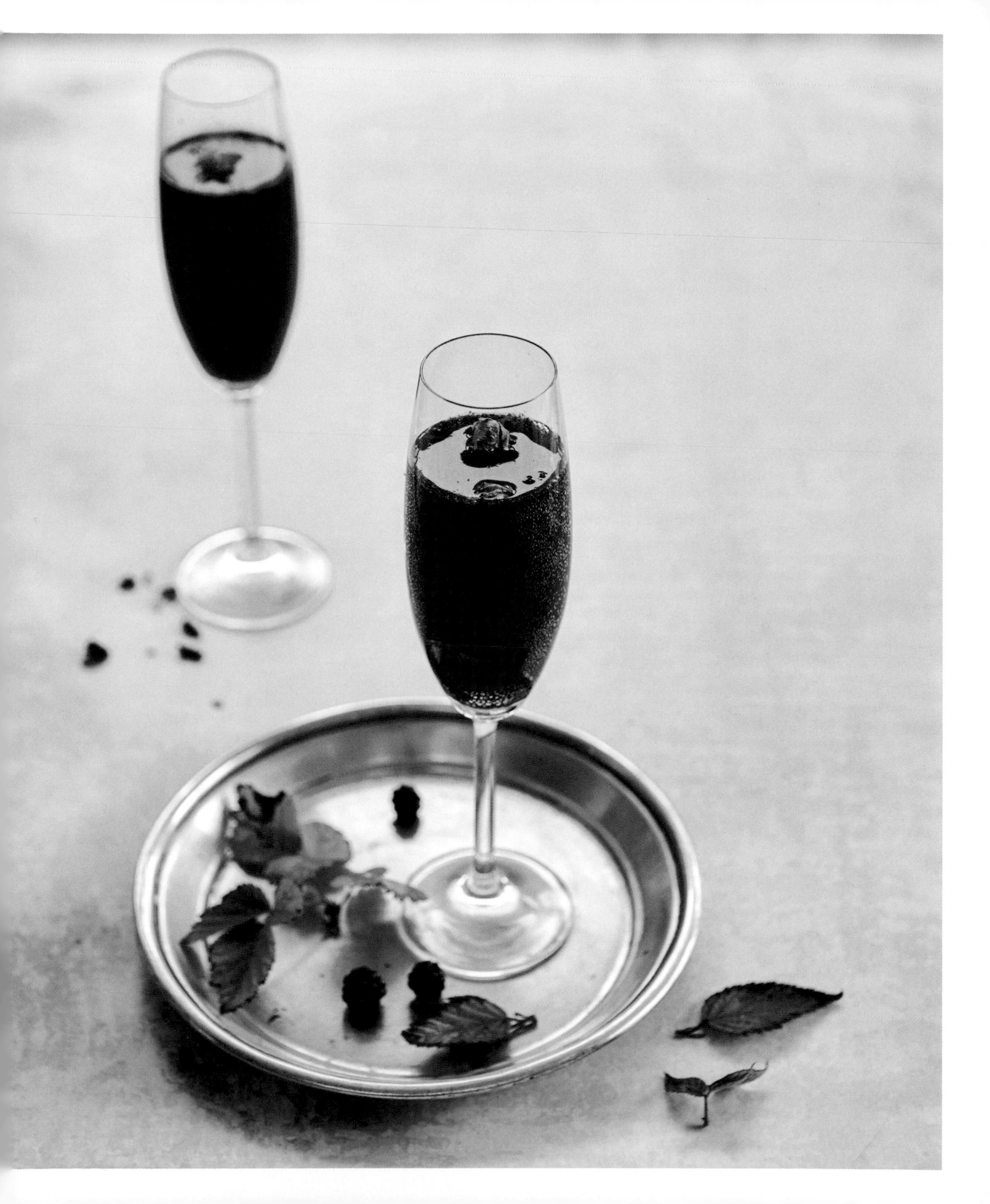

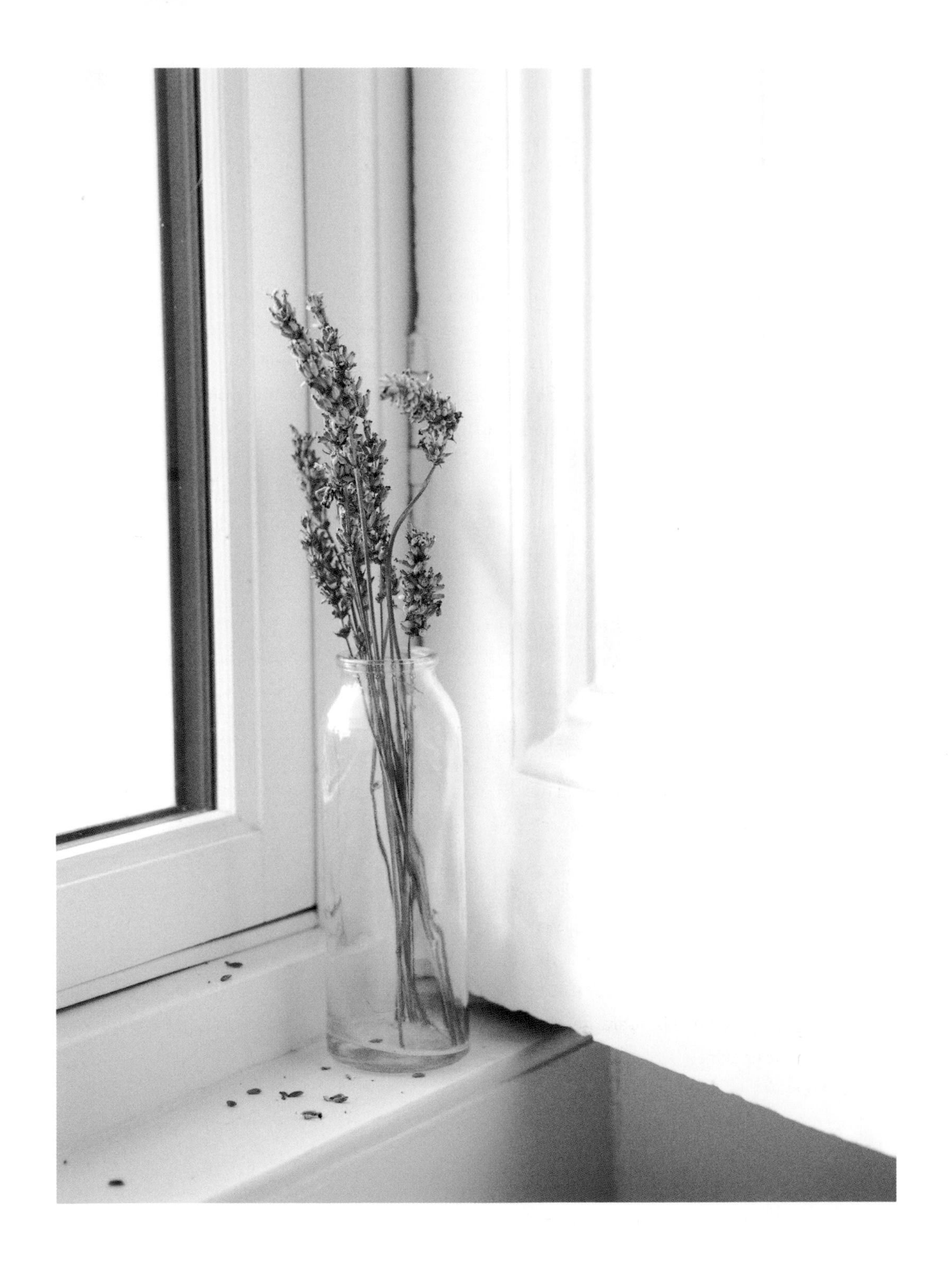

KATE'S TRUSTED BRANDS

◊

Many great products at various price ranges line the shelves. The following are some of my enduring favourites, skincare products I come back to time and time again simply because they work – on my skin, anyway. Every skin is different and it can take time to find those products that really deliver the GLOW for you. So use the ranges below as starting points, whatever your budget, and experiment until you find what really works for your skin. This list is not complete, as there are many more wonderful brands, but I have not yet tried them. Remember to switch up your regime during the different phases of your life and with the seasons, using warmer, more nourishing creams and oils during the colder winter months and lighter, brighter choices over the summer.

- **ALEXANDRA SOVERAL:** alexandrasoveral.co.uk
  Skincare doesn't get more authentic than this boutique range from London's leading skin expert. All of Alexandra's products are pure and free from toxic nasties, and all deliver as promised.
- **AROMATHERAPY ASSOCIATES:** www.aromatherapyassociates.com
  Inspired by the skin-loving benefits of essential oils, this global brand is gentle and nourishing for the face and body. The Hydrating Rose Exfoliating Cleanser and Skin Tonic really do wake up my skin each morning. The Refinery range of men's skincare is great too.
- **BIOLOGIQUE RECHERCHE:** www.biologique-recherche.com
  This trusted French brand is a well-kept secret in this part of the world. The range is extensive, so it is advisable to experience a Biologique Recherche facial to determine what products will work best on your skin.
- **BOOTS PROTECT & PERFECT, RESTORE & RENEW, LIFT & ILLUMINATE:** www.boots.com
  Cutting-edge science is guaranteed with these competitively priced choices, which work best on older skin.
- **DR DENNIS GROSS:** drdennisgross.com
  I chose to use this dermatologist-led range while trialing my four-week plan because many of their vitamin-enriched products are formulated to brighten and renew the skin. I love them all, especially the C + Collagen collection, Alpha Beta Extra Strength Daily Peel and Hyaluronic Marine Moisture Cushion.

- **ELEMIS:** www.elemis.com
  With an ever-expanding range of products – many of which I have not yet tried – my enduring favourite is the multi-award-winning Pro Collagen Marine Cream, which always leaves my skin feeling deeply nourished and glowing.
- **ESPA:** www.espaskincare.com
  This UK brand takes centre stage in spas around the world with a wide range of face and body products. My favourites are the ESPA serums and Tri-Active Advanced Night Booster, which is part of a collection of products formulated to aid sleep.
- **ESTÉE LAUDER:** www.esteelauder.com
  The latest in skin science is guaranteed with many great products available, including my lasting favourite, Advanced Night Repair.
- **ILA-SPA:** www.ila-spa.com
  Every product I have used from this pure plant-based range feels wonderful on my skin, especially the divine Damascena Rose Otto-infused Glowing Radiance Face Oil and the cleanser and toning mist.
- **LA PRAIRIE:** www.laprairieswitzerland.com
  Exceptional research lies behind this cutting-edge Swiss brand, and their use of indigenous mountain plants really does make a difference on the skin. While at a higher price, with La Prairie you get what you pay for.
- **LIZ EARLE:** uk.lizearle.com
  Gentle enough for more sensitive skin, this is the perfect choice for younger skin.
- **PAULA'S CHOICE:** www.paulaschoice.com
  Skincare expert Paula Begoun really knows her ingredients and I recommend all of her products, especially if you have ongoing problems with your skin.
- **PESTLE & MORTAR:** www.pestleandmortar.com
  This hip Irish brand is fast making a name for itself globally. With a limited number of products, Erase & Renew remains my double-cleansing favourite, without exception. The Pure Hyaluronic Serum is excellent too.
- **SARAH CHAPMAN:** www.sarahchapman.net
  This London-based celebrity facialist knows what works on every skin type and her results-driven products speak for themselves. While I have not tried them all, I continue to use those that I have.

- **TATCHA:** www.tatcha.com
  The best of timeless Japanese skincare in a bottle, this authentic brand is great for normal and slightly older skin.
- **THE ORDINARY BY THE ABNORMAL BEAUTY COMPANY:** theordinary.com
  Undoubtedly the best budget skincare brand on the market with products for every skin type and skin mood. Do your research to see what is best for you as the choices are vast.
- **THIS WORKS:** www.thisworks.com/eu
  This leading English brand continues to research the effects that lack of sleep and stress have on skin, and many of their products are formulated to address these key signs of skin ageing.
- **TRI-DOSHA:** tri-dosha.co.uk
  Wonderfully authentic range of Ayurvedic skincare designed to work with individual doshas.
- **VOYA:** www.voya.ie
  This seaweed-based Irish brand uses the best natural, organic ingredients in its wide range of face, body and hair products – all perfect for normal and/or sensitive skin.

If, like me, your skin loves oils, then lather it in a selection of the following pure plant and essential oils to gently nourish and enrich your skin.

- **ALEXANDRA SOVERAL:** alexandrasoveral.co.uk
- **AROMATHERAPY ASSOCIATES:** www.aromatherapyassociates.com
- **ILA-SPA:** www.ila-spa.com
- **KAHINA:** www.kahina-givingbeauty.com
- **MODERN BOTANY:** modernbotany.com
- **ROSALENA BIO-ACTIVE SKINCARE:** www.rosalena.co.uk
- **SOVERAL LONDON:** www.alexandrasoveral.co.uk
- **TAZEKA AROMATHERAPY** www.tazekaaromatherapy.com
- **VOYA SKINCARE BODY OILS:** www.voya.ie
- **WILD WOOD GROVES:** www.wildwoodgroves.com

SELECT BIBLIOGRAPHY

WHAT SKIN NEEDS

Skin Supplements

Ulven, S.M., B. Kirkhus, A. Lamglait, S. Basu, E. Elind, T. Haider, K. Berge, H. Vik and J.I. Pedersen, 'Metabolic effects of krill oil are essentially similar to those of fish oil but at lower dose of EPA and DHA, in healthy volunteers', *Lipids* 46.1 (2011): 37–46.

SKIN STRESSORS

Breaking the Stress–Skin Cycle

Fordham, B., C.E.M. Griffiths and C. Bundy, 'A pilot study examining mindfulness-based cognitive therapy in psoriasis', *Psychology, Health and Medicine* 20.1 (2015): 121–7, http://www.tandfonline.com/doi/abs/10.1080/13548506.2014.902483 (acccessed 18 October 2017).

Sun

Skin Cancer Foundation, 'UVA & UVB', 20 September 2017, skincancer.org, http://www.skincancer.org/prevention/uva-and-uvb/understanding-uva-and-uvb (accessed 18 October 2017).

Skin Cancer Foundation, 'How sunlight damages the eyes', 7 December 2012, skincancer.org, http://www.skincancer.org/prevention/sun-protection/for-your-eyes/how-sunlight-damages-the-eyes (accessed 18 October 2017).

Alcohol

Corrao, G., V. Bagnardi, A. Zambon and C. La Vecchia, 'A meta-analysis of alcohol consumption and the risk of 15 diseases', *Preventive Medicine* 38.5 (2004): 613–19.

GUT AND SKIN

Gut–Brain–Skin Axis

Bowe, W., N.B. Patel and A.C. Logan, 'Acne vulgaris, probiotics and the gut-brain-skin axis: from anecdote to translational medicine', *Beneficial Microbes* 5.2 (June 2014): 185–99, https://www.ncbi.nlm.nih.gov/pubmed/23886975.

Clark, A.K., K.N. Haas and R.K. Sivamani, 'Edible plants and their influence on the gut microbiome and acne', *International Journal of Molecular Science* 18.5 (May 2017): 1070, https://www.ncbi.nlm.nih.gov/pubmed/28513546.

Probiotics

Benyacoub, J., N. Bosco, C. Blanchard, A. Demont, D. Philippe, I. Castiel-Higounenc and A. Guéniche, 'Immune modulation property of *Lactobacillus paracasei* NCC2461 (ST11) strain and impact on skin defences', *Beneficial Microbes* 5.2 (June 2014): 129–36, https://www.ncbi.nlm.nih.gov/pubmed/24322880.

SLEEP AND SKIN

Skin Repair

University Hospitals, 'Estée Lauder clinical trial finds link between sleep deprivation and skin aging', 17 July 2013, uhhospitals.org, http://www.uhhospitals.org/about/media-news-room/current-news/2013/07/estee-lauder-clinical-trial-finds-link-between-sleep-deprivation-and-skin-aging (accessed 18 October 2017).

Sounder Sleep Strategies

Ebrahim, I.O., C.M. Shapiro, A.J. Williams and P.B. Fenwick, 'Alcohol and sleep I: effects on normal sleep', *Alcoholism: Clinical and Experimental Research* 37.4 (2013): 539–49.

INDEX

A

acids (AHAs and BHAs) 22–3
acne
  acids and 22, 23
  causes 39, 47, 54
  fatty acids and 83, 89
  Healing Turmeric Face Mask 120
  nettle and 115, 247
  probiotics and 55
  retinol 21, 22
  sea buckthorn oil and 88
  seaweed and 88
  serums and 11
  turmeric and 91, 120
  vitamin D3 26
  witch hazel and 10
alcohol 51, 121
almond milk
  Buckwheat Pancakes with Caramelised Banana Bites 160
  GLOW Banana Bread 152
  Oaty Banana Smoothie 150
  Orange and Almond Muffins 229
  Salted Caramel Smoothie Bowl 155
  Walnut Basil Pesto 168
almonds/ground almonds 83
  Almond and Honey Facial Scrub 135
  Apple, Pear and Blackberry Crumble 223–4
  Citrus Delight Cake 228
  Courgette and Almond Soup 177
  GLOW Banana Bread 152
  GLOW Trail Mix 232
  Orange and Almond Muffins 229
  Spinach and Broccoli Soup with Flaked Almonds 181
antioxidants 24, 26, 47, 73, 74, 75, 88, 114
  oils and 29, 30, 31, 34, 73
  serums and 11, 15, 16
apple cider vinegar (ACV) 72, 130
  Cashew Cream 168
  Tzatziki 171
  Zesty Apple Cider Vinaigrette 165
apples
  Apple, Pear and Blackberry Crumble 223–4
  Double Green 244
  Earthy Goodness 242
  Vital Skin 245
apricot oil 31, 113
argan oil 29, 120, 127, 130, 136
artichokes 56, 114
Autumn: Root Veggie Bowl 217
avocado oil 31, 73, 127, 136
avocados 72–3, 106
  Avocado on Toast - Three Ways 159
  Guacamole 167
  Minted Farro and Three Bean Salad with Goat's Cheese 191
  Nachos with a Twist 200
  Nourishing Avocado Mess (face mask) 128
  Pineapple Punch 244
  Quinoa, Pomegranate and Feta Salad 184
  Skin Soother 243
  Spring: Asian-Style Salmon Bowl 211–12
  Summer: Cauliflower and Baby Spinach Bowl 214

B

bananas
  Buckwheat Pancakes with Caramelised Banana Bites 160
  Cannellini Bean Salad with Marinated Alaria 192
  GLOW Banana Bread 152
  Intense C 243
  Mint Choc-Chip 'Ice Cream' 236
  Oaty Banana Smoothie 150
  Salted Caramel Smoothie Bowl 155
  Summer Surprise Smoothie 156
basil, Walnut Basil Pesto 168
baths/bathing 33, 88, 122
beauty powders 36
beetroot 73
  Autumn: Root Veggie Bowl 217
  Beetroot, Edamame and Orange Salad 188
  Earthy Goodness 242
  Quinoa, Pomegranate and Feta Salad 184
bergamot oil 67
berries
  Apple, Pear and Blackberry Crumble 223–4
  Berry Sorbet 236
  Blackberry Rose 262
  Intense C 243
  Summer Surprise Smoothie 156
  Vital Skin 245
blueberries 73, 92
body
  bathing 122
  brushing 112
  cellulite 113–14

cleansing body scrub 113
exfoliating scrubs 112
seaweed scrubs 122
steaming 109
Booch Mojito 260
borage seed oil 31, 120, 127
breakfast 105
breathing 42, 67
broccoli/broccolini
Autumn: Root Veggie Bowl 217
Broccolini Risotto 198
Spinach and Broccoli Soup with Flaked Almonds 181
Spring: Asian-Style Salmon Bowl 211
buckwheat 77, 78–9
Buckwheat Pancakes with Caramelised Banana Bites 160
Maya's Granola 145

C

caffeine 41, 65, 102
camellia oil 29
Cannellini Bean Salad with Marinated Alaria 192
carrots 74
Autumn: Root Veggie Bowl 217
Earthy Goodness 242
Quick Homemade Vegetable Stock 173
Shakshuka 163
Shepherdless Pie 202
Vital Skin 245
Zesty Cleanser 242
Cashew Cream 168
cauliflower
Moroccan-Style Salmon 208
Summer: Cauliflower and Baby Spinach Bowl 214
celery
Broccolini Risotto 198
Creamy Squash and Red Pepper Soup 174
Earthy Goodness 242
Orange, Walnut and Quinoa Salad 186
Quick Homemade Vegetable Stock 173
Skin Soother 243
Spinach and Broccoli Soup with Flaked Almonds 181
Vital Skin 245
Zesty Cleanser 242
cellulite 112, 113–14
chamomile 67, 120
cheese
Avocado on Toast – Three Ways 159
Broccolini Risotto 198
GLOW Frittata 195–6
Minted Farro and Three Bean Salad with Goat's Cheese 191
Orange, Walnut and Quinoa Salad 186
Quinoa, Pomegranate and Feta Salad 184
Shakshuka 163
Sweet Potato, Pea and Courgette Cakes 197
chickpeas
Summer: Cauliflower and Baby Spinach Bowl 214
Winter: Warming Squash, Red Pepper and Chickpea Curry Bowl 218–19
chocolate
ChocNOlate Chip Cookies 226
Chocolate Orange Energy Balls 231
dark chocolate 74
GLOW Banana Bread 152
Mint Choc-Chip 'Ice Cream' 236
Walnut Brownies 234
circadian rhythms 62
Citrus Delight Cake 228
Citrus Turmeric Salmon 205
coconut, desiccated
Citrus Delight Cake 228
GLOW Trail Mix 232
Maya's Granola 145
Oaty Breakfast Bars 149
Orange and Almond Muffins 229
coconut milk
Summer Surprise Smoothie 156
Winter: Warming Squash, Red Pepper and Chickpea Curry Bowl 218–19
coconut oil 30, 130
ChocNOlate Chip cookies 226
GLOW Banana Bread 152
Maya's Granola 145
Oaty Breakfast Bars 149
Shakshuka 163
Walnut Brownies 234
coconut water
Double Green 244
Earthy Goodness 242
Pineapple Punch 244
Skin Soother 243
Zesty Cleanser 242
collagen 8, 14, 15, 16, 19–20, 21, 24, 36
glycation and 49, 50
pollution and 47
skin repair, sleep and 60
vitamins and 91

courgettes
Courgette and Almond Soup 177
Moroccan-Style Salmon 208
Shepherdless Pie 202
Sweet Potato, Pea and Courgette Cakes 197
couscous 50, 79
Moroccan-Style Salmon 208
Creamy Squash and Red Pepper Soup 174
cucumber 122
Double Green 244
Mango, Pomegranate and Cucumber Salsa 171
Skin Soother 243
Tzatziki 171
Zesty Cleanser 242

D

dairy/dairy alternatives 96
dandelion 115
dates, Chocolate Orange Energy Balls 231
dermatitis 33, 88
Double Green 244

E

Earthy Goodness 242
eczema 34, 40, 41, 83, 88, 89, 119
edamame beans 74–5, 92
Avocado on Toast – Three Ways 159
Beetroot, Edamame and Orange Salad 188
Broccolini Risotto 198
Herby Edamame Omelette 143
Minted Farro and Three Bean Salad with Goat's Cheese 191
Orange, Walnut and Quinoa Salad 186
Pea and Edamame Houmous 170
Quick Miso Broth with Edamame 178, 180
Sautéed Spinach with Edamame 189
Spinach and Broccoli Soup with Flaked Almonds 181
Spring: Asian-Style Salmon Bowl 211–12
Spring Medley 183
eggs 75, 92, 130
Avocado on Toast – Three Ways 159
Buckwheat Pancakes with Caramelised Banana Bites 160
Citrus Delight Cake 228
GLOW Frittata 195–6
Herby Edamame Omelette 143
Orange and Almond Muffins 229
Shakshuka 163
Sweet Potato, Pea and Courgette Cakes 197
Walnut Brownies 234
emollients 13, 26
environmental stress 42–8
essential fatty acids (EFAs) 14, 34, 83, 89, 100
oils, EFAs and 27, 29, 30, 31, 33
omega-3 34, 56, 72, 73, 75, 83, 84, 89
sources 34, 35, 72, 83, 88, 106, 158
evening primrose oil 33, 120, 127
exercise 16, 41, 42, 64, 102
eyecare 57, 121–2

F

face/facemasks 13, 108–12
Alexandra Soveral's Honey Cleanse 110
Almond and Honey Facial Scrub 135
Calming Lavender Mist 120
face massage 110–11
GLOW Face Blend 135–6
Healing Turmeric Face Mask 120
Herbal Steam 108
Nourishing Avocado Mess 128
Nourishing Facial Scrub 127
Oatmeal Mask for Oily Skin 109
farro 50, 77, 79
Minted Farro and Three Bean Salad with Goat's Cheese 191
Fennel and Mint 248
fermented foods 56, 75, 257–62
fish, oily 34, 83–4, 96, 100
see also salmon
Flax and Sesame Crusted Salmon with Spinach and Tahini 206–7
flours 97
French beans, Spring Medley 183

G

geranium oil 28, 33, 110, 120
Ginger and Turmeric 252
GLOW Banana Bread 152
GLOW foods 71–92
apple cider vinegar (ACV) 72
avocados 72–3
beetroot 73
blueberries 73
carrots 74
dark chocolate 74
edamame beans 74–5

eggs 75
fermented foods 56, 75
grains 77–81
nuts 83
oily fish 83–4
oranges 84
pomegranates 84
sea vegetables 87–8
seeds 89
spinach 89, 91
tomatoes 91
turmeric 91–2
GLOW Frittata 195–6
GLOW Trail Mix 232
gluten 77–8
goji berries
GLOW Trail Mix 232
Oaty Breakfast Bars 149
grains 77–81, 97
Greek yoghurt
Berry Sorbet 236
Summer Surprise Smoothie 156
Tzatziki 171
Green Tea with Mint 254
Guacamole 167
gut
fermented foods and 56
gut-brain-skin axis 54
intestinal flora 53
microbiome 53–4, 56–7
prebiotics and 56
probiotics and 55
skin and 53–7

H

hair 40–1, 128, 129, 130
herbs 96–7, 114–15
Herby Edamame Omelette 143
honey 29, 49, 91, 109–10, 128, 130
Alexandra Soveral's Honey Cleanse 110
Almond and Honey Facial Scrub 135
Damaged Hair Mask 130
humectants 13
hyaluronic acid 8, 11, 13, 20

I

Intense C 243

J

juices 239
cleansing 115, 242
GLOW 245
healing 123, 243
nourishing 131, 244
juices, recipes
Double Green 244
Earthy Goodness 242
Intense C 243
Skin Soother 243
Zesty Cleanser 242

K

kale
Double Green 244
Minted Farro and Three Bean Salad with Goat's Cheese 191
kitchen essentials 95–7
kiwis
Pineapple Punch 244
Skin Soother 243
Kombucha 257–9

L

labels 101
lavender 33, 88, 108, 113, 120, 136
Calming Lavender Mist 120
Lavender and Rosemary 248
lecithin 35, 75, 92, 243, 245
leeks
Courgette and Almond Soup 177
GLOW Frittata 195–6
Quick Homemade Vegetable Stock 173
Quick Miso Broth with Edamame 178, 180
Spinach and Broccoli Soup with Flaked Almonds 181
Lemongrass, Ginger and Mint 247
lentils, Shepherdless Pie 202
liver cleanse 114–15

M

Mango, Pomegranate and Cucumber Salsa 171
maple syrup 51, 57
Buckwheat Pancakes with Caramelised Banana Bites 160
ChocNOlate Chip Cookies 226
GLOW Banana Bread 152
Maya's Granola 145
Oaty Breakfast Bars 149
Orange and Almond Muffins 229
Walnut Brownies 234
marinade, teriyaki 212
Marinated Alaria 193
marula oil 29–30
masks see face/facemasks
Matcha Mint Latte 252
Maya's Granola 145
meat 101
meditation/mindfulness 41, 65–6
mint
Double Green 244
Mango, Pomegranate and Cucumber Salsa 171

Mint Choc-Chip 'Ice Cream' 236
Minted Farro and Three Bean Salad with Goat's Cheese 191
Pineapple Punch 244
Skin Soother 243
Tzatziki 171
Zesty Cleanser 242
monoi oil 30
Moroccan-Style Salmon 208
mushrooms, Quick Miso Broth with Edamame 178, 180
Mustard Dressing 165

N

Nachos with a Twist 200
nettle 115
Nettle and Ginger 247
nut butter 13
Oaty Banana Smoothie 150
Salted Caramel Smoothie Bowl 155
nuts 83, 97
Apple, Pear and Blackberry Crumble 223–4
Cashew Cream 168
Citrus Delight Cake 228
Maya's Granola 145
see also almonds/ground almonds; walnuts

O

oats 79–80
Apple, Pear and Blackberry Crumble 223–4
ChocNOlate Chip Cookies 226
GLOW Banana Bread 152
Maya's Granola 145
Oaty Banana Smoothie 150
Oaty Breakfast Bars 149
Overnight Oats with Seasonal Berries 146
oils
cleansing oils 107
essential oils, using 33, 66–7
healing oils 120, 121
nourishing oils 127
skin oils 27–32, 96, 97
onions
Broccolini Risotto 198
Courgette and Almond Soup 177
Creamy Squash and Red Pepper Soup 174
Orange, Walnut and Quinoa Salad 186
Quick Miso Broth with Edamame 178, 180
Shakshuka 163
Spring Medley 183
Winter: Warming Squash, Red Pepper and Chickpea Curry Bowl 218–19
oranges 84
Beetroot, Edamame and Orange Salad 188
Chocolate Orange Energy Balls 231
Citrus Delight Cake 228
Creamy Squash and Red Pepper Soup 174
Intense C 243
Orange and Almond Muffins 229
Orange and Mint Iced Green Tea 254
Orange, Walnut and Quinoa Salad 186
Sunshine Skin 245
Zesty Cleanser 242
Overnight Oats with Seasonal Berries 146

P

pears, Apple, Pear and Blackberry Crumble 223–4
peas
Autumn: Root Veggie Bowl 217
Broccolini Risotto 198
GLOW Frittata 195–6
Minted Farro and Three Bean Salad with Goat's Cheese 191
Pea and Edamame Houmous 170
Spring Medley 183
peppermint oil 33, 107
peppers, red
Moroccan-Style Salmon 208
Shakshuka 163
Shepherdless Pie 202
Summer: Cauliflower and Baby Spinach Bowl 214
Winter: Warming Squash, Red Pepper and Chickpea Curry Bowl 218–19
peptides 11, 15, 16, 21
pesto, Walnut Basil Pesto 168
pineapple
Pineapple Crush 260
Pineapple Punch 244
Skin Soother 243
plan
morning mantra 105–38, 107
week one: cleanse 107–17, 242, 247
week two: heal 119–25, 243, 248
week three: nourish 127–33, 244, 252
week four: glow 135–8, 245, 254
pollution 40, 41, 47
pomegranates 84

Intense C 243
Mango, Pomegranate and Cucumber Salsa 171
Minted Farro and Three Bean Salad with Goat's Cheese 191
Quinoa, Pomegranate and Feta Salad 184
prebiotics 56
prickly pear seed oil 30, 136
probiotics 55, 55–6
processed foods 49–51
psoriasis
almonds and 83
EFAs and 88
meditation and 41
oils and 31, 33
omega-3 fatty acids and 84
sea weed and 88
stress and 40
Vitamin D3 and 26

Q

Quick Homemade Vegetable Stock 173
Quick Miso Broth with Edamame 178, 180
quinoa 77, 80–1
Autumn: Root Veggie Bowl 217
Orange, Walnut and Quinoa Salad 186
Quinoa, Pomegranate and Feta Salad 184

R

raisins, Cannellini Bean Salad with Marinated Alaria 192
red kidney beans, Nachos with a Twist 200
Reynolds, Dearbhla 257
rice 81, 82
Broccolini Risotto 198
Spring: Asian-Style Salmon Bowl 211–12
Winter: Warming Squash, Red Pepper and Chickpea Curry Bowl 218–19
rosacea 88, 89, 91, 121
rose oil 28, 30–1, 127, 128
rose water 110
Rosebud Brew 255
rosehip oil 31, 127, 128, 136

S

salmon 34, 83
Citrus Turmeric Salmon 205
Flax and Sesame Crusted Salmon with Spinach and Tahini 206–7
Moroccan-Style Salmon 208
Spring: Asian-Style Salmon Bowl 211–12
Salted Caramel Smoothie Bowl 155
Sautéed Spinach with Edamame 189
sea buckthorn oil 88
sea vegetables/seaweed 87–8, 122
Cannellini Bean Salad with Marinated Alaria 192
Marinated Alaria 193
Quick Miso Broth with Edamame 178, 180
seasonal foods 100
seeds 89, 97
Apple, Pear and Blackberry Crumble 223–4
Beetroot, Edamame and Orange Salad 188
ChocNOlate Chip Cookies 226
Flax and Sesame Crusted Salmon with Spinach and Tahini 206–7
GLOW Trail Mix 232
Intense C 243
Mango, Pomegranate and Cucumber Salsa 171
Oaty Breakfast Bars 149
Pineapple Punch 244
Skin Soother 243
Summer Surprise Smoothie 156
Shakshuka 163
Shepherdless Pie 202
skin 7–8
barrier-strengthening foods 92
better skin tips 99–102
dehydrated 71
gut and 53–7
microbiome 54
sleep and 59–67
skin cancer 43
Skin Soother 243
skin stressors 39–51
alcohol 51
environmental stress 42–8
processed foods 49–51
stress 39–42
sugar 49–51
skin supplements
essential fatty acids 34
krill oil 34
lecithin 35, 75, 92
probiotics 35–6
vitamin D 35
vitamin E 35
skincare
in 20s 14
in 30s 15
in 40s 15–16
in 50s 15–16
in 60s+ 16
ageing and 14
body cleansing 112–14

cleansing 9–10, 61, 107–14
daily 138
emollients 13, 26
exfoliation 10, 15, 108
humectants 13
monthly 138
nightly skin regime 61
nourishing 11, 13, 61
peels 10
probiotic 55–6
scrubs 106, 112–13, 122, 127
serums 11, 61
sun protection 10, 14, 15, 16, 43–4, 46
toners/toning 10, 33, 110, 255
weekly 138
see also body; face/facemasks
skincare ingredients 19
acids 22–3
collagen 19–20
hyaluronic acid 20–1
niacinamide 27
peptides 21
retinol 21–2
skin oils 27–8
vitamin C 24
vitamin D 24–5
vitamin E 26
sleep
apps 65–6
breathing exercise 67
circadian rhythms 62
meditations 65
skin and 59–67
soothing sounds 67
strategies 64–7
sleep-inducing foods 65
Soveral, Alexandra 109–10
spinach 89, 91
Beetroot, Edamame and Orange Salad 188
Double Green 244
Flax and Sesame Crusted Salmon with Spinach and Tahini 206–7
Minted Farro and Three Bean Salad with Goat's Cheese 191
Pineapple Punch 244
Quinoa, Pomegranate and Feta Salad 184
Sautéed Spinach with Edamame 189
Shakshuka 163
Spinach and Broccoli Soup with Flaked Almonds 181
Spring: Asian-Style Salmon Bowl 211–12
Summer: Cauliflower and Baby Spinach Bowl 214
Sweet Potato, Pea and Courgette Cakes 197
Winter: Warming Squash, Red Pepper and Chickpea Curry Bowl 218–19
Zesty Cleanser 242
Spring: Asian-Style Salmon Bowl 211–12
Spring Medley 183
squash
Creamy Squash and Red Pepper Soup 174
Winter: Warming Squash, Red Pepper and Chickpea Curry Bowl 218–19
stimulants 65
stock, Quick Homemade Vegetable Stock 173
stress 39–42
breathing and 42
hair, effects on 40–1
skin, effects on 39–40
stress-skin cycle, breaking 41–2
warning signs 41
see also environmental stress
stress hormones 39, 50, 59, 74
sugar 49–51
Summer: Cauliflower and Baby Spinach Bowl 214
Summer Surprise Smoothie 156
sun 64
protection from 10, 14, 15, 16, 43–4, 46
UV radiation 42–3, 46
UVA/UVB 43
Sunshine Skin 245
sweet almond oil 31, 33, 113, 127
sweet potatoes
GLOW Frittata 195–6
Shepherdless Pie 202
Sweet Potato, Pea and Courgette Cakes 197
sweetcorn, Moroccan-Style Salmon 208

T

tahini
Flax and Sesame Crusted Salmon with Spinach and Tahini 206–7
Oaty Banana Smoothie 150
Pea and Edamame Houmous 170
Tahini Dressing 166
tea tree oil 107, 108, 120
teas
cleansing 115, 247
GLOW 254, 255

healing 123, 248
nourishing 131
teas, recipes
Fennel and Mint 248
Ginger and Turmeric 252
Green Tea with Mint 254
Lavender and Rosemary 248
Lemongrass, Ginger and Mint 247
Matcha Mint Latte 252
Nettle and Ginger 247
Orange and Mint Iced Green Tea 254
Rosebud Brew 255
tinned foods 97
tomatoes 91
Autumn: Root Veggie Bowl 217
Creamy Squash and Red Pepper Soup 174
GLOW Frittata 195–6
Guacamole 167
Minted Farro and Three Bean Salad with Goat's Cheese 191
Moroccan-Style Salmon 208
Nachos with a Twist 200
Quinoa, Pomegranate and Feta Salad 184
Shakshuka 163
Shepherdless Pie 202
Summer: Cauliflower and Baby Spinach Bowl 214
Winter: Warming Squash, Red Pepper and Chickpea Curry Bowl 218–19
turmeric 91–2
Citrus Turmeric Salmon 205
Dukkah 214
Ginger and Turmeric 252
Healing Turmeric Face Mask 120
Moroccan-Style Salmon 208
Turmeric Tonic 107
Vital Skin 245
Winter: Warming Squash, Red Pepper and Chickpea Curry Bowl 218
Tzatziki 171

V
Vital Skin 245
vitamins
vitamin A 11, 21, 74
vitamin C 11, 13, 15, 24, 27, 73, 74, 84, 87, 92
vitamin D 24, 26, 35
vitamin E 26, 29, 30, 31, 35, 83, 89, 136

W
walnuts 83
Apple, Pear and Blackberry Crumble 223–4
Beetroot, Edamame and Orange Salad 188
Chocolate Orange Energy Balls 231
GLOW Banana Bread 152
GLOW Trail Mix 232
Minted Farro and Three Bean Salad with Goat's Cheese 191
Orange, Walnut and Quinoa Salad 186
Quinoa, Pomegranate and Feta Salad 184
Sweet Potato, Pea and Courgette Cakes 197
Walnut Basil Pesto 168
Walnut Brownies 234
Winter: Warming Squash, Red Pepper and Chickpea Curry Bowl 218–19

Y
ylang-ylang 33, 67, 120
yoga 42, 67

Z
Zesty Apple Cider Vinaigrette 165
Zesty Cleanser 242